http://connection.LWW.com

Get Connected!

Connect into a one-of-a-kind resource!

connection

Access everything you need for your studies at connection

- **E-mail updates** notify you of recent changes on the site and of content updates to the texts.

- **Chat rooms** enable on-line discussions for you to efficiently discuss specific topics with your peers and professor.

- **Message boards** make communication a snap.

And just for the student...

- **Useful tips** and "how to" instructions for every chapter.
- **Internet links** direct you to online resources for additional information.

Register in 3 easy steps...

1. Simply log on to the **connection** website and access the Resource Center for Thede: **Informatics and Nursing, 2nd Edition**.

2. Enter your name and e-mail address, and set-up a user name and password.

3. Now you have immediate access to all the benefits of **connection**.

Connect today.
http://connection.LWW.com/go/thede

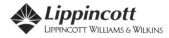

Lippincott
LIPPINCOTT WILLIAMS & WILKINS

SECOND EDITION

INFORMATICS
and NURSING
Opportunities
& Challenges

SECOND EDITION

INFORMATICS *and* NURSING

Opportunities & Challenges

Linda Q. Thede, PhD, RN, BC

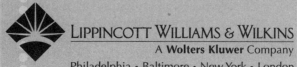

LIPPINCOTT WILLIAMS & WILKINS
A **Wolters Kluwer** Company
Philadelphia • Baltimore • New York • London
Buenos Aires • Hong Kong • Sydney • Tokyo

Acquisitions Editor: Margaret Zuccarini
Managing Editor: Barclay Cunningham
Editorial Assistant: Helen Kogut
Project Editor: Frank Musick
Senior Production Manager: Helen Ewan
Art Director: Carolyn O'Brien

Manufacturing Manager: William Alberti
Indexer: Victoria Boyle
Compositor: Lippincott Williams & Wilkins
Printer: Maple—Binghamton

Edition 2

Thede, Linda Q.
  Informatics and nursing : opportunities & challenges / Linda Q. Thede.--2nd ed.
    p. ; cm.
  Rev. ed. of: Computers in nursing. c1999.
  Includes bibliographical references and index.
  ISBN 0-7817-4020-7
  1. Nursing--Data processing. I. Thede, Linda Q. Computers in nursing. II. Title.
  [DNLM: 1. Medical Informatics. 2. Nursing. WY 26.5 T375i 2003]
  RT50.5 .T483 2003
  610.73'0285--dc21
                                                                      2002041047

9 8 7 6 5 4 3 2 1

Care has been taken to confirm the accuracy of the information presented and to describe generally accepted practices. However, the author and publisher are not responsible for errors or omissions or for any consequences from application of the information in this book and make no warranty, express or implied, with respect to the content of the publication.

The author and publisher have exerted every effort to ensure that drug selection and dosage set forth in this text are in accordance with the current recommendations and practice at the time of publication. However, in view of ongoing research, changes in government regulations, and the constant flow of information relating to drug therapy and drug reactions, the reader is urged to check the package insert for each drug for any change in indications and dosage and for added warnings and precautions This is particularly important when the recommended agent is a new or infrequently employed drug.

Some drugs and medical devices presented in this publication have Food and Drug Administration (FDA) clearance for limited use in restricted research settings. It is the responsibility of the healthcare provider to ascertain the FDA status of each drug or device planned for use in his or her clinical practice.

LWW.com

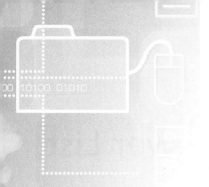

Contributor List

Margaret Allen, MLS-AHIP
Library Consultant
Wisconsin Area Health Education Centers
CINAHL Information Systems, Inc.
Instructor and Developer of Medical Library Association
    Continuing Education Courses
Stratford, Wisconsin

Susan T. Pierce, EdD, MSN, RN
Associate Professor
College of Nursing
Northwestern State University
Shreveport, Louisiana

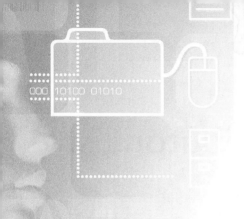

Reviewer List

Rita Axford, RN, C, PhD
Professor and Chair of Distance Learning
Regis University
Denver, Colorado

Jacqueline L. Rosenjack Burchum, DNSc(c), MSN, APRN, BC
Assistant Professor of Nursing and Family Nurse Practitioner
The University of Memphis, Jackson Center
Jackson, Tennessee

Joy H. Fraser, RN, PhD
Associate Professor
Centre for Nursing and Health Studies
Athabasca University
Athabasca, Alberta, Canada

Janet S. Hickman, RN, BSN, MS, EdD
Professor of Nursing
West Chester University
West Chester, Pennsylvania

Karen S. March, MSN, RN, CCRN, CS
Assistant Professor of Nursing
University of Pittsburgh at Bradford
Bradford, Pennsylvania

Mary M. Meighan, RNC, PhD
Assistant Professor of Nursing
Carson-Newman College
Jefferson City, Tennessee

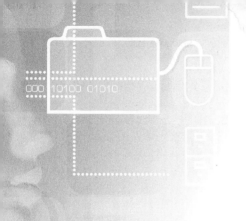

Preface

As the title says, informatics presents nursing and healthcare with many opportunities. As with any innovation, it also presents many challenges, some involved in adapting the innovation to our needs, others due to new issues that informatics brings. When asked, "What is informatics?" some people may say, "Oh, that's just computers." To people familiar with informatics, that's like saying, "Auscultation is just stethoscopes." Stethoscopes are the tool for auscultation, but can hardly be used to define it. In the same way, computers are the tools for informatics, but do not describe the field. Simply defined, informatics is about managing information.

In earlier times, it was possible to manage information in healthcare manually. Today the superabundance of information in healthcare has made this impossible. The goal of informatics is to assist in this task. To meet this challenge, nurses and other healthcare professionals must learn enough about the tools of informatics to use them to effectively manage information.

The first chapter in this book presents an overview of informatics in nursing and healthcare and briefly explores some theories from which informatics borrows. The rest of Unit One, Nursing and Informatics: The Basics, focuses on the tools of informatics necessary as a background to develop computer fluency. This includes a look at computers themselves, an overall view of software, and a discussion of the basics of computer communications. The final chapter in this unit presents some concepts useful in working with computers.

Unit Two, Informatics: eHealth, explores the impact of electronic communication on healthcare, healthcare professionals, and informatics including the new field of consumer informatics.

Personal productivity tools are explored in Unit Three, Informatics: Personal Productivity. Each of the three chapters addressing word processing, presentation programs, and spreadsheets not only presents uses of these programs, but also provides information about some of the premises upon which the programs are based but which are not learned with step-by-step instructions.

Clinical informatics is explored in Unit Four, Informatics: Clinical Information Systems. Nursing informatics is examined as a field and a career, standardized terminologies are explored, and clinical information systems are addressed.

Unit Five, Informatics: Professional Tools and Issues, looks at the role of information in healthcare. This unit includes an introduction to the use of knowledge by nurses and healthcare workers and the use of databases to uncover secrets in clinical data as well as for managing administrative tasks. Another chapter addresses the use of bibliographic and factual databases by healthcare professionals. The book ends with a look at some of the overriding issues in informatics, including security, ergonomics, and user interfaces.

A Web page accompanies this book, which contains additional features that I would have liked to include but had to omit owing to space limitations. I believe that you will find many resources on this page that will be helpful in understanding the book. It contains a glossary of bolded key terms found throughout the text. Additionally, it contains a number of "how-to's" that could not be included. The URL is http://connection.lww.com/go/thede.

The following features are **new to this edition:**

▼ A new chapter—Chapter 15, Other Facets of Informatics: A Wide Impact
▼ Expanded information in Chapter 1, Introduction to Nursing Informatics: Multiple Foci; Chapter 8, Telehealth: Now and in the Future; Chapter 12, Informatics Nurse Specialist: A Specialty in Two Disciplines; and Chapter 19, Informatics: Challenges and Issues.

Additionally, all chapters have been revised to reflect the most current practices in nursing informatics. The accompanying Web site will be updated frequently to maintain the most current and accurate resource.

The opportunities afforded by informatics in nursing and healthcare range from improving patient care through making our professional lives easier to recognition of the value that nursing adds to healthcare. Like all opportunities, these will not be reached without meeting the challenges of working with information and adapting it to nursing rather than adapting nursing to the needs for information.

Linda Q. Thede, PhD, RN, BC

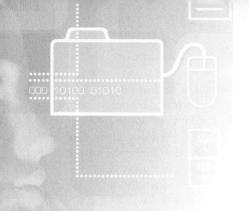

Acknowledgments

With the abundance of knowledge in today's society, it is impossible for one person to be an expert in many areas. This is especially true in writing a book. There are many people who patiently answered my many questions and encouraged me in this process. It would be impossible to mention everyone, but a few deserve special mention. **Peg Allen** not only wrote Chapter 17, but corroborated on Chapter 15 and edited Chapters 6 and 7. **Karen Elberson**, PhD, RN, arranged for the picture in Chapter 8 and put me in touch with **Regina Saiid**, BSN, RN, who heads the University Health Home Service and reviewed the information about their service, while **Jennifer Schute**, BSN, RN, cooperated with Karen to arrange for the picture. **Gail Keenan**, PhD, RN, answered many questions about their project at the University of Michigan, and **Debbie Konicek**, BSN, RN, straightened out my information about SNOMED for Chapter 13. **Mimi Hassett**, MS, RN, BC, updated the information on clinical systems as well as editing what I wrote, while **Teresa Numbers**, MSN, RN, and **Carol Petrusky**, BSN, RN, both carefully reviewed Chapter 14 to see if we had included all necessary information. **Judi Hornbeck** contributed her information about a typical day for a nurse informaticist while **Lynn Geren**, another informatics nursing specialist, shared her knowledge of the computer skills needed by today's nurse. **Jim Quiggle** helped me to understand XML. **Susan Pierce**, EdD, RN, who teaches informatics, not only provided the organizing framework for Chapter 15, but was the impetus for adding this information to the book. **Kathleen Stevens**, PhD, RN, FAAN, reviewed the information about evidence-based practice and graciously gave us permission to use her "Ace Star Model of Evidence-Based Practice.

My many friends, who understood my commitment and relieved me of some of my other obligations while I worked on the book, also deserve special thanks. I also want to voice my appreciation of my husband, **Dexter**, who laboriously reviewed several of the chapters getting me to make needed changes. His patience in never complaining when I was preoccupied and sometimes forgot things, or when I constantly talked about how to approach various topics in the book deserves a special tribute. To all those individuals and to others too numerous to mention, I can only say a heartfelt, "Thank You!"

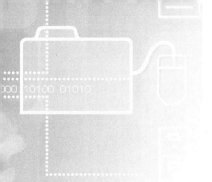

Contents

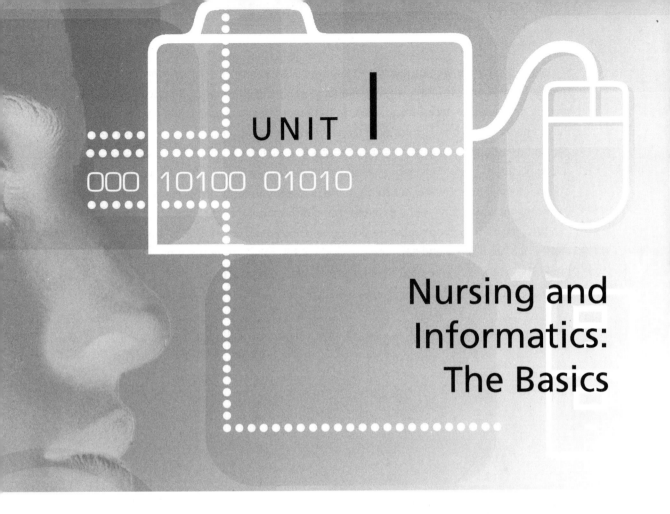

UNIT 1

000 10100 01010

Nursing and Informatics: The Basics

ONE challenging need in adapting informatics to nursing and healthcare is becoming computer fluent. Unit 1 provides some of the basic information needed to meet this challenge. The purpose of informatics is to manage data, the primary tool to do it the computer. Computers today are a mainstay of modern life. We use them to run our cars, microwave ovens, and telephones as a matter of course. Using them directly (and not as part of another function), as practitioners do in healthcare, requires understanding their basic characteristics if we are to achieve our purpose of managing information. Although it is easy to think of a computer in terms of just a combination of hardware and software, the most important part of a computer system is the human who uses it. This unit focuses on providing some introductory material to enable nurses and other healthcare professionals to form an intelligent partnership with the computer, which will allow the computer to do what it does best, but with an understanding of when its limitations have been reached.

Chapter 1 provides an introduction to informatics including theories on which informatics is based and providing some definitions of nursing informatics. Chapters 2 to 5 provide a foundation necessary to become computer fluent. Computer fluency means that someone is not only comfortable with current computer applications, but that the person has enough understanding of the basics to adapt to and learn new programs and applications easily. This background is provided by information that addresses not only hardware and software, but some of the principles about which users are often unaware, but which can greatly ease use of the informatics tool.

A Web page for the book provides additional information, and includes "how to" exercises that are more useful when one is sitting at the computer rather than reading a book. The web page can be found at http://connection.lww.com/go/thede

Introduction to Nursing Informatics: Multiple Foci

Objectives
After studying this chapter you will be able to:

1. Discuss the changes needed in information management.

2. Define nursing informatics.

3. Interpret the changes in healthcare that informatics can make.

4. Discuss factors supporting the need for informatics.

5. Describe five theories on which informatics relies.

6. Discuss the need for nurses to be computer literate.

Information is the structure on which health care is built. Except for procedures done for purely technical clinical reasons (of which there are few, if any), a healthcare professional's work revolves around information. Is the laboratory report available? When is Mrs. X scheduled for surgery? What are the contraindications for the drug prescribed? What is Mr. Y's history? What orders did the physician leave for Ms. Z? Where is the latest radiology report?

The manner in which information is handled and processed has a considerable effect on both the outcome of those who purchase the services of healthcare workers and the economics of healthcare itself. Manually recording and filing information and face-to-face communication are inadequate today if they are the only techniques used to manage the data in a case. As a group, we have made some attempts to use technology to manage information, but these efforts often fall short because of our inexperience in grasping the sources where information originates, how it is used clinically and administratively, and how it can be used to improve practice. The need to study our information needs and to use technology effectively to manage these needs has never been stronger.

 ## The Need: Managing Information

In 1850, it was possible for all the medical knowledge known to the Western world to be put into two large volumes. It was possible for one person to read and assimilate all this information. Today, if physicians read two journal articles every day, by the end of the first year they would be

800 years behind in their reading (McDonald, 1994). Given that the amount of scientific knowledge is estimated to double every 2 years (Zielstorff, Hudgings, & Grobe, 1993), it is impossible for one person to even begin to know everything. Additionally, current knowledge in some fields is constantly changing: one can expect much of one's knowledge to be obsolete in 5 years or less.

In healthcare, the increase in knowledge has led to the development of many specialties: respiratory therapy, neonatology, and gerontology and to the growth of subspecialties within each. As these specialties have proliferated, they have spun off many miraculous healthcare treatments, but as a result, healthcare has too often become fractionalized, causing difficulty in gaining an overview of the entire patient. The pressure of accomplishing the tasks necessary for a patient's physical recovery and safety usually leaves little time for studying a patient's record and putting together the bits and pieces so carefully charted by each discipline. Even if time *is* available, there are simply so many data, in so many places, that it is difficult to merge the data we find with the knowledge that we can remember, as well as with new knowledge we've gained, to provide the best patient care. We are drowning in data but lack the time to channel them into useful information or knowledge.

The challenge of improving the transformation of data into useful knowledge for healthcare practitioners has led to development of a relatively new field: **healthcare informatics**. This field is concerned with the identification, acquisition, manipulation, storage, and presentation of data so that they can be transformed to information. Besides knowledge from healthcare disciplines, health informatics borrows knowledge from many other fields including information science and computer science.

An Information Management Tool: Computers

The development of the computer as a tool to manipulate data can be seen throughout its history. Although not technically a computer by today's terminology, the first attempt to mechanize the task of data manipulation resulted in the abacus about 3000 BC. Although when one had developed the skill, real speed in calculation was possible, the operator of the abacus still had to manipulate data mentally. All the abacus did was store the results step by step. Slide rules came next in 1632, but like the abacus, they required a great deal of skill on the part of the operator.

The first machine to work by itself was Blaise Pascal's "pascaline," a machine that could add and subtract. The first "computer" to be a commercial success, however, was Jacquard's weaving machine, which was built in 1804. Its efficiency so frightened workers at the mill where it was built that they rioted, broke the machine apart, and sold the parts. Despite this setback, the machine proved a success because it introduced a cost-effective way to produce goods.

The Difference and Analytical engines, early computers designed by Charles Babbage in the mid 19th century, laid the foundation for modern computers. The machines, however, were never built. The first time that an automatic calculating machine was successfully used was in the 1900 census. Herman Hollerith (whose company later became IBM) used the Jacquard loom concept of punch cards to create a machine that enabled the results of the 1900 census to be compiled in 6 weeks (Computers: History and Development, 1997) versus the 7 years it had taken to compile the 1890 census results.

The first computer that we would recognize today was the Electronic Numerical Integrator and Computer (ENIAC) built by researchers at the Moore School of Engineering at the University of Pennsylvania in partnership with the U.S. Government. When finished in 1946, it required 18,000 vacuum tubes, 70,000 resistors, and 5 million soldered joints. When it was running, it consumed enough energy to dim the electric lights in an entire section of Philadelphia (Moye, 1996).

Progress in hardware since then has been phenomenal; today's hand-held computers have more processing power than the ENIAC did. This progress was led by the transistor, invented in 1947, which led to the "second generation of computers." Development of the integrated circuit (IC) in 1958 and the subsequent ability to fix it to a flat wafer of silicon developed in 1959 paved the way for the personal computers that we know today. The progress of more powerful and simultaneously smaller and smaller, processing units continues. When properly harnessed, today's computing power can meet information needs. It is informatics that assists in harnessing this tool.

What Is Informatics?

The term **informatics** was derived from the Russian word *informatika* (Sackett & Erdley, 2001) A Russian book, *Oznovy Informatiki (Foundations of Informatics)*, published in 1968, is credited with the origins of the general discipline of informatics by describing information science within the context of computers (Hogarth, 1997). Medical informatics was the first term used to identify informatics in healthcare. It was defined as those information technologies that are concerned with patient care and the medical decision-making process (Hogarth, 1997). Another definition stated that medical informatics is the complex data processing by the computer to create new information. As is the case in many healthcare enterprises, debate went on about whether the term *medical* referred only to informatics focusing on physician concerns, or whether it referred to all healthcare disciplines. Increasingly, it is seen that other disciplines have a body of knowledge apart from medicine, but part of healthcare, and the term **healthcare informatics** is becoming more commonly used. In essence, informatics is the management of information, using cognitive skills and the computer.

HEALTHCARE INFORMATICS

Healthcare informatics focuses on achieving these ends in healthcare. It is an umbrella term that describes the study of the retrieval, storage, presentation, sharing, and use of biomedical information, data, and knowledge for providing care, solving problems, and making decisions (Shortliffe & Blois, 2001). The purpose is to improve the use of healthcare data, information, and knowledge for supporting patient care, research, and education (Delaney, 2001). The focus is on the subject, information, rather than the tool, the computer. The distinction is not always obvious due to the need to master computer skills to enable one to manage this information. The computer is used in acquiring, organizing, manipulating, and presenting the information. Without, however, human direction in how the data will be treated, interpreted, and manipulated the computer is useless. Informatics provides that human direction.

NURSING INFORMATICS

Healthcare has many disciplines, thus it is not surprising that healthcare informatics has many specialties of which nursing is one. **Nursing informatics** is also a subspecialty of nursing and, since the fall of 1992, a specialty in which one can be certified (Newbold, 1996). Nursing informatics has as its focus managing information pertaining to nursing. Specialists in this area look at how nursing information is acquired, manipulated, stored, presented, and used. In jobs in clinical areas, nursing informatics specialists work with practicing nurses to identify the needs of nurses for information and support, and with system developers in the development of systems that work to complement the practice needs of nurses. Nursing informatics specialists bring to the study a viewpoint that supports the needs of the clinical end user so that the resulting system is not only user friendly for data input but also provides the clinical nurse with needed information in a manner that is timely and useful.

DEFINITIONS OF NURSING INFORMATICS

The term *nursing informatics* was probably first used and defined by Scholes and Barber in 1980 in their address to the MEDINFO conference in Tokyo. There is still no definitive agreement on exactly what the term comprises. As Simpson (1998) says, defining nursing informatics exactly is difficult because it is a moving target. The original definition stated that nursing informatics was the use of computer technology in all nursing endeavors: services, education, and research (Scholes & Barber, 1980). Another early definition that follows the broad definition of Scholes and Barber was written by Hannah, Ball, and Edwards (1994). They defined nursing informatics as any use of information technologies in carrying out nursing functions (Hannah, Ball, & Edwards, 1994). Like the Scholes and Barber definition, these other definitions focused on technology and could be interpreted to mean any use of the computer from word processing to the creation of artificial intelligence for nurses as long as the process involved the practice of professional nursing.

The shift from a technology orientation in definitions to one that was conceptually oriented started in the mid-1980s with Schwirian (Staggers & Thompson, 2002). She created a model to be used as a framework for nursing informatics investigators (Schwirian, 1986). The model consisted of elements arranged in a pyramid supported by a base of nursing informatics and aimed at the top of the pyramid, the objective. The other elements were raw material (nursing-related information), technology (the computer), and users (nurses and students). The model was intended as a stimulus for research.

The first widely circulated definition that moved away from the technology to concepts was given by Graves and Corcoran (1989). They defined nursing informatics as "...a combination of computer science, information science and nursing science designed to assist in the management and processing of nursing data, information and knowledge to support the practice of nursing and the delivery of nursing care" (p. 227). This definition secured the position of nursing informatics within the practice of nursing and placed the emphasis on data, information, and knowledge (Staggers & Thompson, 2002). Many consider it the seminal definition of nursing informatics.

Turley (1996), after analyzing previous definitions, added another discipline, cognitive science, to the base from which nursing informatics grew. Cognitive science emphasizes the human factor in informatics. Cognitive science itself is interdisciplinary, drawing ideas from psychology, linguistics, philosophy, and neuroscience. Its main focus is the nature of knowledge, its components, development, and use. Goossen (1996), thinking along the same lines, used the Graves and Corcoran definition as a basis and expanded the meaning of nursing informatics to include thinking that is done by nurses to make knowledge-based decisions and inferences for patient care. Using this interpretation, he determined that nursing informatics should focus on analyzing and modeling the cognitive processing for all areas of nursing practice. Goossen also stated that nursing informatics should look at the effects of computerized systems on nursing care delivery.

Currently, there is a trend to create role-oriented definitions (Staggers & Thompson, 2002). The first American Nurses Association (ANA) definition in 1992 followed this approach by adding the role of the informatics nursing specialist to the Graves and Corcoran definition. The 2001 ANA definition states that nursing informatics combines nursing, information, and computer sciences to manage and communicate information to support nurses and healthcare providers in decision making (American Nurses Association, 2001). Information structures, processes and technology are used to provide this support.

Staggers and Thompson (2002), who believe that the evolution of definitions will continue, point out that in all the current definitions, the role of the patient is underemphasized. Some early definitions included the patient, but only as a passive recipient of care. With the advent of the Internet, more and more patients are taking an active role in their healthcare. This factor changes not only the dynamics of healthcare but also permits a definition of nursing informatics that acknowledges that patients, as well as healthcare professionals, are users of healthcare information and that patients may be participating in informatics by keeping the information in their medical records current. Staggers and Thompson also point out that the role of the nurse as an integrator of information has been overlooked and should be considered in future definitions.

Computers and Healthcare

Informatics originated in healthcare as management of financial information with the computer healthcare applications that began in the late fifties and early sixties. By the sixties, however, a few patient care applications began to appear in computer systems (Saba, Johnson, & Simpson, 1994). By the late 1960s, some hospital information systems were starting to include patient diagnoses and other patient information as well as care plans based on physician and nursing orders.

Historical Aspects

It was the amendment of the Social Security Act to include Medicare and Medicaid in 1965 that accelerated the use of computers in healthcare. This legislation proved to be a boon to nursing information systems because nurses were required to provide data to document the care that was delivered (Miller, 1993; Saba, 1983). The demand by the federal government and other regulatory agencies for more data continues to be a primary driving force behind the use of computers in healthcare.

One interesting early use of the computer in patient care was the PRoblem Oriented Medical Information System (PROMIS) begun by Dr. Lawrence Weed at the University Medical Center in Burlington, Vermont (McNeil, 1979) in 1968. The importance of this system lies in that it was the first attempt to provide a totally integrated system that included all aspects of healthcare including patient treatment. It used as its framework the problem-oriented medical record (POMR) and was oriented toward patients. It was originally implemented on a gynecology unit in 1971, and then completely redeveloped for use on a medical unit.

PROMIS provided a wide array of information to all professions involved in healthcare including the cost of procedures and laboratory tests. Documentation was focused on the problem list. Practitioners from all healthcare disciplines recorded their observations and plans on this list, breaking down barriers between disciplines. The PROMIS system also made it possible to see the relationship between conditions, treatments, costs, and outcomes. This system did not have wide acceptance. To embrace it meant changing the structure of the provision of healthcare, something that did not begin to happen until the advent of managed care in all its variations in the 1990s, reinvigorated a push toward more patient-centered information systems.

IMPACT ON HEALTHCARE

Healthcare is an information-intensive industry, yet most healthcare providers often consider management of their information as an onerous, unappreciated task (Korpman, 1990). Poorly organized and implemented documentation systems tend to hinder the process of finding and using the information needed to provide high quality care. By adding to that the frequent need to enter data twice, or even three times, as well as the time spent trying to locate given pieces of information and records, and the reasons for dissatisfaction become clear.

As healthcare informatics moves to solve these problems, the need for interdisciplinary, enterprise-wide, information management becomes clearer. Improvement of information technology coupled with the evolution of the **electronic healthcare record** will create a steady progression to this end. Integration, however, is not without its perils. Any discipline that is not ready for such integration may find itself lost in the process. For nursing to be a part of healthcare informatics, individual nurses must become familiar with the value of nursing data, how it can be captured, the terminology needed to capture it, and methods for analyzing and manipulating it to improve healthcare. True integration of healthcare data will improve both patient care and the patient experience, as well as enable economic gains.

CHANGES IN INFORMATICS

Besides introducing changes toward increasingly interdisciplinary care, informatics itself is changing. Original computerized information systems were oriented toward process. Put another way, they were implemented to computerize a specific process, for example, order entry or recording results of laboratory reports. This led to the creation of software systems that were not intended to and could not share data which necessitated multiple data entry. Writing the code to allow an interchange between these systems is a difficult and sometimes impossible task. The results are often disappointing to the users and leave negative impressions of computerization in the minds of many.

The move today in informatics is to data orientation with a patient-centered focus. A system organized by data is designed to use one item of data many times. The primary design is based on how data are gathered, stored, and used in an entire institution rather than in terms of a specific process. When a medication order is placed, the system will have access to all the information about a patient including diagnosis, age, gender, weight, and allergies as well as the medications currently being taken. The order and patient information will be matched against knowledge, such as what drugs are incompatible for simultaneous use with the prescribed drug, the correctness of the dosage of the drug, and the appropriateness of the drug for this patient. The system will deliver warnings at the time the medication is ordered to allow any difficulties to be dealt with at the time of order entry. The same information will be available to the dietician in planning the patient's diet as well as to the nurse doing care and discharge planning, thus providing a more complete picture of a patient. Additionally, access to the current knowledge base about a given condition in the form of practice guidelines will be easily accessible. Practice guidelines will be accessed from a distant computer and kept up to date by professionals whose job is to synthesize research and produce these guidelines. These new systems will not only save time but will also reduce errors caused by the necessity for multiple data entry and the previous inability of professionals to have at their fingertips all the latest patient data and information.

Systems that incorporate these features require a new way of thinking. Instead of having all one's knowledge in memory, one must be comfortable both with needing to access information and with changing one's practice to accommodate the new knowledge. Additionally, this system requires computers that are powerful enough to process and direct the data so that information is created on as as-needed basis. Data from a physical assessment must be combined with data from laboratory tests to provide an up-to-date picture of a patient's condition. Next, this information must be linked to current knowledge bases. During the 1980s, clinical systems that were based on this model were tried but failed because of a lack of a computer powerful enough to process the necessary data. Today, such computing power is readily available.

Computerization will affect healthcare professionals in different ways. Some jobs will change focus. As nurses, we may find that our job as patient care coordinator has shifted from transcribing and checking orders to accessing this information on the computer. To preserve our ability to provide full care for our patients, and as an information integrator for other disciplines, we will need to make our information needs known to those who design the systems. To accomplish this, we all need to be aware of the value of both our data and our experience and to be able to identify data we need to perform our job, as well as to appreciate the value of the data that we add to the healthcare system.

Theories That Lend Support to Informatics

Informatics relies on principles from other disciplines such as change theory, systems theory, organizational development, learning theory, and information theory. In this introduction to informatics, four of these theories are briefly reviewed: change theory, information theory, system theory, and learning theory.

CHANGE THEORY

No matter which agency experiences computerization of information, and whether it is an entirely new experience, or an update to an ongoing system, change is involved. It may be a simple change such as a minor upgrade to a system, or a major change such as moving from a paper-based record to a completely paperless electronic system. Whether affected workers perceive the change as minor or major varies from person to person. "What will this mean to me?" is always the question uppermost in everyone's mind when faced with change. Change can be looked at in terms of planned or unplanned change. Unplanned change is represented by Roger's diffusion of innovation theory and planned change by Lewin's change theory.

Roger's Diffusion of Innovation Theory

Rogers' theory examines the pattern of acceptance that innovations follow as they spread across the population of people who adopt it. It was based on depression-era rural research that studied how Midwestern farmers learned to plant hardier strains of corn. This theory is still timely in North America and developed countries with the same culture, but it is doubtful whether it applies to the areas of the world with different cultures.

In this theory, adopters are divided into five categories. *Innovators*, who readily adopt the innovation. They constitute a very small percentage, about 2.5% of the population. (Anderson, 2001).These people, who are often seen as disruptive by those who are averse to risk taking, are not able to sell others on the innovation. This job is left to the *early adopters* who comprise 13.5% of the population. They are respectable opinion leaders who function as promoters of the innovation. The next group are the *early majority* (34%) who are averse to risks but will make safe investments. The *late majority*, who make up another 34% of the adopters, need to be sure that the innovation is beneficial. They may adopt the innovation not because they see a use for it, but because of peer pressure. The last group, comprising 16% are termed *laggards*. They are suspicious about innovation and change and are very intractable. They see their resistance as rational and must be certain that the innovation will not fail before they are willing to adopt it. This group, instead of being discounted, should be listened to. They may grasp those weaknesses that others have failed to recognize.

Lewin's Change Theory

When planning changes in how documentation is done, if they are to be successful, this planning must also take into account preparing users for this change. Lewin's change theory models the processes that occur in a planned change. He divides these changes into three stages: unfreezing, moving, and refreezing. Ways of moving a group from the first to the last stage need to be part of a plan for implementation of a system.

Unfreezing.   This stage is based on the idea that human behavior is supported by a balance of driving and restraining forces that create an equilibrium. When a driving force toward change occurs, a countering restraining force often develops to allow the maintenance of equilibrium. Thus, to unfreeze, it is necessary to reduce the restraining forces and allow the driving forces to become dominant. Restraining forces are often personal psychological defenses or group norms, whereas driving forces can be involvement in the process, having one's opinion respected, and continuous communication during the process.

Moving.   In this stage, the planned change is implemented. This is not a comfortable period. Anxieties are high and if they are not successfully dealt with, the change may be unsuccessful. Additionally, it is important to recognize that in this stage movement may occur in the wrong direction. This is especially likely to happen if the new system has many problems or is not supported by administration. Thus, it is important to gain the support of administration in the planning process, involve users so that the system serves them instead of creating more work, test the system thoroughly before implementation, provide adequate training, and deal with any implementation problems immediately.

Refreezing. In this stage, the planned change becomes the norm, but it is surrounded by the usual driving and restraining forces. For this state to occur the people involved need to feel confident with the change and feel in control of the procedures involved in the new methods. A well-designed help system that can provide answers to frequent procedures as well as those that a user may only use occasionally will assist in this process as will recognition by the organization of new skills. If too strongly reinforced, this stage can become a problem to the next change.

INFORMATION THEORY

Graves and Corcoran (1986), in their seminal article on nursing informatics, based the theory of nursing informatics on Blum's taxonomy (as cited in Graves & Corcoran, 1986) and definitions of data, information, and knowledge. These three entities are regarded as the core concepts of informatics. **Data** are discrete elements that have not been interpreted, **information** comprises data that has some type of interpretation or structure, and **knowledge** is a synthesis of information. Using this taxonomy, data are combined to produce information and information is collected to produce knowledge. For example, the number 37 is a datum (the singular of data, from the Latin meaning *a given*). It is the smallest unit that can be processed. If we combine the number 37 with the datum that this is a Celsius-scale reading of a body temperature for a person, we now have some information. Combining this still further with the information that this is normal body temperature, we have a small piece of knowledge. **Wisdom**, or knowing when and how to use knowledge, was added to this taxonomy by Nelson & Joos (as cited in Joos, Whitman, Smith, & Nelson, 1992). It requires people to combine their values, knowledge, and experience with the three types of data (Fig. 1-1).

The general idea of information theory is that the move from data to knowledge is a progressive process that follows given steps. Figure 1-1 is greatly simplified; in practice one often finds that the lines between each of these entities are blurred and that the process is iterative. In informatics, the processes of converting data to knowledge are formalized and include manipulations such as capturing, sorting, and organizing the data to give them meaning and produce information. To produce knowledge, the relationships between the data and information are formalized. Wisdom is added by the person using the information.

GENERAL SYSTEMS THEORY

General systems theory is a method of thinking about complex structures such as an information system. The original theory was introduced by von Bertalanffy in 1932 (Schuster & Ashburn, 1992). It was developed in part as a reaction against reductionism, or the reducing of entities to small parts, studying each, and ignoring the actions that each part stimulates in other parts. In systems theory, the focus is on the interaction among the various parts of the system instead of the individual parts. It is based on the premise that the whole is greater than the sum of its parts.

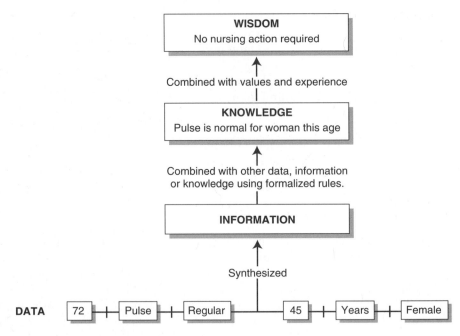

Figure 1-1 • Progression of data to wisdom.

A simplified description of systems theory holds that any change in one part of a system will be reflected in other parts of the system. A computer system, as any informatics person will tell you, is a living example of a system. Making a change in one area invariably affects other sections in ways that were never envisioned. This explains why it is often not a simple matter to make desired changes in systems.

To be part of a system, a phenomenon must be able to be isolated from its surrounding area for analysis yet be part of the functioning of the whole system. Systems are described as being either open or closed. An open system continually exchanges information with the environment outside the system itself. This tends to produce what is called *negentropy*, or higher levels of complexity in the system. Closed systems, however, are isolated from the environment and receive no input from outside. This can result in entropy, or the random and disorganized breakdown of a system. This classification really exists more along the path of a continuum than as an absolute.

Other concepts in systems theory are concerned with the feedback process, which consists of input, throughput, and output, all of which are important functions in information systems. *Input* involves adding information to a system. *Throughput* is the processing that the system does with the information. *Output* is the information or process that results from the processing of input. An example would be the inputting of a patient's temperature into a computer system, the system processing that datum with the order that if this patient's temperature is over 101° F, a specific medication should be given, and presenting such information to the nurse in a manner that specifies any action that needs to be taken. Another example is physiological body processes that are governed by hormones.

COGNITIVE SCIENCE

Cognitive science includes topics such as mental models, skill acquisition, perception, and problem solving. It adds to informatics an understanding of how the brain perceives and interprets a screen (Turley, 1996). Characteristics such as color, font, and screen display are processed by the inputter along with the data and can affect clinical judgment. The amount of information that a person can absorb into a useful pattern is also of concern in cognitive science. Principles from these theories provide a guide to developing systems that allow users to concentrate on the task at hand, rather than requiring cognitive tasks to deal with the computer interface. Cognitive theory can also aid an informatics nurse specialist in understanding the information processing done by a nurse in decision making and facilitate the design of tools to support these processes (Staggers & Thompson, 2002).

LEARNING THEORIES

Learning theories can be applied in informatics to help individuals learn to use computer applications. Many theories explore human learning; the theory into practice database currently lists 50 (Kearsley, 2000). It is impossible to categorize them, but most either fall somewhere on a continuum between stimulus-response, as represented by behaviorism, and self-learning, as represented by constructivism/cognitivism (Table 1-1). Some of the theories not on this continuum may assist one in deciding from which end of the continuum to select teaching methods. These include theories that look at attributes such as developmental age, ability, social influences, and learning style. In preparing learning activities, it is likely that principles from more than one theory will be used. There is truth in all these theories; the best choice therefore depends on the learning situation.

Behaviorism/Objectivism

Behaviorism is a theory of animal and human learning that focuses on objectively observable behaviors. Learning is defined as the acquisition of a new behavior. Developed early in the 20th century with the aim of applying scientific principles to learning, it was a reaction against psychodynamic theories that focused on mental activity and unconscious motivations. These invisible actions were seen as unscientific (Schuster & Ashburn, 1992). The theory holds that all learning is controlled by the environment. Behaviors that are reinforced will recur whereas behaviors that elicit a negative reinforcement will be extinguished. Behaviorism emphasizes breaking subject matter down into the smallest unit for learning; hence, it is often termed *reductionistic* in approach. This theory could be useful in teaching the parts of a procedure that require rote learning, such as how to enter or retrieve data in a system.

Constructivism

In constructivism, learning is seen as a process that occurs when a learner attempts to interpret the world. The result is that knowledge is seen as a personal belief, rather than an independent, verifiable entity. Using this theory, it is assumed that individuals create their own mental structures composed of knowledge and beliefs, which are used to make sense of experiences. Learning, therefore, consists of either adjusting one's model or creating a completely new model. Of the two, the latter involves considerably more work. Frustra-

TABLE 1-1 ● *Comparison of Constructivist and Objectivist Assumptions*

Elements	Objectivist	Constructivist
	Ends of the Continuum	
Reality	The world is a real, structured entity. Its structure can be modeled for and acquired by learners (Jonassen, Wilson, Wang & Grabinger, 1993). Reliable knowledge exists about the world (Jonassen, 1992).	Reality is a result of mental activity that is determined by the experiences and interpretations of the learner (Jonassen, et al. 1993). It is in the mind of the knower (Jonassen, 1992).
Mind	The mind's purpose is to mirror reality by manipulating symbols that represent reality (Jonassen, et al. 1993) through thought processes (Jonassen, 1992).	The mind's role is to interpret experiences and construct meaning from them (Jonassen, et al. 1993). These interpretations are a personal and individualistic knowledge base filtered by one's mind (Jonassen, 1992).
Thought	Learners replicate the interpretations of others (Jonassen, et al. 1993). Thought processes are analyzable and decomposable (Jonassen, 1992).	An individual constructs his own thoughts from his perception of reality (Jonassen, et al. 1993).
Meaning	Meaning reflects reality and is external to the learner (Jonassen, et al. 1993).	Meaning is determined by the learner, and is dependent on an individual understanding that may or may not rely on the structures of the world. (Jonassen, et al. 1993). We all conceive of the world somewhat differently (Jonassen, 1992).
Purpose of instruction	The purpose of instruction is to enable learners to replicate the reality of the instruction in their own minds (Jonassen, et al. 1993).	Instruction should facilitate learners' construction and interpretation of conceptually functional, meaningful, representations of the world (Jonassen, 1992).
Role of instruction	Instructions should interpret and simplify events for learners (Jonassen, 1992, Jonassen, et al. 1993).	Instructions facilitate self interpretation and evaluation of events. They are based in tasks that are both meaningful and able to accommodate constructivistic applications (Jonassen, 1992).
Emphasis	Knowing information (Jonassen, et al. 1993).	Process of learning (Jonassen, 1992, Jonassen, et al. 1993).

From Thede, L. Q. (1995). *Comparison of a constructivist and objectivist framework for designing computer-aided instruction.* Unpublished dissertation, Kent State University, Kent, OH.

tion often occurs when people realize that their current mental structure will not fit a new situation, and they attempt to organize the new data and information to produce a new mental model. These principles explain why people with no computer skills find it very difficult to learn to use a system. They have none of the knowledge structures that a computer user has, hence have no mental model into which to place the new information. This results in a lack of understanding of the material being presented and the inability to implement what is being taught. Individual help for these people can assist them to build the new mental structure needed to use the system.

Adult Learning Theory

Knowles' theory of adult learning, often referred to as andragogy, is an attempt to develop a theory specifically for adult learning. It should probably be considered closer to constructivism than behaviorism but with added information about the characteristics that one might expect in adults. The theory emphasizes that adults expect to take responsibility for decisions and that they are self-directed (Kearsley, 2000). This theory makes the assumptions that adults need to know why they need to learn, they need to learn by doing, they approach learning as a problem-solving exercise, and they learn best when they believe the topic is of immediate value to them. Thus, when using these principles, the process of learning is emphasized over the content learned. Adult learning theory is probably best used as the basic theory for education of healthcare personnel about using computers but it ought supplemented with other theories when the learning requires this.

 ## Benefits of Informatics

Informatics offers many benefits for healthcare. They can be seen in the ability to create and use **aggregated data**, to prevent errors, and to provide better medical records.

BENEFITS FOR HEALTHCARE IN GENERAL

One of the primary benefits of informatics is that data that were previously buried in inaccessible records becomes usable. Informatics is not just about collecting data, but about making it useful. When data are captured electronically in a structured manner, they can be retrieved and used in many different ways, both to easily assimilate information about one patient and as aggregated data. **Aggregated data** are the same piece or pieces of data collected from records of many patients. Table 1-2 shows some aggregated data for postsurgical infections. When aggregated data are examined, patterns can be seen that might otherwise take several weeks or months to become evident or might never become evident. When patterns such as the prevalence of infections with staphylococcal bacteria for Dr. Smith emerge (see Table 1-2), investigations into what these patients have in common may begin. Caution, however, should be observed. The aggregated data in Table 1-2 are insufficient for drawing conclusions, they only serve to indicate a problem and suggest clues about where to start investigating. Aggregated data may be a type of knowledge, but wisdom may dictate that it is incomplete knowledge.

Informatics can also improve patient safety. The Leapfrog Group, which was started by the Business Roundtable in response to the 1999 report by the Institute of Medicine that found up to 98,000 preventable hospital deaths, has started a campaign to improve patient safety (Fact Sheet, 2001). This group is composed of the chief executives of leading corporations in the United States who are interested in reducing their healthcare costs by improving patient safety. Based on the finding that computer physician order entry (CPOE) reduces serious prescribing errors by 50%, this group has as one of its primary objectives the installation of CPOE in all institutions from which they purchase healthcare.

Members of the Leapfrog Group intend to educate their employees about patient safety and the importance of comparing healthcare providers. They will offer financial incen-

			TABLE 1-2 ● *Data in the Aggregate*		
First Name	**Last Name**	**Unit**	**Surgery**	**Physician**	**Pathogen**
Charles	Johnson	3 West	Cholecystectomy	Black	E. coli
Jack	Hearn	4 West	Appendectomy	Black	Strep
Georgette	Brandt	4 West	Tonsillectomy	Black	Strep
Gloria	Grant	2 East	Cholecystectomy	Greene	E. coli
John	Neilson	2 East	Herniorrhaphy	Greene	E. coli
Gloria	Grant	2 East	Cholecystectomy	Greene	Strep
Susan	Susan	3 West	Tubal ligation	Jones	Strep
Ken	Peterson	2 East	Cholecystectomy	Smith	E. coli
Florence	Munson	4 West	Herniorraphy	Smith	E. coli
Ken	Peterson	2 East	Cholecystectomy	Smith	Staph
Florence	Munson	4 West	Herniorraphy	Smith	Staph
Carolyn	Jones	3 West	Hysterectomy	Smith	Staph
George	Jensen	3 West	Open reduction, lt femur	Smith	Staph
Barbara	Danforth	2 East	Herniorraphy	Smith	Staph

tives to their covered employees for selecting care from hospitals that meet the group's standards. Without information systems in place, healthcare providers will have a difficult time in providing the information that these healthcare buyers demand.

Additional benefits for healthcare in general include making the storage and retrieval of healthcare records much easier, providing quick retrieval of test results from many locations, experiencing fewer lost charges due to easier methods of recording charges, and producing printouts of needed information. The computerization of administrative tasks such as staffing and scheduling will also save time and money.

BENEFITS TO THE NURSING PROFESSION

Each healthcare discipline will benefit from its investment in informatics. In nursing, informatics will not only enhance practice but also allow nursing science to develop (Fitzpatrick, 1988). Informatics will improve documentation and, when properly implemented, can reduce the time spent in documentation. Estimates of the time nurses spend in charting vary from 25% to 50% (Dick & Steen, 1991). Duplicate data entry (Iowa Intervention Project, 1997), such as entering vital signs both in nursing notes and on a flow sheet, wastes time and invites errors. In a well-designed clinical documentation system, these data will be entered once, retrieved, and presented in many different forms to meet the needs of the user.

Paper documentation methods create many problems, such as inconsistency and irregularity in charting and a lack of standardized data for evaluation and research. An electronic clinical information system can remind users of the need to provide data in areas apt to be forgotten and provide a list of terms that can be used to enter data. The ability to use patient data for both quality control and research is vastly improved when documentation is complete.

Despite Florence Nightingale's emphasis on data, for much of nursing's history, nursing data have not been valued. They have either been buried in paper patient records that make retrieving them economically infeasible, or worse, have been discarded when a patient is discharged. Hence this information is unavailable for strengthening nursing science. With the advent of electronic clinical documentation, nursing data can be made a part of the electronic healthcare record and become available to researchers for building practice-based nursing knowledge.

The First Step: Computer Fluency

In the previous half-century, the progress in computer processing power has been phenomenal, but healthcare professionals, including nurses, have been slow to take advantage of this (Saba, 2001). A report prepared by the National Advisory Council on Nurse Education and Practice (NACNEP) states that practicing nurses are generally not computer literate and nurses do not fully use computer technology (NACNEP, 1997) Among the categories of nursing informatics needs that they identified were the need to identify and incorporate informatics skills and competencies at all levels of nursing education. To meet these needs, nursing schools must teach information seeking and evaluation skills and must integrate nursing informatics into nursing science, practice and education. One of NACNEP's goals is to provide all nurses with basic computer skills in using computer applications (e.g., word processing and presentation programs), as well as preparing them to use information in the clinical areas. These concepts are based on the belief that if nurses are to provide quality care they need to view the computer as just another professional tool.

As with all nursing skills, technology changes rapidly. Perhaps a better perspective on computer use can be gained by thinking in terms of computer fluency rather than literacy. The term *computer fluency* implies that a person has a life-long commitment to acquiring new skills for the purpose of being more effective in work and personal life (Committee on Information Technology Literacy, 1999). This necessitates a goal of gaining sufficient foundational skills and knowledge to enable one to acquire new skills independently.

Simpson (1998) points out the need for nurses to master computers to avoid becoming extinct. A computer is a mind tool that frees us from the mental drudgery of data processing, just as the bulldozer frees us from the drudgery of digging dirt. Like the bulldozer, however, it must be used intelligently or damage can result.

Given the breadth of careers now open to nurses, learning the physical tasks associated with using a computer for managing information is a necessity. Knowing how to use graphic interfaces and application programs (e.g., word processing, spreadsheets, databases and presentation programs) prepares students and practicing nurses for professional careers. Just as anatomy and physiology provide a background for learning about disease processes and treatments, computer fluency skills are increasingly being seen as a good springboard for more complex informatics concepts (McNeil & Odom, 2000) and as a solid base for learning clinical applications (Nagelkerk, Ritolo, & Vandort, 1998).

Many people, starting with Ronald and Skiba (1987), have looked at the computer competencies required for nurses They identified three levels of competencies: informed user, proficient user, and developer. The informed user should be familiar with basic computer terminology, identify common nursing applications, and be able to operate a computer system. Using the computer as a tool to solve nursing problems, communicating nursing needs for a documentation system, and being able to analyze the relationship between patient outcomes and nursing actions by using a computer to manage data are some of the behaviors required for a proficient user. The top level, a developer, would have the ability to analyze and design systems.

Staggers, Gassert, and Curran (2001) defined four levels of informatics competencies for practicing nurses.

1. A beginning nurse should possess basic information management and computer technology skills. Accomplishments should include the ability to access data, use a computer for communication, use basic desktop software, and use decision support systems.
2. An experienced nurse should be highly skilled in using information management and computer technology to support his or her major area of practice. Additional skills for the experienced nurse include being able to make judgments based on trends and patterns within data elements and to collaborate with nursing informatics nurses to suggest improvements in nursing systems.
3. An informatics nurse specialist has advanced preparation in nursing informatics. The informatics nurse specialist focuses on meeting the information needs of practicing nurses by integrating and applying information, computer, and nursing sciences.
4. An informatics innovator also has advanced preparation in nursing informatics. The informatics innovator's skills include conducting informatics research and generating informatics theory.

The need for basic computer and information management skills in all nurses becomes more evident every day. With pushes from the private sector, such as the Leapfrog Group's initiatives, and federal rules from the Health Insurance Portability and Accountability Act (HIPAA), those who do not understand both the benefits and limitations of a computer are in danger of being lost. In an information age, if data are not included in a computer, the concepts or functions that the data represent are not used in creating the information and knowledge that guides practice and creates policy. For data from nursing to be included, the profession must unite and agree on which data are important and what terminology should be used to represent these data.

Like nursing informatics, the level of computer fluency needed by nurses to work with nursing informatics in their practice may mean different things to different people. In this book, computer fluency is stressed. Background information is presented to provide a grounding in computers as a tool to serve as a springboard to using informatics in professional life both on and off a clinical unit and to adapt to changes in technology. These principles are built on to provide nurses the beginning informatics skills needed in a practitioner, such as the ability to find and evaluate information from electronic sources, understand the need for clinical information management, and work with nursing informatics specialists in providing effective information systems (Display 1-1).

 ## Summary

As knowledge continues to expand logarithmically, tools for information management become mandatory. Healthcare informatics is the science that healthcare uses to manage this information. Comprising knowledge from at least three disciplines, computer science, information management, and healthcare science (and quite probably a fourth, cognitive

---

Display 1-1 • COMPUTER SKILLS REQUIRED BY TODAY'S NURSES AS SEEN BY AN INFORMATICS NURSE SPECIALIST

In today's environment at an absolute minimum, they [nurses] need to have knowledge of word processing, spreadsheet, and e-mail applications as well as knowledge on how to obtain info online. They should also have an understanding of legal and ethical considerations for general computing and specifically for patient information. To reach for the sky—the ideal person would understand how databases function (helpful in grasping concepts of how clinical applications work) and how to work in a networked environment.

Lynn Geren, RN, MSN, CNOR
NMIS Coordinator
Harris County Hospital District
Information Technology—Shared Services—Education
2525 Holly Hall
Houston, TX 77054

---

science), informatics will assist in improving patient care and experiences. Computers are an informatics tool, just as a stethoscope is a healthcare tool. Their use in healthcare started in the 1960s, mostly in financial areas, but with the advance in computing power and the demand for clinical data, computers are being used in clinical areas more and more. With this growth has come a change in focus for information systems from providing solutions for just one process, to an enterprise-wide patient centered system that focuses on data to provide many uses for these data and multiple functionality. To understand and work with clinical systems, as well as to fulfill other professional responsibilities, nurses need to become computer fluent.

connection—ᴗ For definitions of bolded key terms, visit the online glossary available at http://connection.lww.com/go/thede.

CONSIDERATIONS AND EXERCISES

1. What examples can you think of in which your current knowledge had to be replaced with new knowledge?

2. Using the definitions of nursing informatics in this chapter or from other resources, create your own nursing informatics definition that would apply to your clinical practice.

3. When Jacquard invented the weaving machine the workers, fearful of losing their jobs, rioted and broke the machine. How does this relate to today's climate?

4. Dr. Weed's PROMIS system was a radical departure from healthcare organizational thinking. The current healthcare climate, however, is undergoing radical changes. Give reasons why or why not the PROMIS system would be better accepted today?

5. Pressure to improve safety in the healthcare system is now coming from outside healthcare. What implications does this have for healthcare as a profession? (See http://www.leapfroggroup.org/.)

6. The theories supporting informatics are not confined to this field.

   a. In adopting a computer, in which category of Roger's diffusion theory would you place yourself?

   b. Think of planning a change for an organization. What are some of the restraining forces? The driving forces? How would you proceed?

   c. Develop a path of progress for a piece of data, for instance, a number, from raw data to wisdom.

   d. Think of some of the various organizations with which you are familiar. Where would you classify them on the open closed continuum of systems theory? Give your rationale for this classification.

   e. Look at the difference between the objectivist and constructivist assumptions in Table 1-1. On which end of the continuum would you place a recent educational experience?

7. What implications for nursing does healthcare informatics have?

8. Think of the act of giving medication. Which data would you tell a systems developer are needed for this act? How should the data be processed? (Save this answer and compare it with an answer you write after studying Chapter 15.)

9. What computer skills do you possess? What skills do you need to learn to be able to productively use a computer in your career?

REFERENCES

American Nurses Association (2001). *Scope and Standards of Nursing Informatics Practice.* Washington, D. C: American Nurses Publishing.

Anderson, D. (2001). *Diffusion of innovation.* Retrieved January 9, 2002 from http://riccistreet.net/port80/charthouse/present/diffusion.htm.

Blum, B. L. (Ed.). (1986). *Clinical information systems.* New York: Springer.

Committee on Information Technology Literacy, National Research Council (1999). *Being Fluent with Information Technology.* Retrieved May 28, 2002 from http://www.nap.edu/catalog/6482.html.

Computers: History and Development, in *Jones Telecommunications and Multimedia Encyclopedia.* Retrieved January 8, 2002 from http://www.digitalcentury.com/encyclo/update/comp_hd.html.

Delaney, C. (2001). Health informatics and oncology nursing. *Seminars in Oncology Nursing, 17*(1), 2–6.

Dick, R., & Steen, E. B. (Eds.) (1991). *The computer-based patient record.* Washington, DC: National Academy Press.

Fact Sheet (2001) The Leapfrog Group for Patient Safety. Retrieved January 10, 2002, from https://leapfrog.medstat.com.

Fitzpatrick, J. (1988). Nursing: How do we know, what do we do; and how can we enhance nursing knowledge and practice. In *Nursing and computers, proceedings of the third international symposium on nursing use of computers and information science* (pp. 58–65). St. Louis: C.V. Mosby.

Goossen, W. T. F. (1996). Nursing information and processing: A framework and definition for systems analysis, design and evaluation. *International Journal of Biomedical Computing, 40*(3), 187–195.

Graves, J. R., & Corcoran, S. (1986). The Study of nursing informatics. *Image: Journal of Nursing Scholarship, 21*(4), 227–231. Also available at http://www.nih.gov/ninr/vol4/research/Overview.html.

Hannah, K. J., Ball, M. J., & Edwards, M. J. A. (1994). *Introduction to Nursing Informatics*. New York: Springer.

Hogarth, M. (1997). *Medical informatics: An introduction*. Retrieved January 7, 2002 from http://informatics.ucdmc.ucdavis.edu/Concepts/intro.htm.

Iowa Intervention Project (1997). Proposal to bring nursing into the information age. *Image: Journal of Nursing Scholarship 29*(3), 275–281.

Jonassen, D. H. (1992). Evaluating constructivistic learning. In T. M. Duffy, & D. H. Jonassen (Eds.) *Constructivism and the technology of instruction* (pp. 138–148). Hillsdale, N. J.: Lawrence Erlbaum Associates.

Jonassen, D. H., Wilson, B. G., Wang, S., & Grabinger, R. S. (1993). Constructivist uses of expert systems to support learning. *Journal of Computer Based Instruction, 20*(3), 86–94.

Joos, I., Whitman, N. I., Smith, M. J., & Nelson, R. (1992). *Computer in small bytes*. New York: National League for Nursing Press.

Kearsley, G. (2000a). *Explorations in learning & instruction: the theory into practice database*. Retrieved January 9, 2002 from http://tip.psychology.org/index.html.

Kearsley, G. (2000b) *Andragogy*. Retrieved January 9, 2002 from http://tip.psychology.org/knowles.html.

Korpman, R. A. (1990). Patient care automation the future is now: Introduction and historical perspective, part 1. *Nursing Economics 8*(3), 191–193.

McDonald, M. D. (1994, March/April). Telecognition for improving health. *Healthcare Forum Journal,* 18–21.

McNeill, D. G. (1979). Developing the complete computer-based information system. *Journal of Nursing Administration 9*(11), 34–46.

McNeil, B. J. & Odom, S. K. (2000). Nursing informatics education in the United States: Proposed undergraduate curriculum. *Health Informatics Journal 6*, 32–38.

Miller, L. P. (1993). Nursing, computers and quality care. *Medical-Surgical Nursing Quarterly 1*(3), 102–116.

Moye, W. T. (1996). *ENIAC: The army-sponsored revolution*. Retrieved January 8, 2002 from http://ftp.arl.army.mil/~mike/comphist/96summary/.

Nagelkerk, J, Ritolo, P. M., & Vandort, P. J. (1998). Nursing informatics: The trend of the future. *Journal of Continuing Education in Nursing, 29*(1), 17–21.

National Advisory Council on Nurse Education in Practice (NACNEP). (1997). *A national informatics agenda for nursing education and policy*. Retrieved January 10, 2002 from http://bhpr.hrsa.gov/dn/nacnep/informatics.htm.

Nelson, R. & Joos, I. (1989). On language in nursing: From data to wisdom. *PLN Visions, Fall,* 6–7.

Newbold, S. K. (1996). The informatics nurse and the certification process. *Computers in Nursing, 14*(2), 84–86.

Ronald, J. & Skiba, D. (1987). *Guidelines for basic computer education in nursing*. (NLN Pub No 41-2177.) New York: National League for Nursing.

Saba, V. K. (1983). How computers influence nursing activities in community health. In *First national conference: Computer and technology and nursing*. (NIH Publication No. 83-2412.). (pp.7–12). Washington, D. C: U. S. Government Printing Office.

Saba, V. K. (2001). Nursing informatics: Yesterday, today and tomorrow. *International Nursing Review, 48,* 177–187.

Saba, V. K., Johnson, J. E., & Simpson, R. L. (1994). *Computers in nursing management*. Washington, DC: American Nurses Association.

Sackett, K. M., & Erdley, W. S. (2001). The history of healthcare informatics. In S. Englebart & R. Nelson (Eds.), *Healthcare informatics from an interdisciplinary approach* (pp. 453–477). St. Louis: Mosby.

Scholes, M. & Barber, B. (1980). Towards nursing informatics. In D. A. D. Lindberg, & S. Kaihara (Eds.) *MEDINFO: 1980* (p. 7–73). Amsterdam: North-Holland.

Schuster, C. & Ashburn, S. S. (1992). *The process of human development: A holistic life-span approach* (3rd ed.). Philadelphia: J. B. Lippincott.

Schwirian, P. (1986). The NI pyramid—A model for research in nursing informatics. *Computers in Nursing, 4*(3), 134–136.

Shortliffe E. H., & Blois M. S. (2001). The computer meets medicine: Emergence of a discipline. In Shortliffe E. H., & Perrault L. E. (Eds.), *Medical informatics: Computer applications in healthcare* (pp. 3–40.) New York: Springer.

Simpson, R. (1998). The technologic imperative: A new agenda for nursing education and practice, part 1. *Nursing Management, 29*(9), 22–24.

Staggers, N., Gassert, C. A. & Curran, C. (2001). Informatics competencies for nurses at four levels of practice. *Journal of Nursing Education 40*(7), 303-316.

Staggers, N., & Thompson, C. B. (2002). The evolution of definitions for nursing informatics: A critical analysis and revised definition. *Journal of the American Medical Association 9*(3), 255–261.

Thede, L. Q. (1995). *Comparison of a constructivist and objectivist framework for designing computer-aided-instruction.* Unpublished dissertation, Kent State University, Kent, OH.

Turley, J. (1996). Toward a model for nursing informatics. *Image: Journal of Nursing Scholarship, 28*(4), 309–313.

Zielstorff, R. D., Hudgings, C, I., & Grobe, S. J. (1993) *Next-generation nursing information systems: Essential characteristics for professional practice.* (Pub No. NP-83). Washington, DC: American Nurses Association.

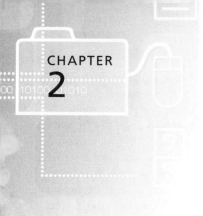

The Hardware: Meet the Computer

Objectives

After studying this chapter you will be able to:

1. *Refute some common computer myths.*

2. *Explore ways to overcome computer anxiety.*

3. *Differentiate uses for various types of computers.*

4. *Identify uses for unique input and output computer devices*

5. *Define selected computer terms.*

Introducing the use of a stethoscope precedes learning how to listen to heart and lung sounds. If a clinician is to be effective in using the stethoscope, it is necessary to know when to use the bell and when to use the diaphragm. In the same way, it is imperative to have some understanding of how and when to use the tool of informatics, the computer.

A complete computer system is the integration of human input and information resources using **hardware** and **software**. In computer terms, *hardware* refers to objects such as disks, disk drives, **monitors**, keyboards, speakers, printers, mice, boards, chips, and the computer itself. **Software** includes programs that give instructions to the computer that make the machine useful. *Information resources* are data that are manipulated by the computer. *Human input* refers to the entire spectrum of human involvement including deciding what is to be input and how it is to be processed as well as evaluating output and deciding how it should be used. In this chapter, we look at the computer itself, in the next chapter at software.

 ## Computer Myths

Some difficulties that many people face when starting to use computers result from computer myths that have collected over time. Three of the most common are:

1. Computers can think.
2. Computers require a mathematical genius to use.
3. Computers make mistakes (Perry, 1982).

Computers cannot think, and they are not smart. Incidents like the one in which Deep Blue (the nickname given to an IBM computer specially designed to play chess) won a game of chess against world champion Garry Kasparov led to such misperceptions. Consider the game of chess. Although there are many possible combinations, there are a given set of moves, rules, and goals that make it a perfect stage to displaythe potential of computers. Deep Blue is a very powerful computer, capable of analyzing hundreds of millions of possible moves each second. It made use of these qualities to beat Kasparov. It did not use thinking in the human sense.

The myth that only mathematical geniuses can use computers, although just as false, continues to flourish. This belief is linked to the development of the first computers as a means to "crunch numbers," or process mathematical equations. Hence, in colleges and universities, many computer departments are still housed in, or closely related to, departments of mathematics. It did not take experts long to translate the mathematical concepts into everyday language, an accomplishment that made the computer available to everyone, regardless of level of proficiency in math.

The last myth, that computers make mistakes, makes it a wonderful excuse for human error. This was well illustrated by a cartoon in the early 1990s that showed a man saying, "It's wonderful to be able to blame my mistakes at the office on the computer, I think I'll get a personal computer." Computers act on the information they are given. As one humorist said, "Computers are designed to DWIS, or Do What I Say." As many a user will tell you, they resist with great determination any inclination to DWIM, or "Do What I Mean!" Unlike a colleague to whom you only need to give partial instructions because the person is able to fill in the rest, a computer requires complete, definitive, black-and-white directions. Unlike humans, it cannot perceive that a colon and semicolon are closely related, and in many cases, a computer believes that an upper case letter and a lower case letter are as different as the letter A from the letter X. There are no "almosts" with a computer.

Computer Characteristics

A computer accomplishes many things that are impossible without it. When programmed properly, it is superb in remembering and processing details, calculates accurately according to its input and instructions, prints reports tirelessly, facilitates editing documents greatly, and spares uers may repetitive tedious, tasks, which frees us to use our time in more productive endeavors. However, remember that computers are not infallible. Being electronic, they are subject to electrical problems. Humans build computers, program them, and enter data into them. For these reasons, many situations can cause error and frustration. Two of the most common challenges with computers are "glitches" and the "garbage in, garbage out" principle (GIGO).

Anyone, who has been using a computer when it **crashed** or "went down" may have experienced a guilty feeling that she or he did something wrong. If the person actually did create the crash, unless she or he were purposely engaged in something destructive, that person did not cause the crash; she or he just found a flaw in the system, which was inadvertently created by the programmer(s).[1] There are times, however, when crashes occur for

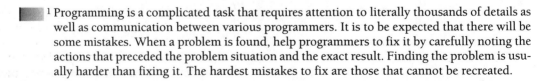

[1] Programming is a complicated task that requires attention to literally thousands of details as well as communication between various programmers. It is to be expected that there will be some mistakes. When a problem is found, help programmers to fix it by carefully noting the actions that preceded the problem situation and the exact result. Finding the problem is usually harder than fixing it. The hardest mistakes to fix are those that cannot be recreated.

seemingly no reason. Computers, regardless of their manufacturer, will at some time, for unknown reasons, perform in a totally unexpected manner (Perry, 1982).

Overcoming Computer Anxiety

The attitudes people have toward computers range from complete dislike and frustration to curiosity and excitement. Although the mass media and personal acquaintances convey both perceptions, people seem to remember the negative points more clearly. As with all new experiences, becoming acquainted with a computer or a new computer application can produce anxiety. The breadth of this problem only in relation to nursing can be seen by looking at some of the many studies that have analyzed computer anxiety and attitudes in nurses (Simpson & Kenrick, 1997; McBride & Nagle, 1996; Jayasuriya & Caputi, 1996; Focus, 1995). It is highly likely that the same type of anxieties were present when the general population found it necessary to learn to drive. There are, however, no known studies of this phenomena dating from that time (Display 2-1).

Addressing these fears takes time for both a trainer and the individual experiencing the fears. One-on-one sessions for the person affected may be necessary and save time in the long run by preventing frantic calls to the help center. Studies show that the learning patterns of those afraid of computers can be improved by treating the bodily symptoms of anxiety and providing distracting thought patterns (Bloom, 1985). Techniques, such as teaching relaxation techniques before starting any hands-on training, often helps, as does giving the anxious trainee something to repeat internally such as, "You're in control, not the computer."

Other helpful techniques include recognizing and accepting fears. Having trainees check off from a list of possible feelings (e.g., panicky, lost, curious) those that apply to themselves can help them face up to their fears. Inherent in all these terrors is the fear of failure and of looking incompetent in front of their peers. This may be especially evident in people who see themselves as having a high degree of competence in their profession, and to whom people look for answers. Placing themselves in a learning situation can be very threatening to their self-image.

Types of Computers

The progress in computers is measured by generations, each of which grew out of a new innovation (Table 2-1). Computer sizes vary from supercomputers intended to process large amounts of data for one user at a time to small palmtop computers. Each type has its niche in healthcare. However, it is becoming increasingly difficult to classify the different types of computers, because smaller ones take on the characteristics of their bigger brothers as the amount of space needed for processing lessens.

SUPERCOMPUTERS

Technically, **supercomputers** are the most powerful type, if power is judged by the ability to do numerical calculations. Supercomputers can process hundreds of millions of instructions per second. They are used in applications that require extensive mathematical calculations, such as weather forecasts, fluid dynamic calculations, and nuclear energy research. Supercomputers are designed to execute only one task at a time; hence they de-

My great-great-grandmother rode a horse but was afraid of a train. My great-grandmother rode the train but was afraid to drive a car. My grandmother drove a car but was afraid to fly. My mother flies in an airplane but is afraid of computers. I use a computer, but am afraid to ride a horse....

What we fear is most often what we are unfamiliar with, or something with which we have had a bad experience. It is not unusual to be unfamiliar with computers, and it is quite possible that some of you have had a less than pleasant encounter with a computer. Unpleasant experiences with computers are often related to a lack of meaningful help when trying to figure out how to accomplish a task. Not too long ago, documentation for software provided information about a function, but neglected to say how to perform it. Fortunately, today's online documentation has progressed to a point where it is much more helpful.

Another thought that can impede one's using a computer fully is a fear that one will break the computer. In truth, it is very difficult to break a computer; unless of course you dump a cup of coffee or other liquid on it, throw it out the window, or hit it with a baseball bat.[1] At times, everyone has been tempted to do at least one of these things. Computers can be frustrating! Breaking the computer or erasing an entire system by means that do not involve physically attacking it, such as by pressing a key, is not something users can do accidentally in a well-designed system. In the rare instance that this should happen it is not the user who has created the problem. It is the software (or hardware) producers who have failed to produce a robust system. Creating good software involves trying to anticipate all the various ways that a user could act when she or he misunderstands what is required and providing *error traps* to assist the user in these instances. An error trap is a programming sequence that responds to erroneous keystrokes or actions with feedback that gives information about the difficulty and how to correct it.

Not knowing what to do when using a computer is where we all begin. This also occurs when we learn a new program, or when we need to learn a new version of an existing program. We all stumble and make false starts as we learn new things. We were not born knowing how to walk, read, or write. Yet today, we can do all these things because we learned how. In the same way, anyone who wants to can learn to use a computer. Just as you made many false starts learning to do any of the aforementioned activities, when you are learning to use a computer you will not always accomplish your objectives on the first or even the third try.

One source of frustration in using computers is the machine's inability to discriminate shades of gray. With a computer, an action you perform either produces the desired result or does not. This behavior, however, is no different than that of other technologies with which you are familiar. If you are in an elevator and push the number five, the elevator will stop at the fifth floor whether you really wanted to go to the fifth floor or not, even when you realize you made a mistake and then push six for the sixth floor. This exactness, however, produces a machine of great predictability, which is the same characteristic that makes the computer functional. A given command produces a given function. Period! Almost is not a computer parameter.

When you think of learning to use a computer, think trial and error. It is this process that produces the knowledge and competency that you are seeking. If you perform an action and what you expected to have happen does not, observe what has happened. Then try again. It may be necessary to use any of the help systems available to you before you gain your goal. *Try to look at your situation as though you made a discovery, not a mistake.* This, of course, is not the model of learning with which most of us are familiar (Simpson, 1996). Prior experience has led us to fear "mistakes" and regard them as a sign of failure.

Educational experience has often conditioned us to expect a teacher to impart the knowledge we need to function. In learning to use a computer, didactic information can only give a small part of the picture. As thinking human beings, we need to apply this information by actively experimenting, observing the results of our experimentation, and reflecting on this information.

Additionally, try to remember that as humans we cannot open our heads and have information or skills poured in. We have to work at learning. Senge (1994) tells us that real learning only occurs when we struggle with feeling incompetent and ignorant. You need to accept the fact that you will make many "discoveries" before you feel comfortable. You will feel frustrated at times too. A good rule of thumb to follow is to take a break when frustration threatens to disable you. Many problems are solved when an individual takes a break and lets the subconscious work. When your frustration level gets high, take a break and remember that you have learned to ride a bike and drive a car, both potentially far more dangerous to your health than using a computer. You can also learn to "drive" a computer.

References

Computer shot dead by frustrated owner (1997, July 12). *Cleveland Plain Dealer*, 8A.

Senge, P. (1994). *The Fifth Discipline: The Art and Practice of the Learning Organization.* New York: Currency Double Day

Simpson, R. (1996). Creating a true learning organization. *Nursing Management 27*(4), 18; 20.

---

[1] There was one frustrated owner who, forgetting that the computer was inhuman, or maybe because of it, shot his computer "dead." He put four bullets into the hard drive and one into the monitor, whereupon he was taken to a mental hospital for observation (Computer shot dead, 1997).

TABLE 2-1 ● *The Five Generations of Computers*		
Generations	**Dates**	**Innovation**
1	1940 – 1956	Vacuum tubes
2	1956 – 1963	Transistors
3	1964 – 1971	Integrated circuits
4	1971 – present	Microprocessors
5	Present and beyond	Artificial intelligence that can produce voice recognition and responses to natural language

From Webopedia (2002). The five generations of computers. Retrieved May 4, 2002 from http://www.webopedia.com/DidYouKnow/2002/April/FiveGenerations.html.

vote all their resources to this one situation. This gives them the speed they need for their tasks.

Mainframes and Minicomputers

Mainframes are designed to serve many users and run many programs at the same time. These computers form the backbone of many hospital information systems. A few years ago, the "computers" found on clinical units were not really computers, but **video-text terminals**.[2] A video-text terminal consists of a display screen, keyboard, and modem or device that connects it to the mainframe. Information is entered on the keyboard and transmitted to the mainframe, which is located somewhere else, often in the basement in a secure, temperature-controlled room. Any processing done to the information is done by the mainframe, which returns the results to the screen of the video-text terminal.

Minicomputers are like mainframes (that is, they are multiuser machines that originally served video-text terminals), but they are smaller and less costly. Today, they may be used as the server for networked personal computers or a **thin client** (today's version of a video-text terminal). Unlike larger mainframes, they do not require a special temperature-controlled room and are useful in situations with fewer users.

Choosing the size of the computer needed is based on the tasks that have to be done. Today, computers come in so many sizes that classifying one as a mainframe or another as a mini is more approximate, a point on a continuum rather than an exact classification. Today one is more likely to see computers that function in this capacity called **servers**.

Personal or Single-User Computers

Personal computers (PCs) are designed for an individual user. PCs are based on microprocessor technology that enables manufacturers to put an entire processing (controlling) unit on one chip, thus permitting the small size. When PCs were adopted in business,

[2] These terminals were sometimes referred to as "dumb terminals" because they did not process information. Processing was done by the mainframe to which these terminals sent and received information. This distinguished them from "smart terminals," such as PCs that were capable of processing information as well as communicating with the mainframe.

they freed users from the resource limitations of the mainframe computer and allowed data processing staff to concentrate on tasks that needed a large system. Today, although capable of functioning without being connected to a network, in businesses including healthcare, personal computers are usually connected or networked to either other personal computers, or servers. They still process information but when networked, they can also share data.

In information systems, PCs often replace the old video-text terminal and handle the tasks of entering and retrieving information from the central computer or server. In addition, they allow personnel to use application programs. Today PCs are often referred to as **desktops**, to distinguish them from other smaller one-person computers.

LAPTOPS/NOTEBOOKS

The original portable computer was more transportable than portable. In the last few years of the 1980s, the transportables were replaced by **laptops**, or computers small enough to fit on one's lap. As technology continued to place more information on a chip, laptops became smaller. They are now referred to as **notebook** computers. Some healthcare organizations use notebook computers for **point-of-care** (POC) data entry at the bedside or anyplace where care is delivered.

Notebook computers do have some drawbacks. The screen is usually much smaller than the one in a desktop and the resolution may not be as crisp. Keyboards are usually smaller. The **mouse**, or pointing and selecting device, can be a button the size of a pencil eraser in the middle of the keyboard, or a small square on the user end of the keyboard, or a small ball embedded in the keyboard. Some users purchase **docking stations** for their notebook computers. Docking stations often contain a large monitor, standard sized keyboard, regular mouse, and a large memory storage device. When inserted into the docking station the notebook user can enjoy the amenities of a desktop without losing the portability of a notebook computer.

HANDHELDS AND PERSONAL DIGITAL ASSISTANTS

Handhelds and **personal digital assistants** (PDAs) are types of even smaller computers (Figure 2-1). They range in size from palmtops, or those small enough to fit easily into one hand, to handhelds, which are a little larger than a checkbook. PDAs originally served as personal information managers (PIMs). In this capacity, they provided users with the ability to enter, organize, and easily access various types of information, such as reminders, lists of names, addresses, and dates. They also often included scheduling and calculator programs. Today, in addition to these functions, some PDAs also function as cellular phones. Some PDAs are capable of faxing, using e-mail, and accessing other Internet features. The tools used to input information into today's PDAs include a small keyboard that folds in half for easy storage but is easily connected to the PDA. Other software provides voice and handwriting recognition and the ability to **download** information from a larger computer. Many users exchange data with their desktop computer, either backing up their PDA or downloading information from their desktop for use in the field. This can be done using a docking station–type device or wirelessly.

PDAs have many uses in healthcare. Not only do they make excellent POC entry devices, but today's PDAs may include a calculator, medication reference tools, and elec-

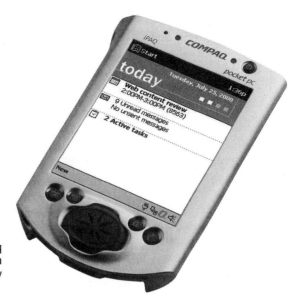

Figure 2-1 • Compaq iPAQ Pocket PC. Compaq logo, iPAQ, and iPAQ Pocket PC product design are trademarks of Hewlett-Packard Company in the U.S. and/or other countries.

tronic textbooks (Criswell & Parchman, 2002), as well as being used to send a prescription to the pharmacy. Software is also available that allows PDAs to deliver real-time information such as MEDLINE journals, a drug information database, and a study guide for nursing rounds (Top Drawer, 2001).

PDAs have also found a use in patient monitoring. For this purpose, the healthcare institution develops a series of questions related to a specific health problem that are programmed into the PDAs (Szynal, 2001). Patients then answer these questions two or three times a week and send the information to the healthcare agency.

THIN CLIENTS

In healthcare, many input and output tasks for information systems do not require the full processing power of a PC. In these cases, a thin client, or a computer without a hard drive and with limited, if any, processing power, fills these needs. Besides costing much less, thin clients do not need to be upgraded when new software is made available because they do not contain any applications. Additionally, older PCs can function in this capacity instead of being retired.

WIRELESS TABLETS

Another type of remote terminal is a wireless tablet. These devices weigh about 2 pounds. They can sit on a lap or table, or hang on a door or bed. All the information storage and processing is done on a remote computer to which the tablet is connected. The screen on the tablet is much larger than the one on a PDA, making it an ideal consideration for use as a point-of-care device.

Personal Computer Systems

Desktop and laptop computers consist of at least three components: a display screen, a keyboard for entering data, and the system components generally housed in rectangular box often referred to as the CPU (i.e., **central processing unit**). These parts provide the input, processing, and output functions needed by a computer.

Computers need a continuous, nonvariable supply of power. Their operation can be affected by a power surge. Although the power surge may be generated by the electrical company, in some homes this can occur when a large electrical device such as an air conditioner comes on. To protect against this, all computers come with some degree of built-in surge protection. When this protection is inadequate, the motherboard may be damaged. For this reason it is a good idea to use a separate, high-quality surge protector. No surge protector, however, will protect from a lighting strike. Some users elect to unplug their computer and monitor altogether during thunderstorms.

PROCESSING COMPONENTS

The system box houses components such as the CPU, **disk drives**, **hard drives**, connectors, and **slots** for special purpose cards. These devices are all mounted on or connected to a **motherboard**. A motherboard is a flat, rectangular board with slots for the **cards** that provide the connectivity for the system components. It may be called the system board. A card is a printed **circuit board** that manages communication between a device such as the monitor and the motherboard or a network and the motherboard.

Central Processing Unit (CPU)

The CPU is the hardware that acts as the heart or brains of the computer; it controls what the computer does. Some computer types such as supercomputers or mainframes may have many CPUs. Personal computers, however, have a single CPU that consists of a single chip called a **microprocessor**. The CPU consists of an **arithmetic logic unit** (ALU), a **control unit**, and some memory registers. The ALU performs all arithmetic and logical operations such as calculating a formula or comparing two items. The control unit directs the flow of information in the computer. It can be thought of as a combination traffic officer and switchboard. It gets instructions from memory, interprets them, directs them, and makes certain they are properly executed. It performs these operations in **nanoseconds** (one billionth of a second) so that to a user the results appear instantaneous.

These chips, smaller and thinner than a baby's fingernail, come in many different varieties. They may be referred to by manufacturer and number or name (e.g., the Celeron or the Intel Pentium 4). All chips with the same number or name are not the same, however. Differences may include power management modifications for battery run computers, or the speed at which the chip accomplishes its tasks. The processing speed is referred to as the **clock speed** of the computer. The clock speed determines how often a pulse of electricity "cycles" or circulates through the circuits, hence how fast information is processed. The more cycles per given time period, the greater the processing speed will be. Clock speed is measured in **hertz**, which is one cycle per second. Most chips today operate in the **megahertz** (MHz) (one million hertz) range although newer chips are capable of speeds in the **gigahertz** (Ghz) range (one billion hertz).

The speed of processing is also affected by what is called "word size." This is not related to a word as we know it in reading, but to the number of **bits** that a computer processes at one time. If a CPU processes 16 bits of information at a time, it is said to be a 16-bit computer, and its word size is 16 bits. A computer that processes 32 bits of information at one time is a 32-bit computer and has a word size of 32 bits. The 32-bit computer, of course, is faster than the 16-bit computer.

Bus

The speed with which the computer returns results is affected not only by the speed of the CPU, but also by the speed and width of a device called a **bus**. Like a bus one sees on a highway, a computer bus is a mode of transportation for data. Physically, a bus is a collection of wires that transmits data from one part of a computer to another, such as from the CPU to the main memory. It also transmits information about where the data should go. Like a CPU, the bus is measured by the number of bits it transfers at one time and the speed of this transfer.

Cards

Many of the functions that a computer performs are regulated by **cards** that are inserted into slots on the motherboard. These cards, which like the motherboard are printed circuit boards, are used for things such as the video display, network connections, and expansion.

HOW A COMPUTER WORKS WITH DATA

A computer does all its work based on whether electronic circuits are on or off. In giving information to the computer, these conditions are represented by a one (1) if the circuit is on and a zero (0) if it is off. Because only 1s and 0s are used, the data are said to be **binary system** data . The decimal system is base 10 whereas a binary system is base 2. Besides the binary system, two other numbering systems may be seen in computers: octal or base 8, and hexadecimal, which is base 16.

Bits and Bytes

The amount of data that can be represented by one circuit is formally called a *binary digit* and is usually referred to as a **bit**. Bits hold only one of two values: 0 or 1. They are the smallest unit of information that a machine can hold. When eight of these bits are combined, there is enough memory, or on-off switches, to represent a letter, number, or other character. This amount of memory is called a **byte**.

American Standard Code for Information Interchange

To make it possible for data to be exchanged between computers, standards were set very early in the evolution of the computer for how the on-and-off switches in a byte would be used for each character. The standard for personal computers is the American Standard Code for Information Interchange (**ASCII**). Under this system, each character on the keyboard is represented by a number.

Types of Data Processing

There are essentially two different types of data processing. Data are processed either interactively or in batch mode. In interactive mode, when a command is issued by the user, the computer responds immediately. In batch processing, information is received and put aside for a time when the computer is not busy. Systems today generally use interactive processing.

MEMORY

Computers need two types of memory: temporary and storage. Temporary memory holds program instructions and data that are being created, edited, or used by a user. This type of memory is kept internally on chips and is formally called memory, or primary memory. *Storage* is the term given to the memory that exists on disks and tape. It is sometimes called secondary memory.

Measurement of Memory

The measurement of memory is based on the byte, or the amount of memory required to store one character. It is expressed by placing prefixes in front of the word byte that denote increments of approximately 1000. A **kilobyte** is 1024 bytes, whereas a **megabyte** is more than 1 million bytes. Although the prefixes in Table 2-2 are from the decimal system, the words they create do not represent numbers divisible by 10 because the amounts are translations from the binary numbering system.

Primary Memory

Internal or primary memory is provided by two types of memory. One is preprogrammed and unchangeable by the user. The other is memory the use of which is determined by the user. It is used by application programs opened by the user and files on which the user is working.

Read Only Memory.   The first type of memory, **read only memory** (ROM), can only be read by the computer; no information can be written to it, and no information can be erased or deleted from it. Users only awareness of ROM may be when they see information flashing on the screen as the computer starts its booting process. The information in ROM is written to before the **chip** containing it is installed at the factory. ROM is used to store critical programs that all computers need such as the program that **boots** (starts) the com-

TABLE 2-2 ● *The Bytes*	
Name	**Number of Bytes**
Kilobyte	1024 bytes
Megabyte	1,048,576 bytes
Gigabyte	1,073,741,824 bytes
Terabyte	1,099,511,627,776 bytes
Petabyte	1,125,899,906,842,624 bytes
Exabyte	1,152,921,504,606,846,976 bytes
Zettabyte	1,000,000,000,000,000,000,000 bytes (approx.)
Yottabyte	1,000,000,000,000,000,000,000,000 bytes (approx.)

puter. It has no relationship to programs installed by a user, or any data that a user creates on the computer.

The **BIOS**, which is an acronym for basic input output system, is usually placed on the ROM chip. The BIOS is built-in software that determines what the computer can do without accessing any additional software. The last instruction that the BIOS executes is to look for an **operating system** and install it. (Operating systems, which are software, are discussed in chapter 3.)

Random Access Memory.   **Random access memory** (RAM) is the working or primary memory of the computer. RAM is temporary memory, or volatile memory which is lost when the power to the computer is lost. RAM is where application programs such as word processing and the documents created with these application programs reside when the computer is on.

A copy of the information needed to function by the application programs is retrieved from secondary storage to RAM each time the user opens the program. Even when the program is in RAM, the full instructions for the application program remain safely on the storage device, usually a **hard drive**. The same is true when users retrieve a file that they created from secondary memory, the original is still on the storage device and the user is working on a copy of the original.

Before shutting off power to the computer, if the user wishes to use the documents he or she created again, he or she needs to store these files, a process called *saving*. The application program does not need to be saved again because the user has not changed those files. If he or she makes changes to the format of the program, the program takes care of saving these when it is shut down before the computer is turned off.

As with processing speeds, the amount of RAM that a computer needs depends on how it is used. For many people, after they purchase a computer, they discover more uses for it than they had originally considered. RAM is contained on a chip that is inserted into a slot. Software specifications usually provide information about the *minimum* amount of RAM required to use a program, but the program may not run as smoothly as a user desires at this minimum level. A good rule of thumb is to buy a little more RAM than you think you may need.

Secondary Memory or Storage

Secondary memory provides storage for user-created files and files needed by application programs when they are not in use or when the computer is turned off. Many devices are used to provide this storage. They employ either magnetic or optical methods of storing data.

Magnetic Disks.   Magnetic disks store information in a magnetized format. Lower-storage-capacity magnetic diskettes consist of a sheet of plastic, whereas larger-capacity disks often have a glass or aluminum core. No matter what material is used to create the core, the base is covered with a thick coating of a magnetizable substance. When in use, the material in this coating is organized so that each bit of information is represented as either magnetized (*on*) or not magnetized (*off*). Because magnetizable material is used, the disk can be remagnetized (i.e., *rewritten*) many times (Figure 2-2).

Before being used, a magnetic disk needs to be **formatted**. Formatting puts the magnetic covering of the disk into a pattern so that the **operating system** with which it will be used can send information or retrieve information from it. This process creates what

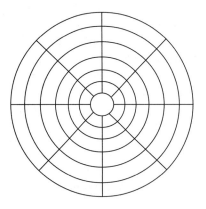

Diskettes are made up of tracks and sectors, which create areas on the disk that can be labeled. The "address" of a sector enables the File Allocation Table (FAT), or table of contents, to locate a file. Large drives may have several layers formatted in this fashion.

Figure 2-2 • Diagram of a diskette.

is called a **FAT**, an acronym for file allocation table. The FAT is the portion of the disk that contains the table of contents of the disk or the area that is used to record the location on the disk of the beginning of a stored file.

Except for the hard drive, most secondary storage formats are portable. To read and or write information to them requires that they be inserted into a computer drive. A *drive* is generally a slot on the front of a computer into which the disk can be inserted. On laptops or PDAs, the drive may be external to the computer and will need to be connected to the computer before it can be used. In each drive is a device called a "read/write" head that is part of the disk drive. This head transfers the information in the form of bits that are either "on" or "off."

HARD DRIVE.   The largest type of a magnetic disk in PCs is the **hard** or **fixed disk**, which is the main form of storage in PCs used today A hard disk consists of several nonflexible disks that are housed along with the read-write head in a hermetically sealed device. It is located inside the box that houses the CPU. Hard disks come in different memory sizes, sizes that are today measured in gigabytes (1 billion bytes), although the day of terabyte hard disks in PCs will come soon. Retrieving data from an internal hard disk is considerably faster than trying to get the same data from other forms of storage.

DISKETTES.   A 3-1/2-inch **diskette** is a common form of a portable magnetic storage device. Although sometimes called a floppy disk because its larger predecessor was flexible, and floppy, currently available diskettes have a hard outer coating. These devices store 1.4 megabytes of data. In practical terms, this is the equivalent of about 300 pages of single-spaced text. Adding tables or any type of graphics (pictures) reduces this number of pages. The number of files also affects the storage capacity because each file includes data needed to name and locate the file. Because they are magnetized and portable, diskettes are subject to environmental hazards (Display 2-2).

Without laboriously using the computer to read the file names on each diskette, it is impossible to tell what an unmarked diskette contains. Organize diskettes by similar contents rather than randomly placing files on them, then carefully label each diskette with a general name for the contents.

Display 2-2 • CARING FOR A DISKETTE

To preserve data on diskettes, keep them 12 to 18 inches from:

1. Magnets (the storage is based on whether a spot is magnetized or not; consequently, any magnet can destroy the memory).
2. Electric motors, including ringing telephones—they give off a magnetic field.
3. Televisions—they, too, give off a magnetic field.

Care for them by:

1. Keeping them dry.
2. Refraining from sliding the protective metal piece covering the read/write surface back and forth. The underneath surface can be scratched.

Reformat them completely before using them to store very important information. (The magnetism in the formatting deteriorates over time.)

ZIP/JAZ DRIVES.   Many people who work with large files find they are too big to transport using a 3-1/2-inch diskette. To meet this need, larger portable diskettes have been developed: **Zip disks** and **Jaz disks**. Zip disks, developed and sold by Iomega Corporation come in two sizes, 100 and 250 megabyte, a 100 megabyte disk holds the equivalent of 70 floppy diskettes. Jaz diskettes are either 1 or 2 gigabytes in size.

TAPE DRIVE (MOSTLY FOR LARGE IS SYSTEMS).   Tape is the least expensive medium for storage and is still used in some systems. The disadvantage to tape as secondary memory is that, like tape in a tape recorder, it is accessed sequentially. Thus, to read a specific block of data it is necessary to read all the preceding blocks, making tapes too slow for general purpose storage. Tapes have a storage rate from a few hundred kilobytes to several gigabytes. On the plus side, a fast tape drive can transfer as much as 20 megabytes per second.

Optical disks.   Optical disks are a storage medium from which data are read and written to by lasers. Data are recorded on optical disks by using a laser to burn microscopic pits onto the surface. Another laser beam is shone on the disk to read them. The holes are detected by changes in the reflection pattern. When a reflection is detected, the bit is on; when there is no reflection, the bit is off. Optical disks have the storage capacity of 630 megabytes of information, which is the equivalent of 700 3-1/2-inch diskettes. Access time, although faster than from a 3-1/2-inch diskette, is generally longer than from a hard disk. Most software sold today is on a compact disk-read only memory (CD-ROM); thus, a CD drive is considered standard equipment on PCs and laptops. CD drives vary in how fast data can be accessed. The speed is expressed as a number followed by an "X". A single-speed CD drive takes 600 milliseconds (or 6/10 of a second) to access 150 kilobytes of memory, whereas a 16× speed drive will access 2.4 megabytes in 1/10 to 2/10 seconds.

In computers, the CD format is being replaced by DVD (digital versatile disk or digital video disk). DVDs can store a minimum of 4.7 gigabytes of information, which is enough for a full-length movie. Newer methods of creating optical disks will continue to enlarge this capacity. Because the data on both CDs and DVDs are burned onto the disks, they are less subject to accidental loss of data than any other portable format. They can, however, be scratched, which can render some data on them unretrievable.

Many computers now come equipped with read/write drives for CDs or DVDs. The technology in these drives has progressed from the ability to read only to the ability to write once and now the ability to rewrite. These capabilities depend on the drive, the software, and the disk itself. Unfortunately, no standard yet exists for DVD read/write, thus what is written to by one computer in one format may not be readable by a computer using a different format.

Nonvolatile RAM.   This type of device does not require an electric current to maintain data in memory. Known as flash memory, it consists of electrically erasable programmable read-only memory (EEPROM) to which data can be written and rewritten. These devices, which are about the size of a pocket flashlight (Figure 2-3), plug into any **Universal Serial Bus (USB) port**, which new computers have. These devices are useful for transporting or saving large files. The amount of data they can hold ranges from 16 megabytes to 1 gigabyte.

Devices for Inputting and Outputting User Information
With a Computer

Many methods are available for getting data into and out of a computer. Some devices are one-way devices, such as a keyboard. Others, such as the disks previously described, function as both input and output devices. Monitors, which are usually assumed to be output devices, function as input devices when light pens, touch screens, and mice are used. Some devices, such printers, are only output devices. The more familiar input devices are explored in Appendix A, the output devices in Appendix B, and those that are both are in Appendix C.

Digital Cameras and Other Imaging Devices.   A newer computer peripheral that has found many uses is a **digital camera**. This device records images digitally on a disk instead of on

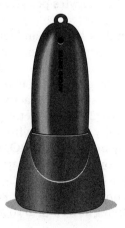

Figure 2-3 • Flash memory device.

film. Using special software and a specially designed disk drive or other connection to the computer, the picture can then be transferred to a computer where it can be placed in a file or a database for easy retrieval, viewed on a computer monitor, printed, or sent via e-mail. The quality of the photo depends on the quality of the camera, resolution of the monitor, and, if printed, the quality of the printer.

Digital cameras are finding a wide variety of uses in healthcare. One outpatient wound center uses them to photograph the wounds at each visit (Brooks & Bryant, 1998, personal communication). The photos are filed in a computer database, then retrieved for comparison at each subsequent visit. This enables the patient and the healthcare professionals to see the progress that has been made and to have evidence of the results of various types of treatment. The photos can also be transmitted to referring physicians as evidence of the patient's progress.

In addition to cameras, imaging devices that can transform images to digital format are useful in inputting data into a computer. Traditional radiology films are being replaced with systems that use digital images. Such images can be transmitted electronically and viewed with sophisticated high-resolution monitors. These monitors produce a higher quality image than traditional film, which may lessen the need for repeat films. Computerized images also reduce costs by eliminating film and requiring much less storage space.

Scanners, too, are being used as input devices for computers. A scanner works like a photocopy machine but instead of printing the image, it sends the image to a computer. Scanned objects are all represented as graphical objects. For text to be manipulated, an **optical character recognition** (OCR) program is necessary. Many healthcare agencies are scanning in documentation to reduce storage space needed. This documentation, however, is in a free text format, which makes it very difficult to aggregate data to make comparisons.

Pen. A cordless ink pen that writes on paper just like an ordinary ball-point pen does but that also enables users to send image data to a computer is a new type of input device. The pen requires a small USB-based receiver attached to the top of the sheet of paper to receive the ultrasonic and infrared signals from the pen. Ultimately, the receiver component will be incorporated into the pen.

Clinical monitoring.   Healthcare systems often make use of specialized monitoring devices that allow patient data such as data produced by fetal or cardiology monitors to be input directly into a computer. This avoids the need for paper strips, which are bulky and can be lost. It also allows the data to be monitored at a central location. The advantage of computerized clinical monitoring is that is allows one person to monitor many patients at once. It may, however, also reduce nurse-patient interaction.

Computerese

Many computer-related terms are used in discussion, instruction, and advertising. Although they are not strictly hardware terms, they can often be confusing. If one watches a computer when it has just been turned on, one will see different types of information flashing across the screen. This information is produced by what is called the "booting" process. **Booting** refers to all the self-tests that a computer performs and the process of retrieving from a disk the software necessary for work to begin. The term **reboot** means to restart the computer. Turning off the computer as a means to reboot should be avoided when possible. The jolt of electricity received each time the computer is turned on may shorten its lifespan. Rebooting the computer without turning it off is known as a **warm boot**. This procedure is often used when a computer **freezes** or crashes. It erases information in RAM, which often eliminates memory conflicts that may have caused the problem. These conflicts can be caused by different programs trying to store data in the same location. If a warm boot fails to notify the programs that it is time to stop fighting for the same space and give control back to the user, the machine must be turned off for a **cold boot**.

A **bug** is a defect in either the program or hardware that causes a malfunction. It may be as simple as presenting the user with a blood pressure chart when a weight chart was requested, or something that causes the entire system to crash.

Compatibility refers to whether programs designed for one chip will work with an older or newer chip, or whether files created with one version of a program will work with another version of the same program. Most computer chips and software are **backwardly compatible**, that is, they will work with older versions of a program or files created with an older version of a program. Some are not, however, "forwardly" compatible. This is particularly true of spreadsheet or database products, and presentation programs.

A **driver** is a software program that allows data to be transmitted between the computer and a device that is connected to the computer. Drivers are generally specific to the brand and model of the device.

Although the term **hacker** originally meant a person who enjoyed learning about computer systems and was often considered at expert on the subject, mass media have turned it into a term to refer to individuals who gain unauthorized access to computer systems for the purpose of stealing and corrupting data. The original term for such persons was **cracker**. Today, differentiations may be made by using the term **white hat hacker** for a person who users his or her computer knowledge to benefit others. **Black hat hacker** is the term used for those who use their computer skills maliciously.

The terms **logical** and **physical** often refer to where data are located in the computer. The physical structure is the actual location, whereas a logical structure is how users see the data. For example, when a user requests information about laboratory tests, he or she may see the indications for the test, the normal values, the cost of a test, and the patient's test results. Although this information may be presented as one screen, which is a logical structure, different pieces may have been retrieved from different files in different locations, which is the physical structure of the information.

A **peripheral** is any external device connected to the computer. Printers, scanners, and digital cameras are peripherals. Setting up peripherals can be a frustrating job. Not only must the correct driver be present, but often jumpers and switches need to be adjusted. These difficulties are being overcome with the use of **plug-and-play**, a concept under which any new device connected to the computer is recognized by the computer, which automatically makes any needed adjustments.

Another potentially confusing computerese term is **object**. Although the more common use of the term "object" is for a physical entity, or at least a picture on the screen, to a computer, an object is anything the computer can manipulate. That is, a letter, word, sentence, paragraph, piece of a document, or an entire document can be an object. Objects can be nested, that is a word is an object nested within a sentence object. A paragraph is an object that is contained in a document. When an object is selected, clicking the right mouse button presents a menu of properties of that object that can be changed.

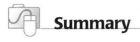

Summary

Understanding how computers function forms the background for a beginning understanding of informatics. Computers are devices, which, although we may anthromorphize them, are still inanimate objects. Computers do not think; they need explicit instructions; and they are incapable of interpreting gray areas. This is not to say that gifted programmers cannot make one think a computer is behaving in a seemingly human manner.

Computers come in many different sizes and shapes—from a simple microprocessor (chip that controls a device) that is found in a watch to a supercomputer. In many cases, the lines between different types of computers are getting dimmer as technology progresses. There are, however, some distinguishing characteristics. Regardless of size, all computers possess some given parts, a CPU, memory and storage devices, and ways to both enter and retrieve data. How many and how much of each of these parts a computer needs depends on the function the computer is intended to serve and often the depth of the owner's pocketbook.

connection——◡   **For definitions of bolded key terms, visit the online glossary available at http://connection.lww.com/go/thede.**

CONSIDERATIONS AND EXERCISES

1. A friend tells you that the defeat of Gary Kasparov by Deep Blue indicated that computers can think. How would you respond?

2. You need to help a colleague who is afraid of computers learn to use one. Outline a plan to help this person reduce his or her anxiety.

3. The unit in which you are working is going to install POC devices. You have been asked to investigate PDAs, thin clients, and wireless tablets and present both their strong points and their weak points as POC devices.

4. To what uses would you put a digital camera in a healthcare situation?

5. What steps would you suggest to overcome the negatives of clinical monitoring systems that allow many patients to be monitored at a central location?

6. Define the following in relationship to computers:

   a. Hacker
   b. Computer crash
   c. Backward compatibility
   d. Plug-and-play

   e. Logical
   f. Physical
   g. Warm boot
   h. Object

REFERENCES

Bloom, A. J. (1985). An anxiety management approach to computer phobia. *Training and Development Journal, 19*(1), 90–94.

Computer shot dead by frustrated owner (1997, July 12). *Cleveland Plain Dealer,* 8A.

Criswell, D. F., & Parchman, M. L. (2002). Handheld computer use in U.S. family practice residency programs. *Journal of the American Medical Informatics Association, 9*(1), 80-86.

Focus. (1995). The impact of computer anxiety and computer resistance on the use of computer technology by nurses. *(1995). Journal of Nursing Staff Development, 11*(3), 172–175.

Jayasuriya, R., & Caputi, P. (1996), Computer attitude and computer anxiety in nursing: validation Validation of an instrument using an Australian sample. Nurses Computer Attitudes Inventory (NCATT) Computer Attitude Scale (CATT). *Computers in Nursing, 14*(6), 340–345.

McBride, S. H., & Nagle, L. M. (1996). Attitudes toward computers: a A of construct validity. Stronge and Brodt's nurses' attitudes toward computerization (NATC) questionnaire. *Computers in Nursing, 14*(3), 164–170.

Perry, W. E. (1982). *Survival guide to computer systems.* Boston: CBI Publishing Company.

Senge, P. (1994). *The fifth discipline: The art and practice of the learning organization.* New York: Currency Doubleday.

Simpson, G., & Kenrick,. M. (1997). Nurses' attitudes toward computerization in clinical practice in a British general hospital. *Computers in Nursing, 15*(1), 37–42.

Simpson, R. (1996). Creating a true learning organization. *Nursing Management 27*(4), 18; 20.

Szynal, D. (2001, August). PDAs come in handy. *Health Data Management, 18,* 20.

Top Drawer Drawer. (2001). University of Virginia School of Nursing and Unbound Medicine Collaborate collaborate to deliver critical nursing information to the point-of-care. *Computers in Nursing 19*(6), 235.

Webopedia. (2002). *The five generations of computers.* Retrieved May 4, 2002 from http://www.webopedia.com/DidYouKnow/2002/April/FiveGenerations.html. (From Table 2-1).

Software:
The Computer at Work

Objectives
After studying this chapter you will be able to:

1. *State the general purpose for each overall type of software.*

2. *Explain the various features that GUIs provide.*

3. *Give examples of defining a clinical nursing problem in preparation for a computer solution.*

4. *Differentiate among proprietary software, shareware, freeware, and public domain software.*

Computer software comes in many varieties, but all of it allows the computer to be used for a specific purpose. In the past, computers were usually purchased without software: today, that is rare. Basic all-purpose packages, including e-mail software and a program to access the World Wide Web, should be included with new computers that are intended for personal use.

Many kinds of software exist. Basically, software manages either the computer system itself or information. Software that manages the computer system includes those programs and utilities that reside in read-only memory (ROM), which enable the computer to boot. System software also includes the operating system that controls the computer and the utilities that allow the user some control over that operating system. Software that manages user information is known as an **application program**. Application programs include information systems in healthcare agencies and off-the-shelf generic applications that can perform a variety of tasks. Examples of the latter include the many Office Suites such as Microsoft Office, Corel WordPerfect Office, and Lotus SmartSuite. Additionally, there is voice recognition software that can convert spoken words to text. There are various brands of each type of software. Although all accomplish the basics of each task, there are differences in how a specific package organizes various the features used with each task.

 Operating Systems

The most important program on your computer is the **operating system**. It coordinates input from the keyboard with output on the screen, responds to mouse clicks, heeds commands to save a file, and transmits commands to printers and other peripheral devices. It is the platform on which application programs run. Application programs are written to work with a specific operating system. Thus, the operating system that you select determines which applications you can run. PCs today and most notebooks use a version of Microsoft Windows. The Apple Macintosh uses a different operating system, as do larger computers. The operating system on personal digital assistants (PDAs), or handhelds, varies, but many use the Windows CE or the Palm operating system.

DOS

Early PCs used the **DOS** operating system, which is an acronym for disk operating system. Although it could refer to any operating system, the term DOS came to mean the operating system developed by Microsoft for PCs. DOS was text based and using it required users to remember a set of commands such as delete, run, copy, and rename. Unlike today's operating systems, DOS allowed only one program at a time to be operational. Transferring information between programs was difficult and time consuming, as was creating anything that was not text. Earlier versions of MS Windows were based on DOS, but today's versions are not. Some older healthcare information systems are still DOS based, but as newer systems are installed, DOS is becoming a historical curiosity.

GRAPHICAL USER INTERFACES

Modern operating systems use what is called a **graphical user interface (GUI)**, which is usually referred to as a GUI (pronounced "gooey"). MS Windows and the Apple Macintosh operating system are both GUIs. A GUI uses computer graphics to facilitate using the computer. Whereas DOS users had to memorize commands, a GUI user simply "points and clicks." *Pointing and clicking* refers to moving a pointer on the screen until it is over the desired object and tapping a button. On PCs, this is accomplished by moving a mouse or mouse alternate in a manner that coincides with the screen movement and tapping the left mouse button. GUIs also use icons (small pictures), a working area called a desktop that has icons on it which are used to open programs and other features, and boxes called *windows* that can be active or inactive. They also feature various types of menus, such as those that drop down from another choice, or pop up when a selection is made.

The symbol that indicates the pointer may vary according to the task and in many cases can be changed by the user. In word processing it is often a vertical "I" bar; in spreadsheets it may be a large plus sign; and in a presentation program, an arrow. Icons are used to represent such things as application programs, files, windows, or commands.

 ## Microsoft Windows

Because GUIs are easy to use, many healthcare information systems are moving to a GUI environment, usually a version of Microsoft Windows. For this reason, as well as the computer fluency demanded of healthcare professionals, it is appropriate to review some basics of using Windows.

OPENING AND EXITING WINDOWS

On most computers, when the computer is booted, Windows starts automatically. Exiting Windows, however, is another matter. Although it is invisible to users, Windows actually works very hard behind the scenes to provide its many functions, as do many of the application programs. To do this, these programs have to remember a great number of things. Often, this is accomplished by creating what are called files, information that the application needs to remember, on the hard disk. These files are temporary and unknown to the users. They are created, changed, and deleted as users change what they are doing. Before quitting Windows, the application programs need to be able to shut these files down. If users do not exit all programs and close Windows properly, these temporary files are left on the disk.

USING PROGRAMS IN WINDOWS*

As with all things in Windows, there are often at least two different ways to open a program—from an icon on the desktop or from the start menu. Which is used depends on the user's preference and computer set-up. To open a program from an icon on the desktop, place the mouse pointer over the icon and click with a left mouse button. To open a program from the start menu click on the start button in the lower left corner of the screen, then click on "Programs" from the resulting menu. Select the program from the list that appears. Some programs that are together in a suite such as Corel Office, Lotus SmartSuite, or Microsoft Office may be on a secondary menu that will be seen when the name of the suite is clicked. Names that lead to other menus are indicated on the Programs Menu by a black triangle mark pointing to the right.

MULTIPLE WINDOWS

In the context of a PC, the term *windows* may refer to the operating system or to the various content boxes that appear on the screen. Each program that is open creates its own window. If a word processor and a spreadsheet program are open simultaneously, two program windows are open. In most programs, a user also may have more than one document or file open. These form windows within the specific program. When needed, there are closing icons for the whole program and for each document within the program window. If a user wishes to close a document within a program, but leave the program open, he or she would click on the closing icon for the document, which is the lower "X" in the upper right hand corner of the screen (Figure 3-1). To close the program itself (after saving all the files that are open), click on the upper "X." One of the hardest things to grasp for those just starting to use GUIs is that not only is it possible to have many different windows open at one time, but using this option is an aid to productivity.

---

[1] This information applies to PC users who are using the MS Windows operating system. Although it is recognized that there are many Macintosh users, the great majority of health agency information systems use Windows-based systems.

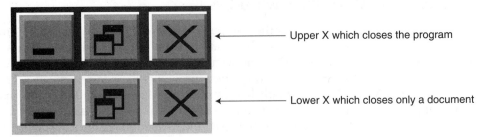

Upper X which closes the program

Lower X which closes only a document

Newer versions of Windows color the top X red and make it larger

Figure 3-1 • Closing documents and programs.

NAVIGATING BETWEEN AND WITHIN DOCUMENT AND PROGRAM WINDOWS

Sometimes when a program is open, the window for that application does not fill the entire screen. If a user wants the window to fill the entire screen, he or she must click on the maximize icon (Figure 3-2). If the desired size is smaller and clicking on the minimize button does not produce a window of the desired size, a user can further resize it by passing the mouse pointer over the borders of the window until it becomes a double arrow. Then the user depresses the left mouse button and drags the window border in either direction until the window is the desired size. Windows, whether they represent a document in a program, or a pop-up window, can be moved anywhere on the screen. To move a window, place the mouse pointer over the title bar, which is the top line of the program and generally colored blue, then depress the left mouse button, and drag the window to the desired location.

It is also easy to switch between windows within a program. Although how this is accomplished varies with the version of the program, it can always be done by clicking on the word *Window* on the top menu line and selecting the desired window from a list of documents that are open within that program. Many times, the name of the desired window will be on the bar at the bottom of the screen and a user will only need to click on the name to open the desired window. It is not necessary to minimize a window before opening another window or program.

Most documents, whether text in a word processor, or data in a spreadsheet or a database, are too large to be seen in their entirety on a display screen. To allow users to scroll to other parts of the document, Windows provides "scroll bars." A vertical scroll bar is on

When this icon is seen in the upper right corner of the screen, it indicates that the document is **maximized**. Clicking on it will minimize the document.

When this icon is seen in the upper right corner of the screen, it indicates that the document is **minimized**. Clicking on it will maximize the document.

Figure 3-2 • Minimize and maximize icons.

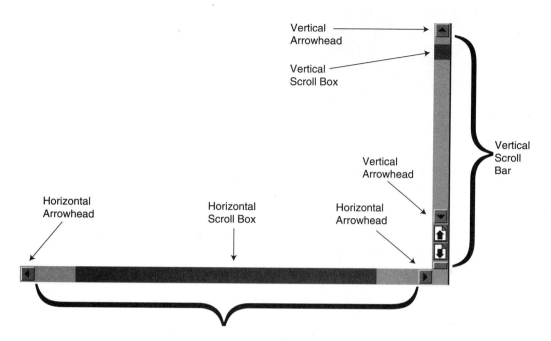

Figure 3-3 • Horizontal and vertical scroll bars.

the right side of the screen, and a horizontal scroll bar is at the bottom (Figure 3-3). To use the scroll bar, place the mouse pointer on the box within the bar, depress the left mouse button, and drag it in the desired direction. It is also possible to scroll in more controlled increments by clicking on the box containing a triangle seen at either end of the scroll bars. The vertical scroll bar serves another function. It allows users to judge where they are in a document by the placement of the box on the scroll bar. If the box is halfway down the bar, the user is in the middle of the document. In many cases, the keyboard can also be used to scroll. The up and down arrow keys move one line up or down, and the left and right arrow keys move one character to the left or right in text programs, or one column left or right in a spreadsheet or database.

When application programs are open, a main menu is on the top of the screen. Other menus become visible as **drop-down menus** when an item on the menu bar is clicked. Pop-up windows appear when users click a selection on a drop-down menu followed by an ellipsis (...), or when an object is selected and, on a PC, the right mouse button clicked.

MENUS AND DIALOG BOXES

Windows is a very interactive system. Menus and dialog boxes offer the ability to invoke features easily. In an application program, the most obvious menus are those at the top of the screen. Each of these, when the mouse pointer is placed over them and clicked, will offer a list of features that can be implemented. Items that are not available at that time are grayed out (i.e., appear faded in gray type). Some of these selections have either a black triangle pointing to the right, or an ellipsis on the right side of the menu. A black triangle in-

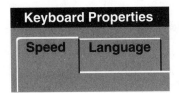
Clicking on a tab labeled "Language" will reveal another dialog box where choices may be made.

Figure 3-4 • Tabs on a dialog box.

dicates that if that selection is clicked, another menu will appear. The ellipsis means that selecting that choice will produce a pop-up dialog box. Dialog boxes may or may not have tabs near the top (Figure 3-4). When tabs appear, clicking on one will provide another dialog box. In this second box, one makes selections to implement the features needed.

Another convention used to facilitate selections is a drop-down menu (Figure 3-5). The small rectangular box will appear to have only one selection, but at the right end will be a black triangle on a gray background. Clicking on this arrow makes a list of choices appear.

Many of these conventions are used in healthcare systems to both save time in data entry and prevent errors. For example, the drop-down box is often used when there are choices, such as smoking or nonsmoking, or clients' gender, that need to be entered into the system. A drop-down menu using the triangle option may also be used. To illustrate, in an intensive care unit, when users click on the black triangle under "tubes," a drop-down list may appear of all the possible tubes or types of tubes that might be used. Clicking on another black triangle, one that indicates drainage, may produce a list of possible drainage tubes. The content of these lists is determined by nurses who work in these areas. Good information systems result from a partnership between the nurses who work in an area with those who are involved with designing and implementing the system.

ACCESSORIES AND UTILITIES

Operating systems usually come with some utilities and built-in software. Certain utilities are helpful with disk maintenance, such as ScanDisk. Additional accessories such as Paint, a simple drawing program, allow a user to create drawings or various shapes, such as circle, square, or triangle in any of the colors available in the program. There are also writing accessories such as Notepad, a product that is useful in creating files in a format that can be read by most programs..

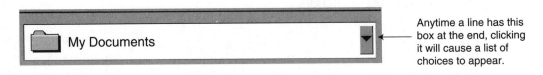
Anytime a line has this box at the end, clicking it will cause a list of choices to appear.

Figure 3-5 • Drop down menus.

Off-the-Shelf All-Purpose Application Software

Beyond use as an information system or for web access, the main uses of a computer today are e-mail and word processing, followed by spreadsheets. To fulfill the these uses, there are several software packages called **office suites** that include at least a word processor, spreadsheet, and utilities such as a scheduler and an address book. Depending on the software publisher, a standard package may also contain a presentation program. To obtain a full fledged database program, one is usually required to purchase the "professional" version of an office suite. All of the major application programs in an office suite are explored in their own chapters.

Software for Computer-to-Computer Communication

As soon as computers could store information in memory, the desire to share this information between computers arose. It was, however, the development of a standard method of computer communication and production of inexpensive modems that made this interaction available to the general public. This software includes e-mail and networking packages.

Groupware

Groupware is software that permits a group discussion. This category was introduced in 1989 when Lotus introduced Lotus Notes (Woolley, 1996), an outgrowth of an earlier product used on the mainframe (Woolley, 1996). The term as currently used refers to software that promotes not only group discussion, but an array of activities such as scheduling and document sharing. There is a wide range in the features that vendors provide in groupware. Some are suites of ready-made applications, whereas others are toolboxes for creating collaborative applications with customizable templates included. These products have been found useful in business and education.

Voice Recognition and Production

Voice input, which involves the ability of a computer to recognize spoken words and translate them into a printed text, has reached new levels. There are two types of voice recognition: discrete and continuous speech processing. Discrete speech processing, which is not used much today, requires the speaker to speak one word at a time pausing briefly after each word. In continuous speech processing, the user can speak at a normal rate.

With the increased power of computers, voice recognition systems have greatly improved. In the past, systems required the user to train the program extensively to understand his or her spoken word. The training consisted of the user's repeating those words the computer would be required to understand, until the word was recognized as spoken by that individual. Some systems today are capable of recognizing the spoken word from different people without this special training, but for optimal use, all require some training (Seymour, 2001). The accuracy of voice software is also affected by the quality of the microphone used for voice input. Several companies have introduced systems that have a large built-in vocabulary that focuses on a specific field, such as radiology (Voice recognition takes off, 1996). Voice recognition is finding many uses in the healthcare system ranging from recording medical histories to nursing documentation.

Other software is also available that will read text and convert it to audio output. The text may be from a file, a document in memory, e-mail, Web page, or text that is being typed. The quality of the voice varies depending on the software, audio card, and speakers, but many of these achieve a human-sounding quality. They will find uses not only with busy people, but also those who are visually compromised.

Creating Software

Software is created using a **programming language**, of which there are many. There are also different levels of languages. These levels depend on the degree to which the language approaches "natural language;" the higher the level, the closer to regular language. The drawback is that as the level of the language increases the flexibility decreases. The lowest level, **machine language**, communicates directly with the zeros and ones that represent bits. The next level, assembly language, uses cryptic names instead of numbers to communicate with the computer. Level three, or the so-called **high-level languages**, include such well-known languages as Cobol, Fortran, and Basic. Fourth-level languages are designed for a specific purpose. Structured query language (SQL) is a fourth-level language designed specifically to query relational databases. Ultimately, no matter which level language is used or which language a program is written in, it must be translated to machine language in a process called *compiling*.

A computer program provides a detailed step-by-step set of instructions to a computer in a manner such that the computer can understand and comply with these instructions. These instructions are called *code*. Before a single line of code is written, it is necessary to define the problem the computer is to solve and develop a flow chart of instructions, which is called an **algorithm**. A flow chart in computer programming is like a flow chart used to model any process. It is a pictorial representation of the process or project being planned. Flow charts provide people with a common understanding of the process. Figure 3-6 shows an example of a flow chart.

As a healthcare professional, a nurse may be called on to assist in defining a problem or testing the proposed solution. Defining a problem with enough accuracy and detail so the computer can be used to solve it is a difficult task. A simple problem such as asking the computer to flag vital signs that require nursing attention requires attention to many details. First, the nurse needs to determine the limits of normal. This may sound easy until the nurse remembers that in some cases, a temperature elevated by 2° F may not be of any concern. In the same way, the nurse also must define "normal" pulse and respiration rates and blood pressures. To do this, the nurse must come up with a set of rules stating what readings need flagging under which conditions.

This information is then programmed using "if-then-else" statements that tell the computer what to do if a certain condition exists. In the situation in Figure 3-6, an if/then statement would have to be part of the code for each of the decisions depicted. When one considers the many variables that impinge on clinical decisions, it becomes easy to see why humans must always evaluate computer output. Evaluation is helped if the nurse knows what limits were placed on each variable. In this example, the user would want to know that the computer flags the blood pressure for a pregnant woman only when the systolic exceeds 140 and diastolic 90. Because it is highly unlikely that every condition can

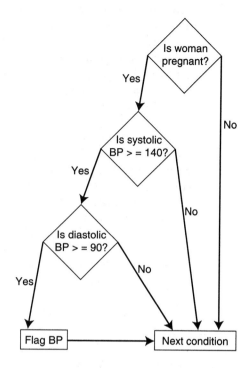

Figure 3-6 • An algorithm in a flow chart.

be programmed, it is imperative that computer users not rely solely on computer output for determining anomalies. There is no substitute for critical thinking by a perceptive healthcare professional.

Open Source Software

Open source software has source code that is made freely available to the general public who may modify it to meet their needs. Early e-mail packages and even Web browsers were open source. An operating system, Unix, that powers many larger computers, is open source software, as is the operating system Linux. The success of open source software is based on the concept that when the code is freely available, other programmers will find and eliminate the bugs in the code. Under this scheme, bugs can theoretically be eliminated and the software can be improved at a much faster rate than when development is subject to the bureaucracy of a corporation. Additionally, users are free to make the software meet their needs, rather than work within limits that may not accommodate their requirements. The downside is that beyond a network of other programmers there is no support for any difficulties that may arise

User Groups

When learning to use a program, sources of help can be extremely useful. Whether using a book, teacher, or other sources of instruction, questions arise for which answers are not readily available. One excellent source of help is a user group, which is a gathering of people who meet regularly for the purpose of sharing information. There are user groups for application programs and information systems. User group members range from novices to those who make a living as a consultant for the program. The level of formal organization varies with the size and purpose of the group. Most user group meetings have an agenda that includes both a question-and-answer session and a presentation by a member or invited guest on some aspect of the group's focus.

There are few geographic areas today in the United States that do not have a computer user group for some type for application programs. In large cities, there may be one umbrella group with smaller significant interest groups (SIGs) that meet independently to learn more about a specific program. For more information about user groups and how to find a group, see the Web site for the Association of Personal Computer User Groups at http://www.apcug.org, or call a local computer store. Computer stores usually have information on the groups in the area. In fact, they may even be the site for meetings.

Like commercial application programs, there are user groups for health information systems. There are two types of information system user groups: internal and external (Simpson, 1990). An internal group consists of users of a system within a given institution, whereas an external group has members from healthcare institutions all over the country (or even the world). Like other software user groups, they share experiences both positive and negative. If a nurse from each unit is not a member of a user group for the information system in his or her institution, the nurse is missing an opportunity to be a powerful advocate for nursing.

 ## Program Copyrights

When selling software, many vendors believe that the users are not buying it but that they are buying a license to use it. In this thinking, breaking the shrink wrap means the user agrees to the conditions of the license. These licenses generally state that the software cannot be sold or given away without the permission of the vendor. Depending on the vendor, users may be told they can install the software on only one computer, or in some cases, on more than one computer if only one copy will be used at a time.

Given the ease of installing software, many people are unaware that not following the license agreement is called **software piracy**. A decade or more ago, most software was "copy protected." Under this scheme, the vendors placed algorithms on the disk that made it difficult to reproduce the program. With the advent of hard disks on which users installed programs, this approach became impractical. Some people mistakenly believe that when the copy protection is removed from programs, so is the copyright. To combat this problem, much software requires users to register the program using a serial number, or other identifying entity. Other programs are designed to no longer operate after a given time frame or number of uses.

The Business Software Alliance estimates that the software industry lost $12 billion in 1999 due to illegal software sharing (Business Software Alliance, n.d.). According to the alliance, *piracy* is defined as the illegal distribution or copying of software for personal or organizational use. This group makes a concerted effort worldwide to find and prosecute those involved in this act. Since their founding in 1988, the Business Software Alliance has filed many lawsuits against those suspected of software copyright infringement.

The Software Copyright Protection Bill, which Congress passed in 1992, raised software piracy from a misdemeanor to a felony (Nicoll, 1994). Penalties of up to $100,000 for statutory damages and fines of up to $250,000 can be levied for this crime, plus the people responsible can be sentenced to a jail term of up to 5 years. Software vendors are very serious about copyright violations. Healthcare and educational organizations are not immune from prosecution. One western university paid $130,000 to the Software Publishers Association when it was found to have illegal software in a laboratory. A hospital in Illinois was fined about $161,000 when they were found engaging in unauthorized software duplication (Chicago Hospital, 1997). Organizations without an enforced software oversight policy are possible candidates for investigation.

Some software is distributed as **shareware**. Software of this type is often found on the Internet. The publishers of shareware encourage users to give copies to friends and colleagues to try out. They request that anyone who uses the program after a trial period pay them a fee. Registration information is included in the program. Continuing to use shareware without paying the registration fee is considered software piracy.

Freeware is an application the programmer has decided to make freely available to anyone who wishes to use it. Although it may be used without paying a fee, the author usually maintains the copyright, which means a user cannot do anything with it other than what the author intended. There are some freeware programs available on the Internet. Software that is in the **public domain** can be used any way the user desires and changes may be made to it. When a user accepts software through any channel but a reputable reseller, they should be certain they know whether the software is proprietary, shareware, freeware, or in the public domain.

Summary

There are many different types of software that are useful in managing information. Yet, it can be said that there are generally two overall types of software: software that manages systems and software that allows people to manage information. Systems software consists of utilities and operating systems. Software that allows users to manage information includes word processors, spreadsheets, database managers, presentation packages, and computer-to-computer communication. There are different vendors for application programs, each of which approaches the task of implementing functions a little differently. Several vendors offer office suites, which consist of a word processor, spreadsheet, presentation package, and database—all designed to work well together.

Programming languages can be classified as machine language, assembly, high-level, or fourth-level languages. Machine language consists solely of zeros and ones, whereas assembly language, which is one level higher, uses some wordlike characters in its code. Fourth-level languages come the closest to natural language.

Most of the software used is proprietary and is copyrighted. Using a copy of a proprietary program for which a user does not hold a license is software piracy. Shareware is software that can be tried for free, but a registration fee should be paid if it is regularly used. Only freeware can be used without cost.

connection For definitions of bolded key terms, visit the online glossary available at http://connection.lww.com/go/thede.

CONSIDERATIONS AND EXERCISES

1. If you have access to a computer with a GUI, experiment with the various options, such as opening more than one program, and more than one document in a program, resizing, moving, tiling, cascading, and closing windows.

2. Write down as many rules as you can think of that define when deviations either above or below the normal temperature of 98.6°F (37°C) are cause for action by a nurse.

3. Create a flow chart of the steps for giving a prn medication. Use a diamond shape for a decision, a rectangle for a process, a parallelogram for data.

4. A friend gives you a CD-ROM with a program on it for you to install. What things should you consider before doing so?

5. You wish to install a program that you have at home on your computer at work. What things need to be considered?

REFERENCES

Business Software Alliance (n.d.) Retrieved January 19, 2002 from http://www.bsa.org/usa/antipiracy/piracyticker.phtml.

Chicago hospital caught pirating. (1997, January). *Healthcare Informatics, 20.*

Nicoll, L. H. (1994). Modern day pirates: Software users and abusers. *Journal of Nursing Administration, 24*(1), 18–20.

Seymour, J. (2001). The truth about voice recognition software. Retrieved January 18, 2002 from http://www.pcmag.com/article/0,2997,s%253D1493%2526a%253D15546,00.asp.

Simpson, R. (1990). What are user groups and how can they help you wield more power? *Nursing Management, 21*(10), 24,28.

Voice recognition takes off. (1996). *Healthcare Informatics, 13*(11), 18.

Woolley, D. R. (1996). *Choosing web conferencing software.* Retrieved January 19, 2002 from http://thinkofit.com/webconf/wcchoice.htm.

Computer Communications: Lightning-Fast Information Dissemination

Objectives
After studying this chapter you will be able to:

1. Discuss innovations that the Internet has created.

2. Differentiate between the Web and the Internet.

3. Identify the parts of an e-mail address and an URL.

4. Identify pros and cons of e-mail.

5. Discuss benefits and drawbacks of the Internet.

A nurse encounters a patient with an unfamiliar disease. From an e-mail message, the nurse learns that a document on a computer in another country has information about caring for patients with this disease. Within 60 seconds of logging on to the Internet, the nurse is printing out the document. This ability to exchange information on a global scale is changing the world. No longer do healthcare professionals have to wait for information to become available in a journal in the country in which they live. Nurses and other healthcare professionals can and do use computers to network with colleagues all over the world.

Networks

Computer networking is not new to healthcare. Since the late 1950s, when healthcare institutions began using mainframes connected to terminals in various offices for financial processing, networking has progressed to the point where institutions are connected to a worldwide network known as the Internet. Computer networks exist whenever two computers share the same data. A network can range in size from a connection between a palmtop and a personal computer (PC), to the worldwide, multiuser computer connection—the Internet.

Variation in network size is often seen in the name used to denote the network, such as a **local area network (LAN)** or **wide area network (WAN)**. A LAN is a network in which the connected computers are physically close to one another, such as in the same department or building. A WAN is a network in which the connections are farther

53

apart. Often, a WAN is an internetwork of LANs. WANs are sometimes referred to as enterprise networks, because they connect all the computer networks throughout the entire organization or enterprise.

Although **peer-to-peer networking** in which each connected computer is a workstation exists, most networks operate under the **client/server** model. This includes most networks in healthcare and the **Internet**. Under this scheme, a connected computer can be either a **client**, a **server**, or both. A client computer has software that allows it to request and receive files from the server. The server has software that can accept these requests, find the appropriate file, and transmit it back to the client (Figure 4-1). When users on a client computer want a file from the server, they request it using the client side of the software. The server uses its special software to accept and implement the request. The client computer then receives the transmission and interprets it. Beyond making the initial request, rarely is any of this process visible to the user, just as when one makes a long-distance telephone call, the process of making the connection is invisible to a caller.

The client computer must have a network card or some sort of **modem** and some type of software to facilitate sending a request for a file and receiving the information. Servers have software that allows them to interpret the request and return the requested file. Besides serving as a repository of files, servers can also function in other capacities, such as managing files sent to a printer by the various computers on the network, or even processing data. Access to a network is controlled by a user ID (sometimes called a login name) and some method of identifying the user, such as a password. Managing networks is an ongoing maintenance task performed by the network administrator.

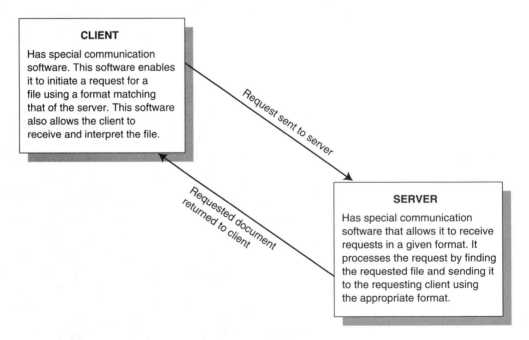

Figure 4-1 • Client-server architecture.

For networks to function correctly, it is necessary that there be agreements known as **protocols**, which prescribe how data will be exchanged between participating computers. These protocols include standards for tasks such as, how the system will check for transmission errors, whether to use data compression, and if so how, how the sending machine will indicate that the message it has sent is complete, and how the receiving machine will indicate that it has received the message.

Wireless Technology

Wireless transmission within healthcare institutions is used successfully today. These transmissions are limited in distance; thus, they do not have to compete with other radio traffic. When a wireless system is installed, receivers are placed at strategic locations throughout the institution, locations that are determined after a thorough assessment of the building. These receivers pick up the signals sent by a user and transmit them to the central server then transmit signals back to the user's computer.

Because it does not depend on the user's being in a given location, wireless technology can offer more efficient use of healthcare personnel's time as well as provide more efficient communication among departments. Assigning each patient a wireless device, such as a wireless tablet that goes with him or her much as the paper chart once did, could make it much easier for personnel to access up-to-date information about this patient.

Several issues about wireless transmissions remain to be resolved. One is interoperability of devices. Certain devices may only work with specific wireless networks. Security is another issue with wireless transmissions (Gardner, 2002). The distance between the sending device and the receiver varies with the wireless technology as does the transmission rate. Some of the technologies vying for use are Bluetooth with a range of 10 meters and speed of 1 **megabit** per second and the IEEE.802.11 family with transmission speeds that vary from 1 megabit per second to 54 megabits per second.

The Internet: A Network of Networks

The Internet is a worldwide, amorphous network of interconnected computers (Figure 4-2). What makes the Internet workable is that each computer connected to the Internet uses specific protocols to communicate. These protocols make it possible for a person using an Apple Macintosh to send a message to a person using a PC or any other type of computer.

The term *Internet* was first used in 1983 to describe the interconnected networks developed by the National Science Foundation (NSF). The Internet, however, traces its beginning to the work of the Advanced Research Projects Agency, which, in 1969, created the Advanced Research Project Network (ARPNET). From those modest beginnings, the Internet has grown to span the world. The result has been a dramatic change in how we communicate, both locally, nationally, and internationally. The Internet provides us many features such as e-mail, teleconferencing, and the World Wide Web (Figure 4-3).

The protocols that are used on the Internet, the **Transmission Control Protocol** (TCP) and **Internet Protocol** (IP), were introduced in 1974. The TCP/IP protocol is actually two protocols. The IP protocol enables computers to find each other and the TCP protocol controls the tasks associated with the data transmission. Although invisible to the user,

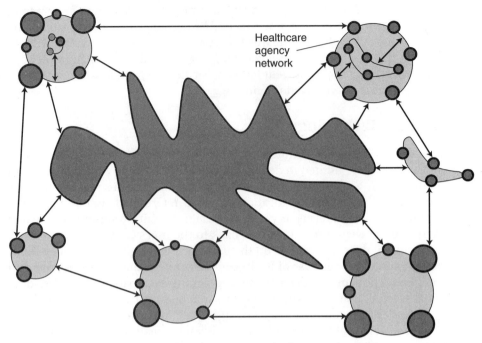

The Internet is millions of connected computer networks that span the globe.

Figure 4-2 • The Internet.

messages sent on the Internet are not sent as a whole. Instead they are broken up into what are called packets. Each packet may even take a different route to its destination. A device called a *router* scans the routes available to the final destination for each packet, selects what looks the shortest and least congested route at that moment, and sends the packet on to another router (Quiggle, 1998. personal correspondence.) for another decision until the packet reaches its final destination.

To make it possible for each computer on the Internet to be located, each has what is called an IP address. Because numbers are difficult for most people to remember, and because they may change over a period of time, each computer is also assigned a name. Each time a message is sent, the Internet **Domain Name System** (DNS), translates the computer name into the IP address. Using this system, only the domain name system must be updated when an IP numerical address change is required. IP addresses can be static or dynamic. A **static IP address** will be the same each time the computer is logged onto the Internet. A **dynamic IP address** changes each time a user connects to the Internet.

Another process used on the Internet is the **file transfer protocol** (FTP). This is the method used to retrieve files from a distant computer, much as one might request a book from a library. Until the early 1990s, this was a manual process and users had to learn commands to do it. Today, Web browsers have automated this process for files that are retrieved from the **World Wide Web** (WWW). People who create pages for the WWW on their own computers use an FTP program to place their files on the server.

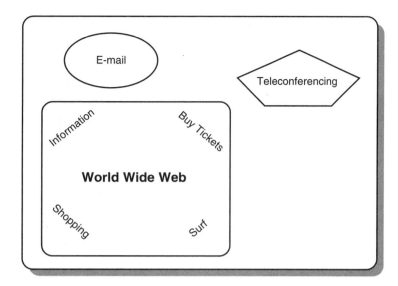

Figure 4-3 • Some parts of the Internet.

INFORMATION RECEIVED FROM THE INTERNET

Several methodologies are used on the Internet to deliver information. **Streaming** is a technique for transferring data that allows the user to start seeing or hearing the file before the entire file has downloaded. This technique is becoming important because of the increase in the number of large files, such as multimedia applications, that users want to download. Its ability to work depends on the receiving computer's ability to collect the data and deliver it in a steady stream, despite the unsteady rate at which data are transmitted on the Internet. Audio files and video clips are sometimes sent in this manner. The plug-in RealAudio provides streaming data.

CONNECTIONS TO THE INTERNET

Computers are connected to the Internet with some type of networking device. The type of device depends on how the connection is made. When institutional networked computers are connected to the Internet, the connection is generally provided at the network level and is invisible to the user. The speed with which a connection to and within the Internet transmits data is referred to as **bandwidth**. The higher the bandwidth, the faster the speed is. Bandwidth varies throughout the Internet.

Telephone Modems

The original method of connecting computers to the Internet was through telephone lines. This system, still used by more than 60% of Internet computers, requires a modem, or a device that will translate computer output (**digital** format) to electronic impulses that can be transmitted over telephone lines (**analog** format). Modems are connected to the computer through a serial port and to the Internet through a telephone line.

Modems vary in speed. The speed with which information can be sent over a telephone line has increased dramatically from the original 25 characters a second (which was measured in baud) to 56,600 **kilobits** a second. Data transmission, however, often does not live up to its full capacity. To attain full speed, the phone line must be clear of noise or interference. More noise on the line slows the connection. Generally, older lines have more noise. Picking up a phone extension while the line is being used for a computer connection and call waiting can also interrupt a regular telephone connection to the Internet. This type of connection, which is known as **plain old telephone service (POTS)**, has probably already reached its top speed.

Higher connection speeds can be obtained with what are called **digital subscriber lines (DSL)**. DSL uses a sophisticated scheme to pack data onto the existing phone lines, which avoids the translation of data to the analog format. This type of connection requires a special modem and a connection that, as this is written, is less than 20,000 feet from the central telephone switching office. DSL lines can transmit data at speeds of up to 32 megabits from the Internet to the client (referred to as **downstream**) and from 32 kilobits to 1 megabit for information sent to Internet (known as **upstream**). DSL transmission uses parts of the telephone line not used in voice communication; hence, unlike POTS service, DSL users can talk on the phone at the same time they are accessing the Internet.

Cable Modems

Cable modems, which share the cable with cable television can attain transmission speeds up of 5 megabits per second (Mbps), but a more realistic speed is 1 Mbps (Cable Internet Basics, n,d,). Like DSL service, downstream transmission speed is faster than upstream.

Wireless Connections

This type of transmission for Internet traffic is still in its infancy, but with the convergence of cell phones and personal digital assistants (PDAs), expect to see this grow. Wireless connections use the wireless application protocol (WAP), which is a specification that allows users to access information instantly with handheld wireless devices such as mobile phones, pagers, two-way radios, and communicators. Devices that access the Internet use microbrowsers, or browsers with small file sizes to accommodate the low memory of PDAs and the low bandwidth of a wireless-handheld network. Although WAP supports the usual Web format, the wireless markup language (WML) is devised especially for handhelds. To provide data using WML, Web servers must have special software. To date, few Web sites provide access for mobile devices. Another disadvantage to wireless Internet services is that they must compete for a share of the unallocated broadcast spectrum.

Satellite

A satellite connection can provide Internet access to rural areas and nations lacking a wired infrastructure. Satellite communication is line of sight. Because the satellites are positioned above the equator, satellite reception demands a clear line of sight in the direction of the equator, that is, south in the northern hemisphere and north in the southern hemisphere. Transmission speeds for this type of connections are about 768 kilobits **downstream** and 128 kilobits **upstream** (Blakely, 2001).

CONNECTIONS WITHIN THE INTERNET

Healthcare agencies, if they are on the Internet, are not likely to use any of these methods. Instead, they will generally have a faster connection such as a T1, T3, or fiberoptic cable connection. Fiberoptic cable provides the fastest connection. It is also used within many healthcare agencies to connect the **nodes** on their networks. The main disadvantage of fiberoptic cable is its expense. Despite this, telephone companies are slowly replacing traditional telephone lines with fiber optic cable, which, with the exception of satellite for underdeveloped areas, may eventually make all of the technologies mentioned here historical artifacts.

Telnet

Telnet, which became a standard protocol in 1983, allows a user to log into a distant computer and use its features. Essentially, it transforms the user's computer into a terminal with all processing done on the distant computer. Some Internet features are still available only by using telnet, but most are being converted to Web features.

INTERNET SERVICE PROVIDERS

Unless connecting to the Internet via an agency which provides Internet connectivity, an **internet service provider (ISP)** is necessary. An ISP is a company that provides access to the Internet. The fee per month varies, but it generally ranges from $10 to $30. An ISP provides users with a username, password, access phone numbers, and at least one e-mail address, often more. Additionally, most ISPs provide between 5 and 10 megabytes of storage on their server, which can be used for a Web page.

There are two types of ISPs: online services and basic ISPs. Online services such as America Online, Microsoft Network, and Earthlink offer not only a connection to the Internet but proprietary content and features that are not available on the general Internet. Basic ISPs, however, may provide fewer busy signals and more readily accessible technical help. To find an ISP, talk with several acquaintances who are Internet users and get their recommendations.

E-MAIL

E-mail, or electronic mail sent and received on the computer, is one of the primary uses of the Internet. Before 1995, users could send e-mail only to those who shared the same network connection. For instance, those using CompuServe as their ISP could only e-mail others who also used CompuServe. Today, with most computer networks part of the Internet, the exchange of e-mail is possible with anyone in the world who has an Internet e-mail address. E-mail, however, does not always have to involve the Internet. Many companies network their computers and provide in-house e-mail without connecting to the Internet.

E-mail offers many advantages to nurses and other healthcare professionals. Most messages arrive at their destination only several minutes after they have been sent, even if the destination is halfway around the globe. E-mail offers a way to avoid "telephone tag" and to create a written message that the receiver can read several times, convert into voice with special software or save. Most mail packages keep a copy of all messages that are sent, so the sender can check to verify that a given message was transmitted. Additionally, all e-mail packages provide some way to preserve incoming mail and organize it into folders for future reference. E-mail is ideal for communicating across time zones, not only because the sender and receiver can respond at times that are most convenient but because it saves postage and telephone expenses.

Care must be taken in what is included in messages that are sent via e-mail. It is very easy for a recipient to either accidentally or purposefully forward your message to someone else. All messages carry headers that can be traced to the original sender making it almost impossible to hide e-mail even if it is deleted (Bennahum, 1999). Additionally, there is no guarantee that e-mail that is sent using an institution's facilities will be private. There is still no definitive case law on whether employees have the right to privacy in e-mail (Atkins, 1998). This includes even situations in which the employer has said that your e-mail is private; if your message can be construed as damaging to the institution, then such promises may be legally invalidated.

Internet E-Mail Addresses

Like all mail, e-mail requires an address. At first, e-mail addresses look forbidding, but as they become more familiar, the rules used to construct them become visible, which makes them easier to use (Fig. 4-4). The first rule is that e-mail addresses never have a space. All Internet e-mail addresses have two main parts, which are separated by the @ sign. The first part, or the letters before the @ sign, is called a **login name** or a **user ID**. These login names are assigned to individuals. The part after the @ is the name of the computer used to access the Internet. The characters after the last dot in an e-mail address indicate the domain or main subdivision of the Internet to which the computer belongs.

E-Mail Address Books

When entering e-mail addresses, it is imperative that they be accurate. To make this job easier, most e-mail software provides an option that allows the user to create an address book for e-mail addresses, or, as they are sometimes called, nicknames. To create such a file, use the help option and follow the directions for the e-mail package to enter the e-mail address and name of any person to whom e-mail is frequently sent.[1] The next time you send this person a message, access the address book, find his or her name, and click on it. Or, in some communication packages, just enter the intended recipient's name. Besides saving time, using this feature prevents errors in typing the e-mail address, which can result in messages that are returned because of an incorrect address.

There are frequently times when one will want to send the same e-mail message to several people, such as when a unit supervisor needs to send an e-mail to all the nurses in the unit. To facilitate this, e-mail software provides the opportunity to create a group, or list of e-mail addresses to which a message will be sent when the name of the group is entered on the address bar. Instructions for creating a group can be found in Outlook Express by clicking on Addresses on the menu bar and clicking on Help. In Netscape, from the main menu bar click on Help, click on Index and enter "Address Book," and select "Creating a mailing list."

E-Mail Etiquette

E-mail is a special form of communication that is not as interactive as the telephone but is more interactive than written communication. Because it often seems very personal and quick, there is a tendency to regard it as a verbal conversation and to forget that the recipient may have been involved in many complicated matters since she or he last sent you

---

[1] Some e-mail packages will automatically place this information in the address book when the e-mail address in a message that has been received is clicked.

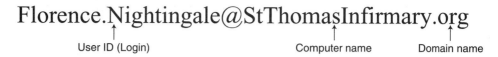

Figure 4-4 • E-mail address.

a message. For this reason, mailers provide an option to include the prior message with the original when you reply. To keep messages from becoming too large and uncommunicative, edit the quoted message when the prior message is included with a reply so that only the parts pertinent to the reply are included. Edit the message the same way that any word processing document is edited. Other forms of etiquette include always including a subject line and signing your messages.

Acronyms and Emoticons

With the informality of much e-mail and the limited typing skills of many who send messages, it is only natural that common acronyms have developed. However, they are valuable only when the recipients understand them (Table 4-1).

E-mail is devoid of the nonverbal commands of face-to-face communication. To meet this need, icons called **emoticons** (emotional icons) were devised by telecommunicators with a sense of humor and knowledge of the difficulties that lack of body language in communication can cause. Sometimes called smileys, these figures are created entirely with characters that can be entered from the keyboard. One that is frequently seen is :-). When tilting your head to the left, which is the position for viewing all emoticons, you can see a smiling face. Like acronyms, they are useful only if the recipient understands their meaning. Use them sparingly, if at all, in business situations.

Unlike with personal conversation, there is low feedback in e-mail, and emoticons have their limits in communicating emotions. In talking, judgments about the intended tone of a message can be made from the sound of the voice, whereas in face-to-face conversations body language is helpful. Additionally, a very short message may come across as curt when not accompanied by anything else and thus could be misinterpreted.

E-mail messages are also different from a letter received through regular mail. These we generally give our full, undivided attention, but a reader who is trying to handle many e-mail messages often does not read the message thoroughly. This can cause problems in

TABLE 4-1 • *Common E-mail Acronyms*	
Acronym	**Meaning**
BTW	By the way
FAQ	Frequently asked questions
f2f	Face to face
FWIW	For what it's worth
<g>	Grin
IMO or IMHO	In my opinion or in my humble opinion
OTOH	On the other hand

relationships. If there is a chance for a disagreement, or e-mail messages seem to be causing disagreements, use e-mail to set up a time for either a person-to-person meeting or a
telephone conversation.

E-Mail Attachments

Many people today exchange not only e-mail, but also files that they have created with an
application program, such as a spreadsheet or a word processor. When sending attachments, it is necessary to understand that different brands of proprietary software create
files that may not be usable by a recipient who does not have that exact software. For example, when a spreadsheet is created with Corel Quattro Pro, it is unlikely that a recipient who only has Microsoft Excel will be able to open the file. Thus, one needs to know
whether the recipient can use an attachment if it is sent. Word processing programs overcome this difficulty by providing a conversion mode known as **rich text format** (RTF).
This is a specification for text files that preserves formatting, while allowing a file created
with Microsoft Word to be opened with Corel WordPerfect or any other word processor.
Instructions for creating RTF files can be found on the Web page for this chapter, on the
book web site at http://connection.lww.com/go/thede.

Attaching files to e-mail messages increases the size of the message, which increases
the time required both to send the message and to receive it. If the attached file is large it
may be advisable to "**zip**" it. Zipping a file involves using a piece of software that com-
presses the file to make it smaller. Files may be zipped individually or as a group. When
the recipient receives the zipped file, he or she will need to unzip it. A zipped file will have
a name that ends in the characters ".zip." One of the better known Internet services, AOL,
will automatically zip file attachments if the subscriber sends or receives more than one
file per message or if the attached file is above a given size (about 40 kilobytes). Zipping
a file works very well with text files, but is not nearly as successful in reducing the size of
graphical files. Several shareware programs are available that will guide a user through
both zipping and unzipping a file. One of the most common is WinZip. It is available for
downloading on the Internet.

World Wide Web

Not since Gutenberg's invention of movable type has there been an innovation that has so
changed the speed with which new information could be made available and the way in
which we access information as the Web. Its short-lived predecessor, **Gopher**, was an early
application to aid users in using information on the Internet. Unlike the WWW, Gopher
permitted only the use of text, although it did feature hierarchical menus that one could
use to access documents.

The WWW can be regarded as a huge, worldwide library. By using it, a user can find
valuable information, such as the latest in cancer treatments, the full wording of bills
pending before Congress, and any information that someone who has a point to make
and access to a Web site wants to publish. Conceived in 1989 and first operational in
December, 1990, the original purpose of the WWW was to enable the sharing of research materials and collaboration between physicists at many different locations. The
WWW is based on providing links to other files in the form of **hypertext**. Hypertext is
a type of cross-referencing in which text that is linked to another file is specially
marked.

WEB BROWSERS

The tool that enables users to retrieve and display files from the Web is called a Web browser, or just a **browser**. Under the client-server model of networking, to retrieve a Web document the browser on the client computer requests a file using a transmission protocol known as the **hypertext transfer protocol (HTTP)**. With this same protocol, the server, using special server software, receives that message, finds the file, and sends it off to the requesting computer. Although there are still text Web browsers such as Lynx, the development of a graphical browser, Mosaic, along with the arrival of graphical user interface (GUI) operating systems that could use a graphical browser, enabled the WWW to take off in popularity. The two most popular browsers today are Microsoft Internet Explorer and Netscape.

MARK-UP LANGUAGES: HTML AND XML

Although referred to as a language, **hypertext markup language (HTML)** is really a system of "marking a document up" by adding **tags** to objects such as text or images to define the manner in which they should be displayed. The tags provide a browser with information about what color to use for a piece of text as well as the font, attributes, and size to use to display the text. The tags also provide instructions for hypertext links to other web pages and instructions for displaying any image files that the document contains. HTML was modeled after SGML (standardized general markup language), which was the original system for organizing and tagging elements of a document. Figure 4-5 shows some of the tags seen in a document that is displayed using HTML, such as <P>. That tag told the browser to display the information following it as a paragraph, whereas the </P> told the browser that the end of the paragraph had been reached and to skip a line before displaying the next object.

Another mark-up language, **XML**, is starting to be used in healthcare. XML is short for eXtensible Mark-up Language. It too is a system of tags, but the purpose of these tags is to define the meaning of the data, thereby making it easier to find information within a document, database, or Web site. Much healthcare information is in a free text or narrative format that lacks any structure (Schweiger, Hoelzer, Altmann, & Dudeck, 2002). Trying to reduce this to a computerized format often results in important information being omitted. However, free text makes it hard to find specific information such as a diagnosis. XML enables tags to be used to identify items such as diagnosis, patient name, gender, and birth date in this free text. XML will prove useful for both exchanging data between incompatible systems and extracting information from free text. Like information in a database, information tagged with XML tags can be displayed in many different ways including on the Web (Quiggle, J, personal communication, 2002.).

USING THE WORLD WIDE WEB

To use the WWW, one must be connected to the Internet and have a Web browser. Whichever browser is used, near the top of the screen a location line appears (labeled the address bar in Microsoft Internet Explorer) that lists the **uniform resource locator (URL)**, or address of the computer that hosts the document that is displayed on the screen. There will also be a way to go to screens that have previously been accessed before (Back) or af-

```
<HTML>
<HEAD>
<META NAME="Generator" CONTENT="Corel WordPerfect 8">
<TITLE>-</TITLE>
</HEAD>
<BODY TEXT="#000000" LINK="#0000ff" VLINK="#551a8b" ALINK="#ff0000" BG

<TABLE BORDER="1" WIDTH="602" CELLPADDING="1" CELLSPACING="1">
<TR VALIGN="TOP"><TD WIDTH="412"><FPMT SOZE="+2"><STRONG>History of th

<P>CERN generously made the WWW tools available to other
interested users. These tools include software to read the files,
called a browser, documents that are specially formatted using a
language called HTML (HyperText Markup Language) and the
use of a transmission protocol called <STRONG>H</STRONG>yper<STRONG>T
<STRONG>P</STRONG>rotocol (HTTP). Using client-server conventions, the
the client software and the computer holding available documents
is a web server.</P>
```

Document formatted with HTML as received from a Web server.

Some of the tags are:
<HEAD> <TITLE>,
<TABLE> <P>
<HEAD> <TITLE>,
<TABLE> <P>
Information seen after the main tag and before the ">" is added formatting information.

History of the WWW

CERN generously made the WWW tools available to other interested users. These tools include software to read the files, called a browser, documents that are specially formatted using a language called HTML (HyperText Markup Language) and the use of a transmission protocol called HyperText Transfer Protocol (HTTP). Using clinet-server conventions, the browser is the client software and the computer holding available documents is a web server.

The same document interpreted by the browser on your screen.

Figure 4-5 • Web documents and HTML formatting tags.

ter (Forward) the current document. Both the forward and back options may be grayed out when the browser is first opened because at this time only one document has been viewed. A button that will allow the user to print the document, find a word or phrase, and request a new document will also be available.

There are several ways to access a Web document. One is to type its address, (the URL) on the location line. All browsers also provide either an open button or a choice on the file menu that presents the user with a dialog box into which an URL can be entered. This option provides the ability to browse, or search for, a file that resides on the same computer, for example if the user downloaded a Web file to his or her computer and now wants to view it.

After a file to retrieve is specified, small objects in an icon in the upper right hand corner of the screen will start moving to indicate the request is being filled. These objects will continue to move until the document requested has been completely downloaded. Unless the file resides on the computer making the request, very seldom is the return instantaneous. Be prepared to wait a minute or two, depending on the document requested, the speed and number of connections between your computer and the one the document is stored on, as well as the traffic on the Internet. A Web document can also be accessed by clicking on an URL that is sent in an e-mail message, if the sender includes the "http://"

in the URL. They can also be accessed from inside some application programs if the URL has been formatted as hypertext, something most word processors do automatically to any entry that looks to them like it is a Web address.

Favorites or Bookmarks

Entering URLs from a keyboard can become very tiresome as well as prone to transcription error. For this reason, browsers provide a way for users to easily record the URLs of sites that are frequently accessed. To access a site that has been recorded, click on **Favorites** (Internet Explorer) or **Bookmarks** (Netscape), select the site from the list, and click on it. To add a site to these lists, with the document displayed click on Favorites (Bookmarks) and select Add. Bookmarks (Favorites) can also be organized into folders.

Error Messages

Occasionally, instead of the requested file, an error message will be received. In general, there are three types of error messages. One type tells the user that the computer matching the name entered in the URL does not exist. Another error message relays that the file requested does not exist. Occasionally, either a site is too busy or Internet traffic is too great and a site will time out; that is, the calling computer will be unable to make contact with the computer called. Table 4-2 provides information about how to react to these errors.

If the user discovers a mistake after a request is made, clicking on the Stop button cancels the command. There are other times when a transfer seems to get interrupted or when only part of the requested file appears on the screen. This problem can sometimes be remedied by clicking on the Reload button, or if the status line says that the document is done, clicking the Back button and then the Forward button.

Web Navigation

Navigation of a Web document is identical to that used for most applications in a **graphical user interface (GUI)** operating system, including the use of the arrow keys, page down and up, and vertical and horizontal scroll bars. There are a few additional properties. Clicking on any area where the mouse pointer changes to a hand with an index finger pointing up will retrieve the document or object to which that item is linked. If the so-called "hot area" is a text word, in a well-designed Web site, that word will be underlined and colored blue. If the hot area is a graphic, moving the mouse pointer over it until it becomes a hand with pointing finger, instead of an arrow, will tell the user that clicking on that graphic will retrieve another file.

After the hypertext feature has been used many times, it is possible to get so far away from the original document that returning to it becomes a lengthy procedure. A feature of browsers, called "History" or "Go," keeps a record of the documents that have been retrieved. To return to a document, click on the appropriate button and then on the name of the desired document on the menu that appears.

Opening a New Browser Window

Sometimes when a link is clicked, a document opens in a new window instead of in the current browser window. In this case, the Back choice on the menu line is grayed out. To return to your original document, click on the browser icon closest to the left on the bottom of the screen. There are times when a user wants to have a linked document open in a new window. To do this, right click on the link and from the menu select "Open in new

TABLE 4-2 ● *Possible Responses to Web Error Messages*

Error	Thoughts on Correcting
	Click on "OK" then:
The computer does not exist. (The server does not have a DNS entry.)	Check the URL you entered, it may be incorrect. Correct and try again. This error can usually be avoided if you copy and paste the URL.
The file does not exist or you do not have access to it. (Error 404). Some Web sites instead of showing this error, have a special page that provides information on locating the file. Some of these automatically retrieve the document from the new URL. (If this URL is in your Favorites be sure to add the new and delete the old!)	1. Check the name of the file. 2. Go up one level in the address and see if you can find the file from there. Do this by deleting the URL in the location (address) line from the right hand end to the next forward slash.
File request has timed out. There is too much traffic at the site or the server is down.	Try once more; usually the best course is to try again at a different time.

window." With this procedure, it is easy to switch back and forth between various documents without having to wait for each to be displayed again.

URLS (WEB ADDRESSES)

All documents on the WWW have an address, or URL. These addresses are often seen in commercials on television or in print advertising. Almost all URLs start with "http",[2] (the acronym for hypertext transfer protocol); a colon; and two forward slashes. Many then follow with "www." The rest of the address varies. Just as with e-mail addresses, URLs may look like a conglomeration of characters when they are first encountered, but there is a pattern to them just as with e-mail addresses (Fig. 4-6). The name of the computer that hosts the document follows either the double forward slash (//) or the dot after www. It includes the **domain name**, which is the letters following the last dot in the name before the leftmost single forward slash (/). The letters after the name of the computer are **directories (folders)** on the host computer. Some URLs have more than one directory name in them. For example, in the URL http://nursingcenter.com/InformaticsNursing/ComputerNetworks/WorldWideWeb/URLs.html, there are three directory names between the name of the computer (nursingcenter.com) and the file name (URLs.html). Directories are organized hierarchically, A forward slash (/) separates each folder from the one above it. The last part of the URL may or may not end with a file name. File names end in a dot and usually the letters "htm" or "html" or "asp."

Non-letter characters may be seen in a URL, such as an underscore (_), a hyphen (-), or a tilde (~). These elements are all integral parts of an address and must not be omitted. When a tilde is in an address, it generally denotes a personal Web page versus an institu-

---

[2] Secure Web sites may have URLs that start with "https."

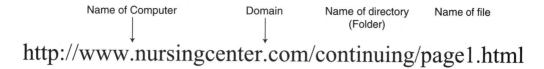

Name of Computer   Domain   Name of directory   Name of file
(Folder)

http://www.nursingcenter.com/continuing/page1.html

To parse this URL back to the home page, starting on the
RIGHT end, delete all the characters back to the "/ " after com.

Figure 4-6 • An URL dissected.

tional one. One thing that all Web addresses (like e-mail addresses) have in common is that they contain no spaces and all slashes are forward slashes. Additionally, the characters in an URL are case-sensitive; that is, if the letter in an URL is uppercase, it needs to be entered in uppercase, if in lowercase, it must be entered in lowercase. Because URLs can become very complicated, whenever you need to enter a complex URL it is best to copy and paste it if you can (see the Web site for this book http://connection.lww.com/go/thede for instructions on how to do this).

Domains

In Figure 4-6, the letters "com" are labeled as the domain. To facilitate locating computers on the Internet, the originators devised a system of naming computers based on their function. In the United States, there were originally six domains, but to accommodate all the organizations and individuals that wish to have a domain name, more domain suffixes have been added (Table 4-3). The domain can also be a country name.

Parsing an URL

One way to discover more information about the organization that provided a given Web document is to parse the URL. In parsing the URL, one places the mouse pointer in the address bar at the far right of the URL and deletes the characters back to a forward slash, then taps Enter to see what displays. Each directory can be displayed in this fashion, or one can immediately delete the letters back to the rightmost single forward slash to see the **home page** of the organization sponsoring the Web page.

Plug-Ins/Helpers

A **plug-in** is a helper program for a browser. Browsers are capable only of interpreting certain types of files, such as those in the html format, or gif and jpeg images. The Internet, however, is capable of transmitting other types of files, such as those created by multimedia authoring languages. Before a user can use these files, his or her computer must have a program that can interpret the file and show it either in the browser or on a separate screen. Plug-ins fill this function.

One of the most common plug-ins is Adobe Acrobat Reader, which is used to read files that are in the portable document format (PDF). Unlike regular Web pages that print according to the dictates of the printer used to output them, PDF files are designed to print in a specified way. This type of file is useful for things like forms that are intended for printing. PDF files, however, are difficult to read online and take longer to download. Most plug-ins intended to display files from the Web, such as Adobe Acrobat Reader, Real Player, Apple QuickTime, or Shockwave, may be downloaded for free.

TABLE 4-3 ● Organization Types as Represented in URLs	
Characters	**Type of Organization**
biz	A business
com	A business
edu	An educational institution
gov	A government source
info	Information
mil	A military computer
name	An individual
net	A network, often an ISP
org	A non-profit organization

SYNCHRONOUS COMMUNICATION

Most communication on the Internet is asynchronous; that is, the interaction does not occur in real time. In the case of e-mail, one sends a message and the recipient reads it anytime after it is received, anywhere from several seconds to several days after it was originally sent. Replies follow the same pattern. In contrast, a conversation on the telephone is synchronous communication, messages are received as they are delivered, and replies are immediate. Synchronous communication is also available over the Internet.

Text-Based Instant Messaging

Instant messaging, or synchronous communication, has become an important feature of Internet use for many people. The original instant messaging was called chat. Originally limited to two people, IRC (Internet relay chat) became available in the late 1980s, making it possible for multiple users to engage in "live" discussions. IRC requires special software on participants' computers and an Internet connection. Today, some ISPs feature chat rooms as one of their features. Unless a meeting is prearranged, users in most chat rooms exchange messages with anyone who is online and in that "room" at that time. At present, chat has mostly been used for socializing and games. The advantage of instant messaging is the instant feedback; many productive relationships have been formed through this method of communication. The downside is that participants have no way of knowing with whom they are "talking." Horror stories abound regarding people who were victimized by relationships with those they encountered through instant messaging.

Telephony

Telephony refers to computer software and hardware that can perform functions usually associated with a telephone. These products are sometimes referred to as Voice over IP (VOIP) or Voice over the Internet (VOI). Using the same technology that forms the basis for voice mail, it is possible for people to communicate using a computer. With this technology, a computer equipped with a sound card, speaker, microphone, and the appropriate software can be set up to function as a telephone (IW Labs, 1996). As this technology improves, voice communication using a computer device and the Internet will become more prevalent.

Teleconferencing via the Internet

Video meetings on the Internet are also becoming more commonplace. Versions of most Web browsers created since early 1997 include software that permits users to conduct a real-time conference.[3] Using a small camera that costs about $100 and an inexpensive microphone, participants can communicate visually as well as by voice. Attendees at these conferences can share files, view a common **whiteboard**,[4] and work collaboratively. Connections for these conferences can be as simple as starting the software and entering the e-mail address of those with whom a user wishes to connect. This technology is currently used by many corporations for business meetings and education. As the bandwidth of the Internet improves, this technology will find a large use in distance education and telehealth.

Issues

No innovation occurs without related issues. Computer networking is no exception. Healthcare networks, even before the age of the Internet, were vulnerable to misuse. Insider abuse, however, is the most prevalent security issue. **Firewalls** are used as one means of protection against outside invaders. These and large network security will be thoroughly explored in Chapter 19.

SECURITY

Internet users who connect using either cable or DSL lines need protection against computer invaders that is greater than those who connect using POTS. A number of protective devices are commercially available for this purpose.

Many Web users shop **online**, giving out their credit card numbers. Web browsers are used by shoppers to determine whether it is safe to provide their credit card number. When a user is at a secure site, this is demonstrated on the bottom line of the screen. In Netscape, a padlock in the lower left corner, which is otherwise open, will close. Windows Explorer indicates a secure site by displaying a lock icon on the bar on the bottom of the screen. If these signs are not visible, providing any personal information is very dangerous. Even with these signs, users should know the reputation of the organization with which they are doing business.

WEB COOKIES

There is a great deal of fear and misinformation about Web **cookies**. Web cookies are a collection of data that are sent to your computer by some Web sites. The browser stores the information in a cookie file, which is an ASCII text file. They may be used when a user fills out a form on the Web that has more than one screen so the browser can remember what was entered (Cookies, 2002). In this instance, they are quite useful. People who shop online are often greeted by their name on return visits, and may find that their login names are remembered. This information came from a cookie. Cookies can also be programmed

---

[3] Netscape conferencing software is CoolTalk whereas MS Windows conferencing software is called NetMeeting.

[4] A whiteboard is a device that allows online participants to write or draw while the other online group members observe the board on their computers.

to remember what a user sees at a site. By categorizing this data, information can be created and used to provide users with information that they might find useful.

When a site places a cookie in a cookie file on the user's computer, this information tells how long the cookie is valid. Some expire when the user leaves the site, some only exist for a given time, but most last forever. Sites identify their cookies by a keyword that allows them access to any information about your visit to the site that they have recorded in the cookie file. Essentially cookies were originally designed as a way for a server to better meet your needs. As with all things, this information can be used in ways that are an invasion of privacy, such as tracking surfing habits or targeting the user for ads that the site believes would be of interest. It is possible to set your browser to refuse all cookies or to ask you each time a site wants to send you a cookie and refuse it if you wish. More sophisticated programs also exist to help you decide which cookies to accept or decline. Newer versions of some Web browsers let you view cookies and provide the ability to delete one or many.

SPAM

Spam is the electronic equivalent of junk mail, except that it shifts the costs of advertising to the receiver. It also fills the Internet with unwanted messages. Few people like it, but owing to the cheapness of the mode it proliferates. Usually spam originates from a false address, so replying is a waste of time. If, however, you receive a spam message from an Internet service provider that you know to exist, such as one of the online services, you can forward it to *postmaster@online.service*. (Substitute the name of the service for "online.service.") Most services and ISPs take a very dim view of spamming and terminate the account of anyone who sends junk e-mail, or if someone's identity has been illegally assumed, it will look for ways to prevent this from happening in the future.

One of the best ways for users to avoid spam is to avoid giving out their e-mail address on the Web. An alternative is to acquire a free mailbox from a site that features these and give that e-mail address when asked for one. All the spam can then be easily deleted when the time is available to visit the free mailbox. Using this address when shopping means that all records of orders will be sent to that mailbox.

CHAIN LETTERS

Like their "snail-mail" counterparts, chain letters have become common in e-mail. A chain letter asks you to forward the letter to a given number of people, and may also ask you to send money to the last individual on the list. If you are accessing the Internet through an account at an institution where you work, chain letters may be prohibited. Penalties can range from a warning to a loss of Internet privileges or even job loss. Anyone choosing to forward a chain letter needs to keep in mind other factors. Many people today do business by e-mail. Most of them have to read and respond to 25 to 200 e-mail messages a day. Few are happy to find a chain letter in their mailbox.

OPT IN/OPT OUT

A concept that theoretically provides user choice is opt in or opt out. Under opt in, people will not be included in promotions or other deals unless they specifically request it. Opt out requires an individual to specifically request *not* to be included. Unfortunately, these choices, especially opt out, are often spelled out in very small print and are difficult to find. Additionally, the default is usually set to opt in so unless users find this choice and make the change manually, they will be considered to have opted in. This practice is endemic on the Web.

Summary

Computer networks are a natural outgrowth of the use of computers to manage information. Very few computers exist today that are not somehow tied into a network, either as part of a local area network or by access to the Internet. From its earliest beginning, the Internet has had a part in distributing data, information, and knowledge. In a relatively short time, the Internet has changed the way we communicate between individual people, communities, and countries.

One feature of the Internet, e-mail, is now such an accepted part of daily life that many people include their e-mail address on business cards. The arrival of the World Wide Web, or software called browsers that read documents formatted with HTML tags and provide hypertext links, has greatly increased the use and popularity of the Internet. Like all innovations, the Internet is not without its drawbacks. When networks are connected to the world, the security of data becomes a vital concern. This is especially true in large networks and personal computers that connect to the Internet using cable or DSL. Many Web sites place pieces of information on users computers called cookies that, although generally helpful, can be used to invade privacy. Spam has proliferated, wasting users' time, and Web users who register at a site need to be careful to read the fine print about whether they wish to be included in offers from the site.

connection For definitions of bolded key terms, visit the online glossary available at http://connection.lww.com/go/thede.

CONSIDERATIONS AND EXERCISES

1. How do you see the rapid communication and availability of knowledge via the Internet affecting society in general? Affecting healthcare?
2. Wireless Internet devices require Web sites to be specially designed to accommodate them. As wireless devices proliferate, what affect do you see this having on Web pages?
3. What advantages can you see to communicating with e-mail? What disadvantages?
4. Look at three e-mail messages that you have sent or received, and evaluate them according to e-mail etiquette as described on the Web site for this book http://connection.lww.com/go/thede.
5. Visit a Web site with many directory names. Parse the URL by working your way backwards until you read the domain name. What did you learn?
6. Add two sites to Favorites (if using Internet Explorer) or Bookmarks (if using Netscape).
7. Add three names and e-mail addresses to an e-mail address book and create a group for those three individuals.
8. How do you set your Web browser preferences to refuse cookies?

REFERENCES

Atkins, L. (1998, Jan 21). Big brother is watching—and reading your e-mail. *Cleveland Plain Dealer*, 11B.

Bennahum, D. (1999, May). Daemon Seed. *Wired*, 10, 12–13.

Blakely, T. (2001) *Satellite internet - What is it?* Retrieved January 23, 2002 from http://www.speedguide.net/editorials/satellite.shtml.

Cable Internet Basics. (n.d.) Retrieved June 17, 2002 from http://www.cable-modem.net/gc/basics.html.

Cookies. (2002). Retrieved January 25, 2002 from http://www.internet-tips.net/Security/cookies.htm.

Gardner, D. (2002). *Wireless insecurities*. Retrieved January 21, 2002 from http://www.infosecuritymag.com/2002/jan/cover.shtml.

IW Labs (1996, June). Internet phones: The future is calling. *Internet World*, 40, 42–46;48–52.

Schweiger, R., Hoelzer, S., Altmann, U., & Dudeck, J. R. J. (2002). Plug-and-play XML. *Journal of the American Medical Informatics Association*, 9(1), 37–62.

Understanding Computer Concepts: Features Common to Most Packaged Software

Objectives

After studying this chapter you will be able to:

1. Use the right mouse button correctly.

2. Apply computer conventions when faced with new situations.

3. Use the "help" option to learn to perform new functions.

4. Select, copy, and move an object on a computer.

5. Use "save" and "save as" functions appropriately.

6. Employ file organizational principles in copying files.

7. Apply safe computing principles.

8. Identify a virus hoax when received as an e-mail message.

Remember the first time you cared for a patient? Everything took a long time and required absolute concentration while you moved through each procedure step by step. By gaining experience, procedures were modified according to each patient's needs. Similarities in tasks became apparent, and these principles were then applied to all patients.

For example, when beginners measure someone's blood pressure, the procedures involved in wrapping the cuff, pumping up the manometer, placing the stethoscope properly, and releasing pressure slowly takes precedence over results. After some experience, blood pressure is viewed as a part of the total assessment picture and the procedure is done automatically. When a nurse is able to judge when to take a blood pressure that is not ordered, the importance of the action exceeds simple required recording of the results. This knowledge is freedom from a dependence on procedures and allows the nurse to practice professionally.

The same thing happens in working with computers. At first, a user may be very concerned about the keystrokes needed to perform each function. As more experience is gained, specific procedures (such as creating headers) become just another tool. In experimenting with different application programs, similarities and differences can be recognized, which makes the task of learning different programs much easier.

Expanding Your Computer Horizons

In learning to use computers, without realizing it, the user internalizes concepts that are transformed into quicker understanding and mastery of other computer tasks. In the hope of facilitating the process of seeing computer use as a whole instead of a series of functions, each requiring a different procedure, it is useful to explore concepts encountered in many different computer applications.

MOUSE USE

One feature that every graphical user interface program has is a mouse, or a device with a similar function that allows a user to move a pointer on the screen by physically moving some real object, such as a track ball or mouse. When a button on the mouse is clicked, the insertion point moves to the place on the screen where the pointer was, or an object[1] is selected. PC mice usually have at least two buttons, each with a different function. The left button selects objects; the right shows features that can be applied to the selected object. When directions are given to "click the mouse," they always refer to clicking the left mouse button. Although there are exceptions, generally one left mouse click selects an object, whereas a double click is required to implement a feature. If the right button is to be clicked, the instructions will specify that. Learning to use a mouse can be trying. Playing solitaire, or one of the games that are packaged with Windows, can help ease this task by allowing the user to become familiar with the mouse in a nonthreatening environment.

TEXT EDITING

All computer programs use similar methods to edit. This includes not only word processors but also e-mail programs, spreadsheets, and databases. When pressed, the backspace key always erases the character to the cursor's left, and the delete key (if there is one on the keyboard) erases the character to the cursor's right, or the one it is under. A computer interprets as characters spaces and "returns" (when the Enter key is tapped to create a new line), allowing them to be erased in the same manner as any other character.

Word wrap, or the ability of the computer to move the text to the next line when the space on the current line is full, is another text-editing feature that is universal in most computer applications. Saving the information that one has entered is managed the same way in most application programs, but in databases this may occur as soon as the user's insertion point leaves the spot ("field") where the data were entered. Tapping the Tab key in a table in a word processor, a cell in a spreadsheet, or an online form automatically takes the user to the next cell or open space on the form, and Shift-Tab will move one cell backward.

SCREEN APPEARANCE

Screen design is very similar in most programs. All programs have title bars, which give the name of the application program that is being used, menu lines, and tool bars (Figure

---

[1] An "object" in cyberspace can be anything on the screen from a character to a page, a part of a graphic, or an entire graphic.

5-1). Many also have a status line on the bottom of the screen. Since the introduction of Windows 95, PCs also have a program bar at the bottom of the screen. This bar shows all the programs that are open at any given time. Clicking on any one of them opens the document that is active in that window at that time. Between the top and bottom lines is the work area, or the place where the user can enter or edit information. There are some variations between programs and operating systems, but generally these elements are available in similar form in all programs.

The area where any document or file is edited is called the *work area*. Its appearance varies with the program, but it is where users enter data and create files, documents, or pictures. In describing the following features, the term **document** is used to denote any item that a user creates that is in RAM. **File** is used to denote any document that has been saved.

MENU LINE

Not only are the screen layouts very similar in most programs, but the features that one will find in each of the menu choices are also similar. On the menu line, most Windows programs place, in the following order, "File," "Edit," "View," "Insert," and "Format." As would be expected, clicking on View will show options that pertain to what is on the screen such as normal (draft) or print view of the document, whereas under Insert one can expect to find features relating to materials that can be inserted into a document. The choices under **Format** usually refer to how the document will look. Relating these names

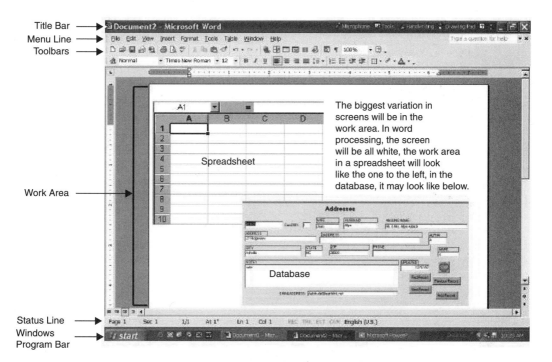

Figure 5-1 • Typical screen.

to concepts makes it easier to "guess" where each feature can be found (Table 5-1). Many features found on a menu have shortcuts, or keys that may be pressed to activate the same function. These are listed on the drop-down menu to the right of the choice. Appendix D gives a list of universal Windows key press shortcuts.

TOOLBARS

As with menus, toolbars also have many similarities. Most start with the same four icons, three of which are usually "Open a new document," "Retrieve a file," and "Save a document." Windows almost always has at least two, if not three, ways that a similar feature can be implemented, thus icons usually represent functions that can also be found as choices on a menu. Some of the more common icons are seen in Figure 5-2. An icon's function is usually revealed automatically in a pop-up label when the mouse pointer is left over it for a few seconds.

STATUS AND PROGRAM BARS

The second line above the bottom of the screen is called the *status bar* or *status line*. The status line gives information about the current document that varies among programs and vendors. In many word processors, this line indicates the page of a document, the line of text on that page, or how far from the left margin the insertion point is located. The status line may also indicate whether the Caps Lock is on or if the user is in insert ("Ins") (any characters entered will make room for themselves) or overtype (a strikeover or typeover status in which entered characters will type over the characters already on the screen) mode. The program line on the bottom of the screen shows an icon for all the programs the user has open at that time. Clicking on any of these icons opens the associated window.

DEFAULT

Another universal concept is the **default** function. Defaults are properties or attributes that may be changed but that are employed by the program unless otherwise specified. For example, when using a word processor, the default mode for entering text is the insert mode. That is, unless this is specifically changed by tapping the insert key, any text entered is in-

TABLE 5-1 ● Common Menu Features					
Menu Item	**File**	**Edit**	**View**	**Insert**	**Format**
Focus of functions found on the menu.	Functions pertaining to a file	Functions that allow you to edit the text.	Functions that affect the screen display.	Functions that can be inserted into the file	Functions that affect how the text will appear.
Some functions found on this menu.	Open a file Save a file Print Exit	Cut Copy Paste Find	Zoom Tool bars that are visible.	Graphics (Pictures) Footnotes Endnotes	Paragraph styles Fonts Attributes

Although there are differences between vendors, these functions are generally found on the drop down menus for all programs.

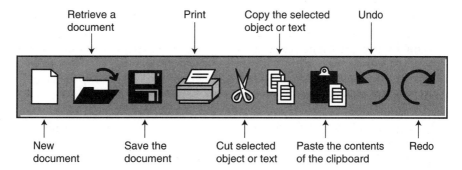

Figure 5-2 • Universal icons.

serted at the location of the insertion point. The new text does not overwrite any text that is already there but instead pushes the text already there ahead of it. Other defaults are margins, which vary from 1 to 1.25 inches, and a default font, usually Times New Roman or Arial.

When a change is made, whatever characteristic is assigned becomes the new default for that document. If the default margin, for instance, is 1.25 inches on all four sides, but a user changes the margins to 1 inch, the 1-inch setting then becomes the default margin for that document. Most of the properties changed will only alter the default for that characteristic for the active document. Very few affect the overall action of the program. If something different from the default is frequently used, such as a 1-inch margin, most programs provide a way to change the default so it will affect all documents. They also provide a way to return all settings to the default.

Many users are not happy with the default tool bars, colors of the screen, or other items. These too can be changed. The terminology used to provide this opportunity varies as does the option on the tool bar where it can be found, but when the word "preferences," "options," or "customize" is seen, selecting this option will allow making some changes. Some of these choices are on the menu bar; others, such as the tool bar, will only be seen when the object is selected and the right mouse button clicked.

UNDO (CTRL + Z) AND REDO (CTRL + Y OR CTRL + SHIFT + Z)

Two commands many applications have, especially word processors, spreadsheets, and graphics programs, are "undo" and "redo." By clicking on the undo icon, the last "edit" or change becomes undone. Clicking once again will undo prior changes in some programs. The number of changes or types of changes that can be undone depends on the program being used. Redo puts changes back in the order in which they were removed.

HELP (F1)

Feeling comfortable using a computer is often a matter of getting help when it is needed. Classes may provide some beginning skills, but when a user tries to use the functions learned or experiment with new functions, problems often may arise. The start menu features help for using Windows itself. There is also a short tutorial that new (and even experienced) users may find very helpful.

For most applications available today, printed manuals no longer come with the program, although one is sometimes available for a fee. Instead, users are expected to use the online help. Most programs provide this form of help, or help that is available by clicking on a word on the menu line or by tapping the F1 key on the top of the keyboard. When one clicks on the Help menu, although the contents of the drop-down menu varies among programs, the menu almost always contains an item that starts with "About." Clicking on the "about" item presents information about the program. This information may contain the serial number of the program, the exact version of the program in use, and possibly how much RAM remains available.

Some application programs feature "Wizards," which are the default mode of accomplishing a task. A presentation program, for example, may assume a user is going to make regular slides, and therefore takes the user step-by-step toward accomplishing this goal without the user's having to make many program-related decisions. Wizards can be helpful, but they can also be limiting because they use only a small fraction of the features a program may have.

Books about the software in use are also helpful. Many texts about popular software products are available; however, there are so many that making a decision about which book to use can be complicated. Some are written for beginners, whereas others are complete references for a program. Keep in mind that the beginning books are very limited in their coverage of a program's functions. They are helpful when one is first starting to use a program, but it might be more cost-effective in the long run to buy a more complete book.

Books can be overwhelming in the material presented. If you are learning a program from a book, one suggestion is to work your way through the book until you feel reasonably comfortable with the program. Then create a document that is needed, referring either to online help or the book when necessary. After becoming a little more comfortable with the program, take the time to peruse the rest of the book, noting what features are available. By knowing what is available, you can plan a document using this information, and learn how to implement the feature when you will use it.

Often the best help is to "read the screen." It sounds obvious, but most of us when we are coping with learning a new feature develop tunnel vision and will not see all the choices on the open window. As explained in Chapter 3, any rectangle with text in it and a triangle pointing down will provide other choices if one clicks on that triangle. Often what cannot be found will be in the list that appears when the triangle is clicked. Many of these drop-down boxes have scroll bars; so scroll up and down before concluding that the feature you want is not available.

If one is using an institutional copy of a program, the way it is licensed may stipulate that only specific people may call the vendor. In these cases, there will usually be a help desk for the program within the institution. Whether learning to use an application program or a healthcare organization's information system, it is important that the user locate the sources of help available and take advantage of them. Asking for help is a sign that the user is serious about learning to employ a program fully.

Selecting, Copying, and Moving Objects

Choices on a menu, as well as objects, are selected by moving the mouse pointer over them and clicking. As the mouse pointer moves over the menu, the selected feature is **highlighted**, which means that the feature changes to a different color scheme. Clicking when the feature one desires to activate is highlighted (selected) implements that feature. The principle of selecting and clicking is used in all computer applications, not only in menus, but also as they apply to many features.

The **objects** that can be selected vary from application program to application program. Note that the word *object* is applied to anything that is selected, as previously mentioned. This can be a letter, word, paragraph, page, entire document, cell or cells in a table or spreadsheet, an image, or pieces of that image. One selects objects to apply **attributes** or features such as delete or copy. Attributes are characteristics such as boldfacing, typeface, thickness, and color of an object. To select text,one positions the mouse pointer at the beginning or end of a passage and holds down the left mouse button while dragging the pointer to the opposite end of the desired text. Holding down the shift key and using the arrow keys to move will also select text.

Selected objects are visible in text by highlighting; in graphics programs, other methods (such as placing a temporary border with markers on the selected object) are used. After an object is selected, an attribute can be applied to it. Clicking the right mouse button on a PC will reveal a menu of features that can be applied to selected objects. Graphical objects are selected by positioning the mouse pointer on them and left clicking.

When text is selected, any key press will replace that text with whatever is pressed. For example, if a sentence is selected and the enter key is tapped the sentence will disappear and a new line will be entered. (Use the undo key to get it back!) This principle holds true in any form, or in a Web browser on the address or location bar. When any text is highlighted indicating that it is selected, one can simply type the replacement without deleting the original.

Selected objects can be "cut," or "copied" and then "pasted." This feature is very useful in editing documents. After an object is selected, it may be dragged to a new location, or cut, or copied and pasted. When a selected object is cut either by clicking on the scissors icon or using cut from the edit menu, the selected object is removed from its present location and placed on the **clipboard**. When an object is copied, the original remains in its current location, but a copy of the object is on the clipboard. Having been put on the clipboard an object can be pasted, or placed, in many places: in another spot in the same document or in another document either in the same or a different program. The object stays on the clipboard until it is either purposely erased or replaced by another object's being cut or copied. Thus, one object may be pasted in many places without copying or cutting it more than once.

 ## Graphics

Graphics, or non-text items, can be inserted in word processing programs, spreadsheets, and databases, as well as presentation or graphics programs. Graphical objects share many similarities with text objects. After they are selected, when the right mouse button is clicked, a list of properties and functions for the selected object is displayed. The properties, however, differ, depending on the program and type of object.

Although drawing and presentation programs present the most options for working with graphical objects, no matter where they are found, many features can be used with a selected objects. The user can cut or copy the object, or resize it. Resizing of an object is done in the same manner as resizing a window; by moving the mouse pointer until it is over one of the squares that indicate that the object is selected, changing the mouse pointer to an arrow, then holding down the left mouse button to drag the side. To resize a graphical object without distorting it, drag one of the corners. Dragging a side will lengthen or widen the object and leave it out of proportion. Graphical objects may also be moved. To move a graphical object, place the mouse pointer over one of the borders of the selected object or inside the border until the pointer becomes a cross with an arrow at each end, hold down the left mouse button and drag the object to the new location.

 ## Documents

Documents are only electronic charges in RAM while they are being created. If the power goes off for some reason, and the document has not been converted to a file by saving, it will be lost. This holds true for all computer programs. The only exception may be when entering data into a database. Databases save data as soon as the user leaves the **field** in which the data was entered.

SAVING

Saving a document in any program involves invoking the save command in one of three ways:

1. Clicking File on the menu line, then Save on the menu
2. Clicking on the disk icon on the tool bar
3. Tapping Ctrl + S.

When a document is saved, a copy of the current document is put on a disk where it can be retrieved for future use. When additional changes are made to the document, these are not recorded on the file on the disk until the document is saved again. Thus, frequent saving keeps users from losing a document in its updated version (Figure 5-3).

The first time that a document is saved, the user is asked to name the file. To make it easier to find the file the next time it is needed, the name chosen should reflect its contents. Names can have up to 256 characters and include spaces. Some characters may not be used in a file name (e.g., the hyphen and the slash). Letters and numbers are always safe to use in file names.

After the file has been saved the first time, each save using one of the three methods above is a repeat save, that is, the new version of the document replaces the one put on the disk by the previous save. There may be times when one wants to preserve the original document but wants to use it as a basis for a new document (Figure 5-4). In this case, a user should select to "Save As." This choice can be found on the File menu on the menu line. After the file has been saved under the new name, all that is necessary to preserve changes is to do a repeat save, which follows the regular saving process. Beginners, sometimes use save each time they save a document. This often results in confusion when they try to determine which is the current version. As a rule, unless you has a good reason for wanting different copies of a document, save the file under only one name, but back it up on another disk.

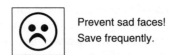

Prevent sad faces!
Save frequently.

Figure 5-3 • Save!

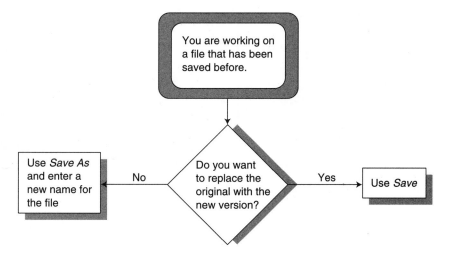

Figure 5-4 • Decision tree for using *Save* or *Save as.*

Sometimes when a file is saved for the first time, the user will receive a message stating that a file by that name already exists. The program also asks whether the existing file by that name should be replaced. Unless the user knows what is in the file on the disk that has that name and does not mind losing that file, the user should click on "No" and select a new name.

Many programs have a provision for an automatic backup. That is, after a given number of minutes the computer will back up one's work without a command being given. Although this can be a life saver, there are some difficulties associated with it. The location of the backup file may be difficult to find (particularly on a network), the feature may not have been activated, or a networked computer may be set to automatically delete all backup files every time it is booted (started). There is no substitute for regular saves and re-saves!

PRINT

Printing is another function that is available in all computer programs. When printing things such as spreadsheets or databases, it is easy to forget that a piece of paper has a finite size. Although this is not usually a problem with word processors because the formatting is tied to paper size, with both spreadsheets and databases, this can present difficulties. It is common with either of those program types to design a document that is wider than any paper a printer can use. When an attempt is made to print the document, the part that is too wide to fit on one sheet may be completely omitted, or it may print on another sheet of paper.

If the spreadsheet or database in question is not too large, there are two possible ways to solve this problem. One is to change the paper orientation from the default **portrait** to **landscape** (Figure 5-5). In landscape orientation, the longer side is horizontal instead of the shorter side. Although this approach can take care of some width problems, it still can-

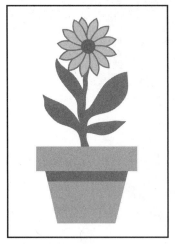

Portrait orientation

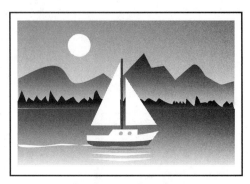

Landscape orientation

Figure 5-5 • Page orientation.

not accommodate all cases. More room can be created by using the font at a smaller point size, but this solution has its limitations in readability. The best solution is to remember paper size when designing any item that will be printed.

 Files

A document becomes a file when it is saved to any disk. The file format, or type of file created, is determined by the program that was used to create the document and save it. Applications from different vendors create files that are often incompatible with other programs, the same applications from other vendors, and even different versions of the same program. Generally software is **backwardly compatible**; that is, a newer version may open files created by an older version, but with the exception of word processors, in most cases the reverse is not true. These two reasons (a program from a different vendor created the file, or a newer version of the software was used), are often the cause when recipients of file attachments are unable to open the attached files. There is, however, a way to save a file in both a different format and in the format used by the older version of the same program (Figure 5-6). In this procedure, any features not supported by the older program will be lost, but this is not often a problem. For example, a database created by Microsoft Access 2002 and saved in the Microsoft Access 2000 format would lose any features that were new in Access 2002.

FILE EXTENSIONS

The name of the program that created the program can be identified by the letters of the file name following the dot. For example, in the file name "Chapter05.wpd," the **file extension** is "wpd" indicating that this file was created with Corel WordPerfect. All pro-

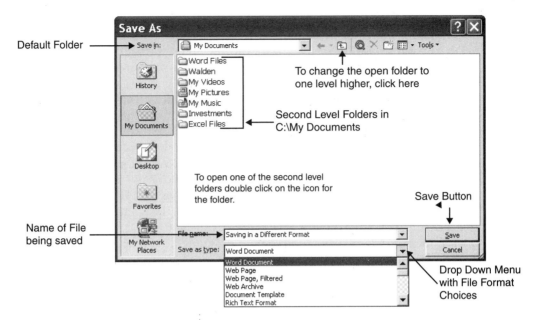

To save a file in a format different than the one used to create it first, save it in its native format in the desired folder. Then click on File on the menu line and click on Save As. In the Save window, near the bottom, is a "Save as type" box. Click on the triangle at the right end of the box, select the appropriate format and click Save. The file will have the same name as the original, but the extension will be different.

Figure 5-6 • Saving a file as a different type.

grams also have icons that can be used to identify the files that belong to them. Microsoft Word uses a blue W. These icons precede the file name. If the computer being used does not show file extensions, this can be changed. Instructions for doing so can be found at http://connection.lww.com/go/thede.

As mentioned already, knowing what program was used to create a file is necessary when opening attachments. Although the rich text format (**RTF**) is usable by many programs, particularly word processors, the one format that is universally accepted by most programs is the **ASCII** format. Files saved in this format have a .txt extension. ASCII contains only text, and each line is regarded as a separate paragraph, which means that subsequent editing of that document will be difficult. Even so, ASCII can be a very useful format for structured data (data organized by rows and columns), because it can be easily opened in a spreadsheet or a database. The universal word processing format, RTF, is a type of ASCII file that does retain formatting information, such as fonts and margins, and is useful when sending word processing files as file e-mail attachments.

DISK ORGANIZATION

Files when they are saved go to a **logical** (that is, one that is visible to the user, but which may have no relationship to the actual **physical** placement of the file) location on the disk. The logical location has a name that starts with the name of the disk drive on which the file is saved and is followed by a colon and one backward slash. For example, if a file is saved to a 3-1/2-inch diskette in drive A, the file name will start with "A:\" Note that this is the backward slash (\), or the one on the key under the backspace key, not the forward (/) found under the question mark. The disk name is known as the **root** of the disk. For the disk in drive A, the root of the disk is "A:\." File names that start with the root of the disk are called **path names**. If a file named Informatics created by Microsoft Word was saved on the A drive, its full path name would be "A:\Informatics.doc."

Files can, of course, be saved on the root of a disk. On storage devices that are larger than a 3-1/2-inch diskette, if every file were saved on the root, finding a file when needed would become a chore akin to finding a particular loose sock in a huge, unorganized sock drawer. To facilitate finding files, disk management allows the creation of **folders**. A folder is a logical entity that users create on a disk to manage their files. The default folder that most Windows programs use is a folder called "My Documents" which is a first-level folder on the root of the C drive. Its full path name is "C:\My Documents." There are many other folders on a hard disk. They contain program files for application programs such as a presentation program or a database and files needed to support the operating system.

When users have only a few files, the folder C:\My Documents may be adequate to organize their files. Eventually, keeping all the files they create in this one folder again becomes the story of finding the sock in the unorganized sock drawer. To avoid this disorganization, users can create folders that are one level lower in the hierarchy than C:\My Documents. For example, students taking Nursing Informatics may create a folder called Nursing Informatics that is a subfolder of C:\My Documents. Its full path name would be "C:\My Documents\Nursing Informatics." Folders are organized the same way as directories on a Web Server. On a PC, however, each folder is separated by the backward slash versus the forward slash on a web server. If a user saved a file created with Word named "Assignment One" to the folder "C:\My Documents\Nursing Informatics" the full path name of that file would be "C:\My Documents\Nursing Informatics\Assignment One.doc."

To illustrate further, imagine that each computer has several large filing cabinets available in which to store files. These filing cabinets have drawers. Files can be placed in folders and folders can be placed in the drawers. If anyone is going to be able to find anything in this filing system, it is necessary to devise some way of naming the various items (Figure 5-7). Because there is more than one filing cabinet, it is necessary to give each a name. One that happens to be a gray color might be called "GRAY." Then to avoid confusion about the drawers, they are also named. The top drawer in GRAY may be called "TOP," the next drawer "MIDDLE," and the bottom drawer "LOWEST." The folders that go into these drawers also need to have names. One of the folders that is placed in the MIDDLE drawer may be named "DIABETES." Inside that folder is a document that is titled "EPIDEMIOLOGY." In describing how this document may be found, one could say to go to the GRAY filing cabinet, look in the drawer named "MIDDLE" for the folder named "DIABETES," and pull out the document titled "EPIDEMIOLOGY." Because the instructions are thorough, this document would be easily located. A shortened way of giving retrieval instructions using the logical organization of a disk would be "GRAY:\MIDDLE\DIABETES\EPIDEMIOLOGY."

Now imagine that although the filing cabinet has a finite size, the number or size of drawers and folders within drawers are not constrained by any physical size beyond the fact that collectively they cannot exceed the overall size of the filing cabinet. Instead, the

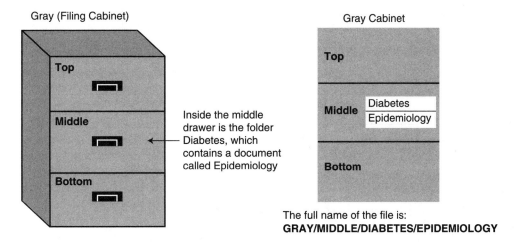

Figure 5-7 • Comparison of filing system.

number of drawers, folders, and files can be increased or decreased to meet current filing needs.

This is a perfect analogy for the way items are named and organized on a disk. Instead of the different divisions' being called filing cabinets, drawers, folders, and documents, the "filing cabinet" is called a disk, the drawers first-level folders, the folder a second-level folder, and the document a file (Table 5-2). Where disk storage varies greatly from a physical filing cabinet is that the folders can increase or decrease in size as needed. If you are using Windows 3.X or DOS, folders are referred to as directories.

This organizational method is hierarchical, that is, the items on top encompass those below them. Look at Figure 5-8. The root directory sits atop the hierarchy. This type of arrangement is called a tree arrangement. The root supports the entire tree and all folders and files take their names from the root.

Why is this important? There are at least four reasons. One, to keep files organized to expedite finding them, files need to be saved to a location that facilitates finding them. Second, files need to be backed up (Display 5-1), so that there are at least two copies,

TABLE 5-2 • *Comparisons of Document in a Filing Cabinet and a File on a Computer Hard Disk*				
	Object	**Name**	**Computer**	**Computer Name**
Root	Gray filing cabinet	Gray:\	Hard disk	c:\
1st level folder	Middle drawer	Gray:\Middle	First level folder	c:\Middle
2nd level folder	Diabetes folder in the middle drawer	Gray:\Middle\Diabetes	Second level folder	c:\Middle\Diabetes
File name	Epidemiology file	Gray:\Middle\Diabetes\ Epidemiology	File	c:\Middle\Diabetes\ Epidemiology

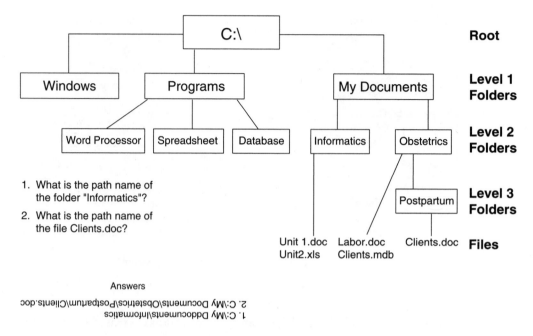

1. What is the path name of the folder "Informatics"?
2. What is the path name of the file Clients.doc?

Answers
1. C:\My Dddocuments\Informatics
2. C:\My Documents\Obstetrics\Postpartum\Clients.doc

Figure 5-8 • Hierarchical disk organization.

each on a different disk. Three, to attach a file to an e-mail message, the file must be located, and four, when files are downloaded, a user must be able to locate them. Understanding how files are organized on a disk greatly facilitates all of these requirements.

Personal style is reflected in how a filing cabinet is organized and how users name their files and folders. In some organizations, protocols for both file naming and folder organization are used by everyone to facilitate finding files that more than one person will use. Creating and using some type of organization will make backing up files to smaller disks a much easier process. For example, the user in Figure 5-8 can probably fit all the files she or he will create under the folder Informatics on one backup device. This enables the user to know which diskette to use if a problem arises. A rule of thumb is to limit the number of files in a folder to a size that can be easily copied to the backup storage device that one is using.

SAVING TO A SPECIFIC LOCATION

The folder into which a file goes when saved, or the folder where the computer will look for a file, is not a random choice. When using the "open file" icon, the files seen are the ones in the current working, or default folder. When users save a file, if they do not enter either the full path name of the file, or change the default folder, the file arbitrarily goes to that folder. In Figure 5-6, the current default or open folder is C:\My Documents whose name can be seen following the words "Save in." Several second level folders are listed in the window. Instructions for changing the folder can be found on the web page for this chapter at http://connection.lww.com/go/thede.

Display 5-1 • WHY BACK-UP FILES?

"Thank goodness that is done," you say as you watch the printer deliver the paper you have spent the last 2 weeks creating. The next day you deliver it to your instructor (or boss, or whomever). About 2 days later you receive a call from this person.

"I'm really sorry," she says, "but when I was cleaning out my office, your paper accidentally got mixed up with the papers that I needed to shred and I shredded it. I need another copy."

"No problem," you reply, "I'll print one out right away." You go to your computer, turn it on, and ask your word processor to retrieve the file. The disk whirs for a while, and to your dismay, delivers only one third of your paper. Not believing this is possible, you try again, and then again. The same thing happens each time. "This can't be happening," you think. You place a call to your favorite computer guru and describe the situation.

"What's the problem?" says the guru, "just use your back-up copy."

"What back-up copy?" you say.

"You don't have a back-up copy of an important document?" exclaims the guru. "That's too bad, I'm afraid that I can't help you."

With your stomach feeling as if it has dropped to your feet, you hang up the phone. "Why didn't I learn to back up files?" you moan. The sign hanging in the computer laboratory comes to your mind as you prepare to redo the paper.

Anyone who does not have a back-up copy of an important document is a disaster waiting to happen.

COPYING OR MOVING FILES

Several different methods exist for copying or backing up a file. The simplest, of course, is to save the file on two different disks. This works fine for one file, but if you need to copy more than one file, or entire folders, this process becomes very cumbersome. Windows provides Windows Explorer to expedite moving and copying files and folders. This is a different program than Internet Explorer. It aids a user in exploring a disk instead of the Internet. Accessed by right clicking on the Start button and clicking Explore, it presents a picture of the logical organization of a disk. Folders are listed in the left window and the contents of the active folder in the right window. Dragging files and or folders from the right window to the folder on the left will move them to that folder if on the same disk, or copy them to that disk or folder if it is on a different disk.

HYPERLINKED FILES

With the popularity of accessing information on the World Wide Web (WWW), many application programs today provide the ability to place a **link** to a Web document in a document in an application program. This area is visible by the use of different attributes, generally the familiar blue underlined text. When a user clicks on the link, if the computer on which the program is being used is online, an Internet browser takes the user directly to the address specified in the link.

Another function many programs provide is creating a document using HyperText Markup Language (HTML) that can be published to the WWW. The exact procedure for each program is different for programs from various vendors, but usually it is available. There are also Web authoring programs that give a Web page creator much more leeway in how a document will look.

MOVING DATA FROM ONE PROGRAM TO ANOTHER

After a block of data has been entered into the computer, it should never have to be entered again. When data are entered properly, they can be transferred between programs. The ease with which data can be moved between programs depends on the type of data. Structured data in a spreadsheet, statistical package, or database can be easily transferred from one program to another to take advantage of features not available in the original program. For example, a user may have data in a spreadsheet that needs statistical analysis or requires manipulation that is more easily accomplished in a database. Often this can be accomplished by using the **export** or **import** feature on the File menu. The export and import feature can change the file format in ways that "save as" cannot. It is very useful when exchanging data between different types of programs and different graphical formats.

Data can also be imported into a computer through the use of **scanners**. Often tests or the answers to research questionnaires are entered onto special (optical mark scan) paper for the purpose of being scanned. The output, besides being printed, can be used to create an ASCII file. This ASCII file can then be imported into a database, spreadsheet, or statistical package for further manipulation. Many hospital information systems will create an ASCII file of data that can be used by nurses or other healthcare personnel in a database or spreadsheet for creating reports or investigating phenomena.

Viruses

Sharing information is vital to the global healthcare system. Unfortunately, a small percentage of this sharing can cause problems. Programs known as **viruses** fall into this category. A program of this type is a small piece of code that is written to alter the way a computer operates without the permission of the computer owner. Although not all the programs of this nature are technically viruses, this tends to be the generic name for this category. In addition to viruses, which spread through infected files, there are **worms** and **Trojan Horses**. Any of these malicious programs can be operated as a **logical bomb**. That is, when certain conditions, (e.g., a date) are met, the program activates.

A virus, in the most correct use of the term, must meet two conditions: it must execute and it must replicate by itself (Symantec Knowledge Base, 1999). Officially, five different types of viruses exist, but basically they infect either a program file (**file infector virus**), the boot sector of a disk (**boot sector viruses**), data files (**macro virus**), or some combination of these three. File infector viruses are spread by opening an infected program. Once the virus is active in the computer, it infects any other program that is opened. These are usually found in **executable programs** the names of which have suffixes such as ".exe", ".com", or ".vbs". Boot sector viruses are spread by booting (starting) the computer with an infected disk. They enter a computer when an infected diskette is in the A drive when the computer is turned on. From then on, any disk including the hard drive that is used on that computer becomes infected. A macro virus is spread when a user opens a file that has a virus macro. Worms are another variant of a malignant program. A worm, unlike a true virus, replicates itself without a host file. Worms are often in the form of a macro inside another file. After being activated, they release another document with the worm that can then use the address book of a user to send itself to every address listed. When a file is opened, many programs detect a macro and ask the user whether he or she wishes to activate the virus. Unless a user knows exactly what the macro is and does, the best course is to say no. Macro viruses can exist in any of the office suite application programs.

A Trojan horse is a file that claims to be one thing but is in reality something else. These programs do not replicate themselves, but they contain code that can cause loss or theft of data. One variant acts as a login program to a network, but in reality captures the user's login name and password for use in accessing the network. These programs usually invade a computer when a user installs a program, particularly one that has been downloaded from an "unknown" site on the Internet.

ANTI-VIRUS PROGRAMS

Keeping copies of all important files is the first step towards protecting one's data. Purchasing and installing a virus protection program is the next step in protecting one's computer against viruses. One of the most important steps in installing an anti-virus program is to update the program on installation. Even when downloaded from the vendor's Web site, the anti-virus programs are not up-to-date. The first update may take several hours if using plain **POTS**; thereafter the updates will download in a few minutes. It is a good idea to update frequently, possibly every week. Some anti-virus programs can be set to update themselves automatically after a given time period. This works only if the computer is turned on and the computer is logged on the Internet at the time when the update is scheduled.

When installing the program, take advantage of the opportunity to create rescue disks. These will be invaluable if despite all efforts at protection, a virus invades the computer. Additionally, one needs to create a clean, write-protected bootable system diskette. If a hard disk has a virus, before it can be eliminated with a virus protection program, the user needs to boot the computer without activating the virus. This diskette will accomplish this task. Most anti-virus programs assist in creating these diskettes. Once this procedure is done, write-protect the diskette or diskettes, label them, and place them in a safe place.

Today, viruses usually enter a computer through the Internet. Downloading and installing a program from anything but a known and reputable source is risky. If this is done, the downloaded file should be scanned with the most updated version of the anti-virus program before being installed. This still does not guarantee 100% protection.

E-mail attachments, however, remain the most popular route for spreading a virus. In most cases, the e-mail message itself is not infected, but the attachment is. Attachments can be any type of a computer file, one that is a program, or a file from an application program that contains a macro. If the attachment contains a computer virus, opening the attachment will activate the virus. A good rule of thumb to follow is to *never* open a file attachment unless you know the person who is sending it, and more important, you know what the file is. When in doubt ask the sender what was sent *before* opening an attachment (Figure 5-9).

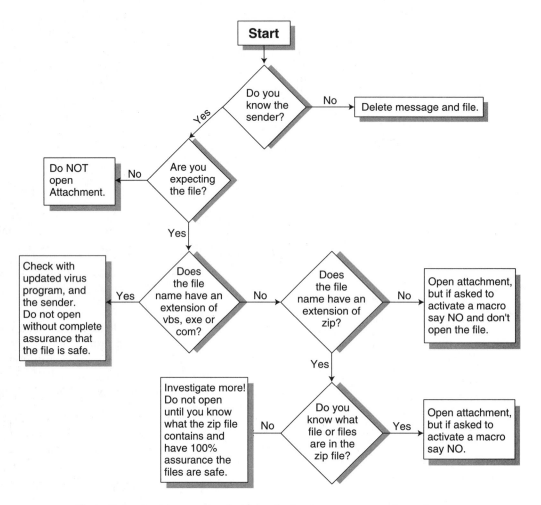

Figure 5-9 • Decision tree for deciding whether to open an e-mail attachment.

VIRUS HOAXES

E-mails that warn of viruses are a hoax 99% of the time. Although, with one exception, these are not harmful, they are a waste of time and clutter up the Internet and internal networks with useless messages. Hoaxes sound very credible, frequently citing sources such as an official from Microsoft or Symantec. They also threaten that the virus will destroy a hard drive or perform other dire computer damage. They always tell the recipient to forward this message to anyone she or he knows. Despite containing the statement that, "This is not a hoax," such messages are. Discard these messages and do *not* forward them. When there is a real virus you are most likely to hear about it in the regular mass media, especially if the virus is new and your anti-virus program does not have any protection against it. There are several web sites where a virus warning can be checked to see if it is a hoax.

There is another type of hoax that is not exactly a hoax, but a malicious practical joke that is also spread by e-mail. A user receives a message saying that if a file named "such and such" is on the recipient's computer the recipient should delete it immediately because it is a logical virus that will execute in so many days and damage the computer, files, and so on. Included are elaborate instructions for how to determine whether the file is on the computer, and equally elaborate instructions for deleting it. When a user searches for this file, it is found on the computer. Not thinking, the user deletes it. Unfortunately, it is a file that is part of the operating system, or other application program on the computer. Deleting the file causes a problem when the system or application program needs that file. Repairing the damage is often a lengthy chore.

If a recipient has any doubt that a message such as the above is a malicious practical joke, after finding the file, he or she should maximize the Find Screen and look at the date that the file was created. Unless the computer is younger than the given time period, the date will be well before the time period stated in the warning. If the file is part of the operating system, the date will be the date that Windows was installed on that computer. As a rule of thumb, except for deleting files that were user-created with an application program, proceed very cautiously in deleting any file. Know exactly what the file that is to be deleted does and be 100% certain that it is not a necessary file.

Summary

Computers are tools used to manage information. The task of learning to use a computer to manage information is facilitated when a user understands some of the computer conventions such as how to use a mouse, edit text, find things on a screen, and use the "Help" function. Help is useful to both beginners who need direction on many things and experts who infrequently use a given function. Many functions such as opening or saving a file, entering text, or printing follow the same principles in all application programs. Similarities also occur in the methods a computer uses with graphical objects, whether they are clip art, a drawing, an object that has been scanned, or the result of a screen capture. Understanding these principles makes transferring knowledge from one situation to another easier.

To make files easily retrievable, files are organized on a disk in a manner similar to files in a filing cabinet. Files are placed in folders, and folders and files can be placed in another folder. A well-organized disk facilitates making copies of files for back up purposes. All important files should be on at least two different disks such as the hard disk and a floppy diskette.

Although they are a real threat, computer viruses and other malicious programs are controllable in personal computers. Viruses are basically of three types and need a host program to spread. Most viruses today come from the Internet, either as a downloaded file or as an e-mail attachment. Although a good virus program will protect against many of these invaders, there is no substitute for a user's running through a series of decisions before opening a file attachment. Virus hoaxes proliferate in e-mail messages and should never be passed on before being checked out at an Internet site that catalogues and describes all hoaxes.

connection ➔   **For definitions of bolded key terms, visit the online glossary available at http://connection.lww.com/go/thede.**

CONSIDERATIONS AND EXERCISES

1. Identify what each icon at the top of a word processing program does by placing the mouse pointer over it and waiting a few seconds.

2. Open a word processing program. Without looking, guess under which of the file menus one would be the most likely to find the following:

   a. Save
   b. Print
   c. Place a file into another file
   d. Place a picture into a document
   e. Check spelling

3. Open several programs at the same time. Compare the options found in the File, Edit, and View menus. Briefly describe the concept on which the options in each menu focus.

4. In a word processor program, type a few words and delete them. Click on the undo icon. What happened?

5. Experiment with the help option.

   a. In the operating system (In PCs, this will be found on the Start Menu).
   b. In an application program.

6. Differentiate between a file and a folder.

7. What is the full path name of the **folder** on the hard disk where you store the documents that you create. (Remember, path names start with the root.) What is the full path name of the last **file** that you created?

8. Open the Windows Explore program and look at the tree structure in the left window. Open and close some folders. Practice using it to copy a file from the C:\My Documents folder to a floppy disk. If a folder is available, copy the entire folder (drag it just as if it were a file).

9. Create a list of computing practices that will prevent you from introducing a virus to your computer.

REFERENCES

What is the difference between viruses, worms, and Trojans? *Symantec Knowledge Base.* Retrieved June 18, 2002 from http://securityresponse.symantec.com/avcenter/faq.html.

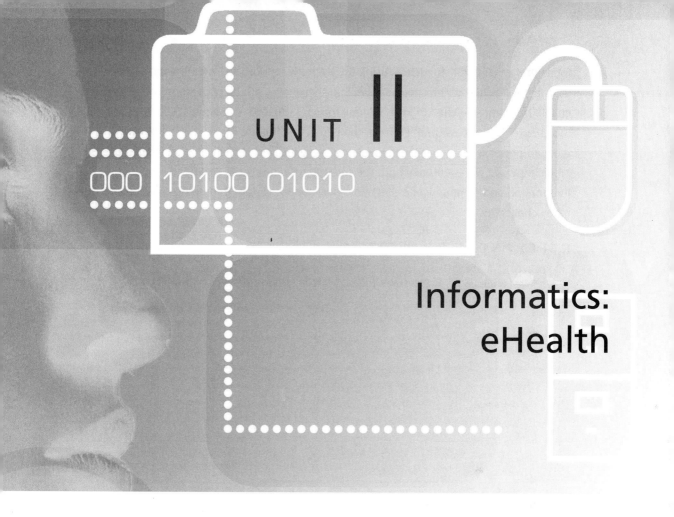

UNIT II

Informatics: eHealth

eHEALTH, the topic of this unit, "... is the use of emerging information and communication technology, especially the Internet, to improve or enable health and healthcare. This term bridges both the clinical and nonclinical sectors and includes both individual and population health-oriented tools" (Eng, 2001, Executive Summary). eHealth is a vast expansion of telehealth, and the term comprises all healthcare services offered over the Internet, including support, information, products, and direct services. eHealth uses the same tools that the Internet delivers to everyone, but uses them to support healthcare. The goals of eHealth are to make healthcare more efficient and to permit patients and professionals to do what was previously impractical or impossible.

Chapter 6 looks at the tools available to eHealth from the point of view of overall use. Information about searching the Web and evaluating Web resources, although it concerns professional tools and could therefore be part of Unit 5, is placed here instead because it has a direct bearing on the use of the Internet in healthcare. Some of the forms that eHealth takes, such as using the Web for support, are examined in Chapter 6. Chapter 7 will examine specific ways that these tools can be used to promote and enable healhcare. Telehealth in its various forms is the topic of Chapter 8. Included in this chapter is a discussion of some of the issues that the growth of this healthcare medium presents, including those involving financing and security. It is be difficult to predict how we will eventually optimize the opportunities presented by the emerging information and communication technologies, but it is certain that doing so will present many challenges.

REFERENCE

Eng, T. (2001). *The ehealth landscape.* Princeton, NJ: The Robert Wood Foundation. Retrieved from the World Wide Web February 3, 2002 from http://www.rwjf.org/.

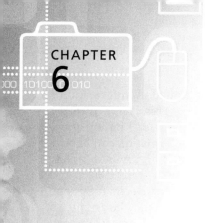

The Internet: eHealth Tools

Objectives
After studying this chapter you will be able to:

1. Select an appropriate search tool for finding information about a given topic.

2. Use search tools to allow narrowing or broadening a search.

3. Evaluate information found on the Internet.

4. Discuss the various forms of online publishing.

5. Compare and contrast the Internet networking entities.

Healthcare depends greatly on communication. Communication between the nurse and patient, communication between healthcare professionals, communication about organizational issues, and communication with the general public. One of the core elements of eHealth is the use of electronic technologies to enhance this communication for the purpose of furthering the goals of healthcare. Face-to-face communication is still important and, in many instances, cannot be supplanted, but communication using electronic means can supplement and enrich these meetings as well as provide an early warning system for threats to the public health. The tools that technology provides such as application programs and those specific to the Internet such as the World Wide Web (WWW), **intranets** and **extranets**, online publishing, and mass communication are useful in both professional and patient education. Like all innovations, however, their effective use requires knowledge.

 ## World Wide Web Documents

As more and more information continues to find its way online, the WWW has provided users with an encyclopedia in their computer. Unlike an encyclopedia, however, the documents that provide the needed information are located all over the world and are not always easily found. Additionally, the WWW provides an outlet to anyone who wishes to share his or her views. Thus, the use of WWW documents puts a burden on the user to become adept not only at finding sources but also at evaluating these sources.

TYPES OF SEARCH TOOLS

The WWW contains all sorts of documents, including, but not limited to, informational documents, advertisements, white papers, and personal opinion. This factor, together with the size of the WWW, which is currently estimated to comprise over 3 billion documents, makes indexing WWW documents in a manner in which information can be provided to those who need it a monumental task. Finding a book in a library is relatively easy because libraries are indexed using a standard vocabulary and some standardized system, such as the Library of Congress subject headings or the Dewey Decimal System. When searching the WWW, the task of finding the correct search term may be as much a matter of selecting the right tool as guessing the best term to use and, of course, some trial and error.

One of the best sources of information is word of mouth. Members of electronic **mailing lists**, **forums**, or **news groups** often post Web sites that they have found to be helpful. **Uniform resource locators** (URLs) for helpful information can also be found in print sources and on television. Many useful sites are also discovered by following links in a document, much as using a reference list in an article can yield helpful resources.

Many **search tools** are available on the WWW. Basically, the searching that they do is done either automatically or by a human who may search the Web, but such a person can also evaluate the information at sites that notify the search tool that they wish to be listed. Although it used to be possible to place search tools into a definite category, today many sites use both methods, although one form generally predominates (Sullivan, 2001). The automatic search tools, often called *search engines*, are powered by a tool called a *spider* that roams the Internet looking for a new site or one that has changed. The information a spider collects from a site varies depending on the dictates of the search tool (Sparks & Rizzolo, 1998)

Search Engines

Basically, these tools have three parts: a spider, an indexer, and software that allows a user to search the index. The spider, or *crawler* as it is sometimes called, visits a Web page, scans it and follows links to other pages within that site. The spider goes to known pages, then follows the links it finds; it is virtually impossible for a page to be indexed by a search engine if it is not linked to a page that is already indexed (U.C. Berkeley, 2001). The spider continually roams the Internet, returning to a page on a regular basis looking for changes. The pages found by the spider are catalogued into an index that contains information about every Web page found by the spider (Sullivan, 2001). What information is indexed depends on the criteria of the search engine. Some index major section headers, others the first lines of text on a homepage, frequently-mentioned words and phrases, or even every word (Sparks & Rizzolo, 1998). Some search engines provide information about how their database is indexed, but most do not. When the spider finds changes in a Web page, the index is updated (Sullivan, 2001). There may be a lag time between the spider's finding a page or any changes and this information's being added to the index. After a page is added to the index, it is available to people who use that search software. The indexes that are compiled vary from search engine to search engine, with some being more complete than others. Google (http://www.google.com/) is one example of this type of search engine.

Metasearchers are search engines that, instead of sending a spider to the Web at large, search the indexes of many search tools and compile the results into one display, often eliminating duplicates. Although they sound like the easy way to search, they are not as effective as a knowledgeable searcher (U.C. Berkely, 2001). One reason is that they do not always search the best search engines or directories, and they only search about 10% of each tool's holdings. Some of these are now organized in directory form. An example is Ixquick (http://www.ixquick.com/)

The human-powered search tools depend on either Web page developers' writing a short description of the site or an editor's finding and writing about a site that he or she has reviewed. Called *directories*, the search software looks only in these descriptions. The pages indexed are organized by categories to help a user limit a search. Changes in Web pages are not reflected in a search of this type of search tool. Yahoo (http://www.yahoo.com) is mainly a directory-type search tool, although it will use Google for some searches.

Specialized Search Tools

There are both directories and search engines that search for Web pages in specialized areas. The directories are often compiled by experts in the field, or librarians who spend time searching the web and evaluating the resources available. Infomine (http://infomine.ucr.edu) and the Academic Info Reference Desk (http://www.academicinfo.net) produce directories in areas of interest to academicians. Although targeted for business, Northern Light (http://www.northernlight.com/), when the Power Search function is selected, will provide a search of many nursing journals. A small description of articles is provided along with the ability to purchase the full-text document. Pricing for most documents is three dollars, with a money-back guarantee.

It is also possible to search only for images. If a user prefixes a search on Alta Vista with the word *image*, a list of URLs for images, instead of documents, will be received. Yahoo has a category devoted to images, and Ixquick provides the ability to search for images. Many images available on the Web require a royalty to use. However, when downloading an image, be sure to comply with copyright laws about its use.

Health-Related Search Tools

Several sites create directories for health-related topics. Medical Matrix (http://www.medmatrix.org/index.asp) provides subscription-based search services for health care professionals. A directory oriented to the lay public is Health A to Z (http://www.healthatoz.com/atoz/default.asp). Other search engines look for health oriented topics. CliniWeb International (http://www.ohsu.edu/cliniweb/), produced by the Oregon Health Sciences University takes the terms a user enters and maps them to terms from the MeSH disease classification (Schloman, 1999). This site also provides links to the National Library of Medicine's PubMed database. Medical World Search (http://www.mwsearch.com) charges users, but provides very powerful searches and links to full-text resources. Some of the fee-based tools may be available through a healthcare or academic library that provides institutional subscriptions for their users. Check with your librarian about this.

The Invisible Web

Only a portion of the offerings on the Web are available using a search tool. Some pages and links cannot be located by search engines, and some are excluded by the policy of the specific search tool. These pages are called the **invisible Web**. There are estimates that the invisible Web is two to three times bigger than the visible Web. There are several reasons for documents being invisible; one is that not all pages are static or permanent. Some are dynamic; that is, created on the fly in response to a question. An example would be a schedule of flights requested by a user or a list of resources from a question asked. Some sites require a password or login, which keeps spiders out because they cannot type.

Sometimes, the type of page prohibits it from being found by the search tool. For example, some sites, instead of using html format for their pages, use the **portable document format** (PDF). Few search engines can access these pages; hence, few include them. Other types of files that may not be found are images, sound files, and streaming files. Many search engines are programmed to avoid any page with a question mark in the URL. A question mark indicates that there is a script in the Web page. Although there are many legitimate reasons for including a script, a script can also be a trap, designed to bog a spider down in an **infinite loop**. Lacking any human judgment, most spiders just back off and ignore these URLs. There are tools that will provide a search of some of these pages. The Invisible Web Searchable Sites (http://library.rider.edu/scholarly/rlackie/Invisible/Inv_Web.html) provides examples of this type of tool.

TIPS IN SEARCHING FOR DOCUMENTS

Like any search of the literature, finding documents that are useful depends on the search strategy employed. For simple topics, using a one-word search may be helpful, but locating all the pertinent information on many topics requires a good preplan. The plan starts by listing all the words that might be associated with the topic (U.C. Berkeley, 2001), including acronyms or abbreviations. If there are any organizations that might have information on the topic, adding their pages to your search may also help. Often, these groups provide links to sources that might otherwise remain hidden. Table 6-1 summarizes some concepts often employed by WWW search tools. Investigating and using the advanced tips for a search tool that is used frequently will save time in searching for pertinent documents.

Finding useful information also depends on selecting the right tool. Tools' appropriateness varies with the information needed. If the topic is very broad, such as diabetes, select a directory tool. If the topic is very narrow, or if the user doubts much information is available, start with a good search engine. Take the time to become familiar with help, hints, tips, or **frequently asked questions** (FAQ), which are options that each search service provides. Some search tools in their advanced features allow the search to be limited to a specific **domain**. For example, when overwhelmed by documents, most of which are not pertinent to the desired topic, one may wish to limit the search to pages sponsored by an educational institution. Thus, the user would limit the search to the .edu domain.

EVALUATING SOURCES

The freedom of publication on the Internet allows an airing of ideas, many of which are not expressed in more mainstream communications. The veracity that we count on in print media with the reputations of various newspapers and journals is not yet available on the WWW. Although we may long for the security of a library in which all material has been vetted to some degree, the fact that yesterday's "far-out idea" may become today's

TABLE 6-1 • *Concepts Useful in Searching the WWW*			
Characteristic of the Term	**Tool to Use in Searching**	**Example Topic**	**How Term Is Entered Into Search Tool**
Several words (known as a phrase).	Quotations to surround the words.	Chronic heart failure	"chronic heart failure"
Two words that need to occur in the document.	Boolean "AND" This is the default for many search tools. Sometimes a "+" (See the advanced help for exact syntax.)	Knee and pain	knee pain knee AND pain Knee + pain
Combination of a phrase and a term.	Treat as though each term were a separate case	Digoxin treatment of chronic heart failure	"chronic heart failure" AND digoxin
Two words often associated, but only one wanted.	Boolean "NOT" Sometimes a "−" (See the advanced help for exact syntax.)	Knee but not running	knee NOT running knee − running
Searching for something that could be expressed in more than one way.	Separate with the Boolean "OR"	Licensed practical nurse or licensed vocational nurse	"licensed practical nurse" OR "licensed vocational nurse"
Term has two possible endings.	Truncations; indicate with asterisk (*) May be called stemming. Not all tools use this. As an alternative, enter both terms using "OR"	Nurses and ethics, could also be nursing and ethics	nurs* AND ethics nursing OR nurses AND ethics
Complex topic.	Sub-searching, a search tool that allows searching within the results.		

newest knowledge would make this undesirable. Additionally, try as hard as we might, evaluation is never 100% objective. The values of the evaluator are always involved.

The great variety of types of information on the Web means that using only one set of yes/no criteria for Web document evaluation is not a valid method. When using an evaluation tool, it is imperative to select one that is appropriate for the document. An evaluation tool for an advocacy document would not be pertinent for a personal Web page. Using an evaluation tool should not replace common sense.

Domain

Even before starting to use a tool, look at the URL and identify the top domain. This provides information about the sponsor of the page. For example, a top domain of ".com" or ".biz", or ".co" in the U.K., tells a user that the supporting site is a business organization. Often professors at educational institutions (.edu) place informative documents on their Web pages that may be helpful. Although they may be based on other sources, these articles ultimately represent the personal opinion of the professor, as do published articles. This fact does not devalue these papers or articles but readers should be aware that no information is value neutral.

Other Criteria

Documents on the Web fall into many different categories, among them advocacy, business/marketing, informational, news, personal, and entertainment. Identifying the type of document will focus the evaluation. A document from the top domain of ".org" may be of the advocacy type and should be evaluated carefully for objectivity, as should any document that is on a site that sells things. Documents from these sites may be very helpful, or very one-sided, or fall anywhere in between. Classifications of type of documents are not exact, and many documents will overlap a classification, but one point in evaluating is to think about which category or categories a document typifies.

Characteristics to Think About

It is important to remember that evaluation is subjective. In conducting an evaluation of a resource, whether on the WWW or elsewhere, besides thinking about the top domain and the type of document, consider how the resource will be used. Criteria that are helpful in evaluating a resource include accuracy, authority, objectivity, currency or timeliness, coverage, and usability.

Accuracy. Evaluating the accuracy of a document is often difficult. There are, however, some items that should be considered when making a judgment. Check for obvious errors in the information. Sometimes you will find excerpts from print material. In these cases, the original print source might have to be examined to evaluate whether the information was used correctly or taken out of context. If terms like "prove" are used, be suspicious. Research results never prove anything; they either lend support to a hypothesis, have no effect on it, or show a lack of support. A plethora of spelling or punctuation errors may indicate a lack of attention to detail, which may also be reflected in the accuracy of the content.

Authority. With print text, authority is often judged by source. If an article is published in *Nursing Research*, we can be reasonably certain that it has undergone extensive review by others with knowledge of the subject (peer review). If it is published on the Internet, it will fall somewhere on a continuum from a peer-reviewed article to someone's highly opinionated soapbox.

Certain criteria can be considered in deciding whether the source is reliable. The most important is the source of the document. What is the reputation of the organization at whose site the document was found? If the document does not reveal this information, parse the URL as described in Chapter 4. If the URL contains a tilde (~), the page is most likely a personal page; however, given the ease of obtaining a domain name in any domain, the absence of this sign does not necessarily mean that the page is not a personal Web page.

Documents without any author listed should be looked at very carefully. If an author is listed, what is the reputation of the author? Initials after the name can give information about credentials. Some authors are linked to their home page, which may list some of their accomplishments. Another avenue is to determine whether the name can be found in a bibliographical database appropriate to the field, for example, *CINAHL* or the *International Nursing Index*, in nursing.

Not finding any of these things does not automatically mean the document is flawed; it just means other criteria need to be used when making a decision. Is the information in the document verifiable? Are thought-provoking statements supported by references to other sources that are reliable? If so, is the reference stated fully enough so that it can be found? Are there outside evaluations of the site? Who made them? Do any of the Web guides list the site? Inclusion in these guides lends some reliability to the document. Is the site or document peer-reviewed or edited? If so, by whom?

Many organizations rate sites and provide a site with the privileges of using their logo on the site and stating that the site is approved by the given group. When clicked on, the logo should provide a link to the home page of the approving organization, where the criteria used to approve the site being evaluated will be found. There are also groups that make awards to various sites. If the criteria used to make the award cannot be easily located, the award may have little meaning.

Objectivity. Information is rarely neutral. Because data are used in selective ways to form information, they are generally synthesized into information in a way that represents a point of view. When evaluating information found on the Internet, it is important to think about any biases that may be present in the document. The popularity of the Internet makes it the perfect venue for commercial and sociopolitical publishing. These documents may be based on highly subjective uses of data.

Try to identify the point of view of the document and decide whether it is acceptable for the intended purpose. A point of view does not render a piece unusable, nor is finding biases necessarily bad. Most of us have opinions on many things. This does not make our writings or speech unacceptable.

Currency or Timeliness. Like print information, data on the Internet can become outdated. However, it is often difficult to tell what the true date of the data is. Well-designed pieces carry the date when they were last updated. What is not stated, however, is what "updated" means. It may mean that a complete review of the document was completed, or that a few items were changed, or just that it was read again. The date the document was first created is the best source of date, but this is available on very few Web documents. Additionally, the date first created and the date the document was placed on the Web may differ. If the document is undated, look at View/Document Information to see if the date that it was last updated is there. Another way to determine the currency of the document is to test the links. Finding many nonfunctional links is a sign that the information is probably old.

Coverage. Criteria in this category are specific to the proposed use of the document. What needs to be determined is whether the depth and vocabulary are adequate for the purpose. A document intended for a lay audience that provides little or no documentation will probably be inadequate as a resource for a professional paper. Conversely, a professional article would probably contain too much depth and technical vocabulary to give to most clients.

User Friendliness. If a document is intended for use with others, several things should be considered. Can the document be accessed directly or must the user access the front door of the site and hunt for the document? What is the download time of any pages that a user has to navigate to reach the document? Consider that most users connect to the Internet with plain old telephone service (POTS), which has varied speeds.

Does the document have any objectionable characteristics? Sound when used simply for effect, can be a nuisance, but if a user wishes to hear breath sounds, it is a necessary accompaniment to the site. Color can contribute to functionality or be a distraction. Graphics that take a long time to download but that are unnecessary for understanding can limit a site's usefulness. Whether it is easy to navigate the site also determines usability. The readability of any document should be evaluated based on the intended audience.

Some Web resources may require a plug-in such as Acrobat Reader or Shockwave. Well-designed pages inform users of this and direct them to a source for this software (which is generally free). Unfortunately, the desire of vendors for dominance in browser use has diminished the push for standardization of **HTML**. Thus, some pages may render differently in different browsers. Additionally, the size of the user's screen may alter the page that is being viewed.

Overall Rating. Arriving at a decision about the use of a document for a given purpose is not easy. It is hoped that the criteria that were discussed will be used as considerations when evaluating items from the WWW, not as an end in themselves. The WWW is a new medium. To deal with it effectively requires critical thinking abilities and a weighting of the criteria that depend not only on the type of document, but also on the presence or absence of some of these criteria. For example, if a document does not have an author, then the credibility of the organization where it is posted needs to be more heavily weighted. A document without references will be more valuable when the reputation of the author lends credence to the validity of its contents.

Use as a Resource in a Paper

Many times one can find resources on the Web that can be used as a reference in a formal paper. One ought to be cautious about this for several reasons. Any resource used as documentation in a paper needs to be examined very carefully. The highest quality resource for this purpose is another paper complete with citations and references. These may be found in some **online journals**, and sometimes on personal pages of academics or other experts. Unless found in a peer-reviewed online journal,[1] all Web documents should be carefully evaluated using the criteria addressed earlier in this chapter. There are times when one may find what one believes to be an excellent resource that is missing citations and references. Although these documents may contain valuable information, it is necessary to exercise careful judgment as to the authenticity of the information.

One difficulty with using Web resources as documentation in a formal paper is the impermanence of Web documents (Display 6-1). To protect yourself, if using any Web document as a resource, print it out and keep a copy. Be sure that the URL on the printed version matches the URL on the version on the Web. When a site uses what are called **frames**, or one file where the URL is represented in the address bar but that places linked files into a portion of this page without changing the URL, the correct URL cannot be seen. To determine whether this is the case, see if the last part of the URL changes as different documents are accessed. When frames are used, keep a record of how the document was accessed. Sometimes one can open the document in another window (Display 6-2) and obtain the correct URL. In this case, test the URL to be certain that the site will let you ac-

---

[1] Unless an online journal states that it is peer reviewed and provides a link to the list of reviewers, assume that it is not peer reviewed.

**Display 6-1 • GUIDELINES FOR USING
A WEB RESOURCE FOR
A FORMAL PAPER**

Refer to a printed source if available.
Print and keep the article and URL.
If the correct URL is not visible in the address bar, keep a record of
    how the document was obtained.
Select articles with a stated author if possible.
Record the date the document was retrieved.
Evaluate carefully using all criteria.
If no date or no author stated, request this information from the
    webmaster. Address is webmaster@name of computer. E.g.
    webmaster@nursingcenter.com
Check with professor or instructor for any guidelines for using Web
    resources.

cess that URL without going through their "front door." When including the URL as a reference (Display 6-3), the best approach is to copy and paste the URL instead of trying to type it accurately.

Accreditation of Health-Related Web Sites

Studies of accuracy of health information on the Web have revealed many problems, even from supposedly reliable sources such as individual practitioners, clinics, and educational organizations. A study of pages with information about managing fever in children revealed that only a few Web sites provided accurate and complete information (Impicciatore, Pandolfini, Casella, & Bonati, 1997). Fallis and Frické (2002) studied the same topic and found that three things correlated with accuracy: displaying the HONcode logo, having an organization domain (.org), and displaying a copyright symbol. Another study examined the information available for a lay person about the treatment of childhood diarrhea (McClung, Murray, & Heitlinger, 1998). Only 12% of the 60 articles examined adhered to the guidelines of the American Academy of Pediatrics (AAP) guidelines on the management of acute diarrhea, and only 20% gave recommendations that came near to following these guidelines. This compliance had no correlation with the source of the information. Sites associated with major academic medical centers were as likely to be deficient as other sources. Additionally, conflicting infor-

**Display 6-2 • OPENING A LINK IN A NEW
WINDOW**

Right click on the link.
Select "open [Link] in New Window" from the pop-up menu.

Display 6-3 • FORMAT FOR AMERICAN PSYCHOLOGICAL ASSOCIATION ELECTRONIC CITATION, 5TH VERSION

Some Common Electronic Citations

WEB DOCUMENT WITH NO AUTHOR
Health On the Net Foundation. (1997). *HONcode Principles.* Retrieved February 9, 2002 from http://www.hon.ch/HONcode/Conduct.html.

ARTICLE FROM ONLINE JOURNAL (NO PRINT VERSION)
Thede, L. Q. (2001, September 30) "Overview And Summary: Telehealth: Promise Or Peril?" *Online Journal of Issues in Nursing.* *6* (3). Retrieved February 9, 2002 from http://www.nursingworld.org/ojin/topic16/tpc16ntr.htm.

ARTICLE BASED ON PRINT SOURCE
Silberg, W. M., Lundberg, G. D., & Musacchio, R. A. (1997). Assessing, controlling, and assuring the quality of medical information on the Internet: Caveant lector et viewor-let the reader and viewer beware [Electronic Version]. *Journal of the American Medical Association, 277,* 1244–1245.

WEB DOCUMENT WITH NO DATE OR AUTHOR
Common FAQ (n.d.). *What is Nursing Informatics.* Retrieved February 12, 2002 from http://www.allnursingschools.com/faqs/informatics.php/?src=goto37.

---

mation on diarrhea was found within various departments of the same academic institution.

Given this situation, it is not surprising that many organizations are trying to address the issue of the quality of health information on the Web. One of the first such attempts was by the Health on the Net Foundation,[2] originally founded to advance the development and application of new information technologies in health and medicine (About Health on the Net Foundation, 1998). The Health on the Net Foundation responded to concerns regarding the varying quality of medical and health information available on the WWW by developing six criteria for medical and health Web sites. Sites that agree to abide by these criteria are entitled to display the Health on the Net Foundation logo (Figure 6-1). The criteria include the provision that only appropriately trained medical professionals give advice, that the advice be scientifically supportable, and that the site not encroach

---

[2] The Health on the Net Foundation is an international nonprofit foundation supported by donations. The Web page can be found at http://www.hon.ch.

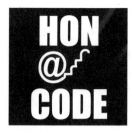

We subscribe to the HONcode principles
of the Health On the Net Foundation

Figure 6-1 • Health On the Net Foundation logo. Used with permission from Health On the Net Foundation, a non-profit international foundation, which can be found at http://www.hon.ch.

on any physician-patient relationship. (Health On the Net Foundation, 1997). Compliance is voluntary, and a site that displays the logo must provide a link to the Health on the Net Foundation page where the criteria are displayed. The decision about whether this logo is warranted, however, is left to site visitors, who are responsible for reporting any deviance from the criteria to the Health on the Net Foundation.

To meet the challenges that consumers face when searching for health information, the Internet Healthcare Coalition (http://www.ihealthcoalition.org/) has created a code of ethics. The code is international, comprehensive, and is focused on ethics, not law (eHealth Code of Ethics, 2000). This code is intended to cover not just Web sites, but also listservs, forums, and chat rooms; in short, any use of the Internet that may be health related. It is aimed at all people who use the Internet for health-related purposes, including vendors, researchers, patients, and healthcare providers.

Other groups are also creating codes of conduct with the goal of providing citizen protection. Different philosophies and approaches are guiding these efforts (Risk and Dzenowagis, 2001). The Risk and Dzenowagis study looked at many codes including, but not limited to, eHealth Code of Ethics, the Health Internet Ethics (Hi-Ethics), TNO Quality Medical Information and Communication (QMIC), DISCERN, and the American Medical Association (AMA): Guidelines for Medical and Health Information Sites on the Internet: Principles Governing AMA Web Sites. They found three different approaches to approval: codes of conduct, third-party certification, and tool-based evaluation. Some advantages for codes of conduct are stakeholder consensus and broad-based participation in their creation. Disadvantages include that there is a potential for misinterpretation of principles so that it is difficult to measure effectiveness. Third-party certification does provide independent validation and education for the provider of the site, but has a high cost and is labor intensive. Tool-based evaluation provides consistency, but may also provide a false sense of security.

As can be seen in the varied approaches, many difficulties are associated with regulating Web sites. For one, the Web is truly world wide, and acceptable healthcare information in one country may not be acceptable in another; even within political boundaries there are differences in opinions about health-related information. Additionally, it is very easy to change a Web page after it has been approved; in fact, it is necessary to make changes to stay current. Thus, Web information will always carry a caveat emptor, just like printed information.

Online Publishing

Online publishing has taken many formats. Although the term *online journal* is often used, this label is not precise. The online field includes "ezines," or what might be termed a newsletter, a Web presence for a print journal, and online journals that are published solely on the Web. Some online publications are free to all users; some, although free, require users to register before viewing; some have fees for use; and some are available only to selected groups.

EZINES

An **ezine** is a regular online newsletter that focuses on a given topic. Most are delivered without charge and supported by advertising. Generally, they address current topics such as career information, jobs, and news items of interest to their audience and are supported by advertisements. Few ezines maintain archives; thus, information on these sites has a very short shelf life. If using an article from an ezine as a reference, be sure to print it and save it. Brian Short's *Allnurses* (http://allnurses.com/) is a biweekly nursing ezine.

WEB PRESENCE FOR PRINT JOURNAL

Most print journals today have a Web presence. The amount of information that is provided, however, varies. Most provide a table of contents for their current issue, and often for back issues. The table of contents may or may not allow access to an abstract, and there may or may not be a way to purchase the article. Some journals will freely place online an article or two, even offering continuing education credit on completion of a test and payment of a fee.

One recent development for publishers is to have both a print and electronic versions of the journal. In many cases, having a subscription to the print version entitles the subscriber to access the electronic version. Many libraries today have agreements with publishers to provide full-text articles online to those served by their **intranet**.

TRUE ONLINE JOURNALS

A true online journal publishes all its articles online with no print version, features peer-reviewed articles, and maintains an archive of articles. At this writing, most online journals are available without charge to anyone with access to the Internet. Some are indexed in the nursing bibliographic databases such as *CINAHL* and even in *MEDLINE*. Most feature articles in HTML format, but some use pdf files, which require the Acrobat Reader to use.

Factors Affecting Online Journals

One of the biggest difficulties with online journals is the perception that the quality of their content is lower than that of print journals. Some bibliographic indexes still categorically refuse to index such journals. Part of this perception may result from the great variability in online journals; part is a belief that only print journals have refereed articles. It is generally believed, especially among academics, that only a peer-reviewed journal has reliable, valid, clinical papers, however, this perception is slowly changing, especially where faculty have technical skills (Schloman, 2001).

Given that most writers are members of academic faculties who need publication in recognized journals to gain promotion, this presents a dilemma. Promotions are made both on the number of articles published and the reputation of the publishing journal. This makes publishing in an online journal risky for nontenured faculty who are seeking tenure. These perceptions can affect the quality of writers, and therefore the quality of the articles these writers produce.

Another difficulty is lack of awareness about online journals. Nurses in all careers need to be information literate, but many today are not. A person who has not learned to use the Web is limited to print journals. Additionally, too many listings of online journals still make no distinction between any of the types, whether an e-zine, a print journal with an online presence, or a true online journal. Seeing a huge list and accessing too many false leads in a search for a real online journal, many users simply conclude that none exist.

Unlike most print journals, which are a product of a publishing house, most online journals have been started with little financial or organizational support. This has resulted in many being started but not nearly as many being able to maintain staying power. It is not unusual to find that an online journal has not had any new articles for several years, or to find that it has disappeared entirely. Although it looks easy to run an online journal, a large amount of work is involved in producing a high-quality journal. Writers need to be found, as well as reviewers; someone must coordinate the progress of the articles; the articles need to be converted to a Web format; and the journal needs to be marketed. All these tasks take time. Without some financial backing, these tasks can become insurmountable. There are also expenses for long-distance phone calls, postage, and other supplies.

 ## Internet Networking

The online environment offers several ways for networking in addition to e-mail. Bulletin boards were one of the first online networking tools, although they did not involve the Internet. Although now mostly history, they served the purpose of providing users with an ability to post and read messages. Bulletin boards have been mostly replaced by news groups, forums, and electronic mailing lists.

NEWS GROUPS

News groups are electronic discussion forums. First established in 1979 at the University of North Carolina as Usenet News, their purpose was to provide a forum for the discussion of politics, religion, and other subjects. They became very popular, and users from all over the world soon joined (Timeline, 1997). Although the term *news* is used for these groups, the news refers to messages sent by *any* person who chooses to do so and replies to those messages. For the most part, these messages are *not* refereed. As originally conceived and distributed under Usenet News, these groups were organized in hierarchical levels under seven different headings. As more groups developed, some did not fit into the seven original categories, and an Alt category was created to house them (Oliver, 1996).

A loose network of computers was established. Their users agreed to carry the messages and replies that had been posted to these groups and make them available to the public. The number of groups grew to cover many different topics, including health-related and nursing-related topics (e.g., sci.med.nursing, alt.npractitioners) for nursing. By 1995, there were more than 12,000 such groups generating 300 megabytes of information a day (Fleishman, 1995). Today, many groups exist that are strictly local and intended for communication about issues of interest only to a small group.

To access news groups requires a special news reader. Most browsers include this software, but more extensive news readers are also available. A good reader keeps track of the messages that have been read and allows one to subscribe to a particular group. A subscription, which is free, just means that the group can be easily accessed without going through the hierarchy to locate it. The reader also provides ways to post messages to the group.

FORUMS

Forums are similar to news groups, but they are sponsored by individual organizations and are usually Web based. Depending on the organization, there may be one or more forums, but the topic of discussion for each will be related to the mission of the organization. To access a forum, visit the Web site of the sponsoring organization. From there, follow the instructions for entering the desired forum. Newcomers are often asked to register by giving their names and assigning themselves a password to use for future visits. After registering, most forums send an e-mail to the new registrant message with the login name and password and instructions to keep the message. Some forums will set a cookie in the registrant's browser, so that this information is read each time this person returns to the forum, relieving the member of the necessity to remember the password and login name.

ELECTRONIC MAILING LISTS (LISTSERVS)

An electronic mailing list is an interactive means of communication between a subscriber and the group. An electronic mailing list group is a different form of network "news." As noted with network news, there are many groups, each of which focuses on specific topics, but instead of using a special reader to read the messages, the messages are sent to subscribers' e-mail addresses. Joining a list is called *subscribing*, and like Usenet news groups, subscriptions are free. After a user has subscribed to a group, copies of any message posted to the group are sent to all members' mailboxes (Figure 6-2). Members can reply to any of the messages or send an entirely new message to the group. The tasks of keeping track of subscribers and sending copies of messages are accomplished by a software program. The original software program that managed these electronic mailing lists was called "ListServ," which is why mailing lists are often called *listservs*.

Lists can be moderated, moderated with editing, or unmoderated. On unmoderated lists, *all* messages posted to the group's address are automatically sent to the group. On a moderated group, messages first pass to the list's "owner," or the person who takes responsibility for the list. This person may post a message or not, depending on the criteria of the group. In a moderated-with-editing group, the messages not only go to the owner, but this person may edit the message before posting. There are advantages and disadvantages to all formats. On an unmoderated list, subscribers receive all messages including

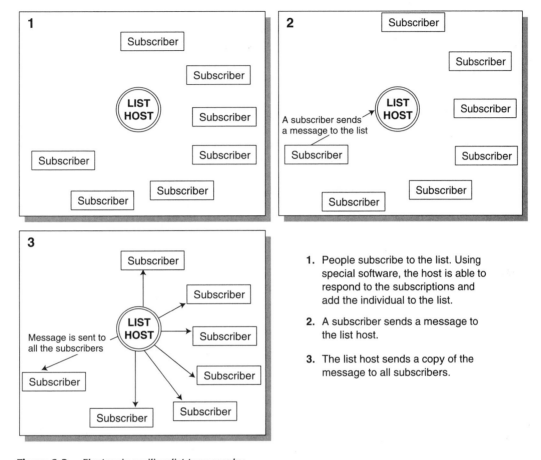

Figure 6-2 • Electronic mailing list topography.

1. People subscribe to the list. Using special software, the host is able to respond to the subscriptions and add the individual to the list.

2. A subscriber sends a message to the list host.

3. The list host sends a copy of the message to all subscribers.

obvious errors or requests mistakenly sent to the group instead of the software that manages the list. However, the messages are posted immediately. On lists that are moderated, the owner does not post obvious mistakes and can keep messages off the list that do not meet the list criteria, but there is usually a delay between when a message is sent and when it is posted to the group itself. A list that is moderated and edited may or may not be refereed but it will usually involve a longer time lag before a message sent to the group is posted for all to read.

Mailing lists can also be private or read-only. A private mailing list is one set up by a group that wishes to exchange information among its members, such as a class or organization. It can serve both as a communication tool and a forum for discussion of issues pertaining to that group. A read-only mailing list is intended only for the distribution of information to a fixed group. Subscribers cannot post messages to a read-only list.

Features
Most mailing list software offers many options for subscribers beyond just sending messages. For this reason, there are two addresses for each group. One manages the list, per-

forming such tasks as subscribing a new member or evoking any of the available options such as temporarily suspending mail from the group, and another address that is used *only* when one posts a message to the group. This information is included in the information that is sent to all new subscribers. Saving this information for use will prevent subscribers from having to ask the entire group how to accomplish a function such as unsubscribe. The message can be either printed or filed in a folder in the user's e-mail software.

Finding an Electronic Mailing List

There are many mailing lists; finding the right one is not always easy. One can always use a search tool, but using a Web site that has a list of current mailing lists is more efficient. Maintaining an up-to-date list of current mailing lists is not an easy job. It is not uncommon for a person to start a mailing list with good intentions, then become bogged down with the tasks associated with running a mailing list and consequently abandon it. One of these tasks is handling error messages that result when subscribers fail to read the welcome message and do not take their responsibilities seriously. Another difficulty is in generating messages and discussions on the list. The most successful mailing lists have an "owner," or a person who takes responsibility for the list, who carefully nurtures the list and seeds it with messages at the beginning, and in general is supportive of the other subscribers. When trying to subscribe to a list from one of the Web sites that catalogue mailing lists, if you find that a list does not exist, it is courteous to notify the owner of the listing Web site so the information shown there can be updated. Information on sites that feature lists of current mailing lists will be found on the Web page for this chapter at the book web site (http://connection.lww.com/go/thede) as will information about listserv etiquette.

Flame Wars

Messages sent to an electronic mailing list go to many people that the poster does not know. They will be read under many different conditions, by people in many different moods. Given these circumstances, it is not surprising that occasionally a member takes umbrage at what another says and posts an overheated message. A message of this sort, called a flame, can easily deteriorate into a **flame war** when others respond derogatorily with other positions on the disputed topic. In most groups, this ends on a conciliatory note when cooler heads prevail. Flame wars can happen in any group but tend to be more common in groups that discuss controversial topics.

Worldwide communication has opened a new chapter in interpersonal relations, one in which we are still learning to see our communications from many different points of view. Rereading all messages before sending and trying to imagine how they will look to others who do not share the same view or background goes a long way toward preventing flame wars. It also opens the door to a real understanding and a rich discussion.

THREADED MESSAGES

When messages are **threaded**, they are organized by the topic of the message. The first message for that topic starts the thread with other messages about the topic following. Often the number of other messages on this topic is in parentheses after the topic of the group. News groups and most forums have threaded messages. Because they arrive as individual messages, mailing lists are not threaded, but any archives of messages are. The threading concept works only when posters preserve the original subject, by either using the reply or reply all function, or placing the exact wording for the original subject on the subject line. It breaks down when posters use the reply function to start a new topic without changing the subject.

 ## Summary

The Internet provides a vast new medium of communication, both one-way and interactive, for use in all aspects of healthcare. For those who know how to search and evaluate Web documents, the WWW provides an encyclopedia in every Internet-connected computer. Online publishing, which is still in its infancy, offers timely newsletters as e-zines, and provides faster publication for articles in online journals because an article can be immediately posted rather than waiting for space in a print journal.

Some issues, however, remain to be solved. The lack of permanence for Web pages creates problems for those who wish to refer clients to a page, or for their use as references in a paper. At present most Internet resources are still free, with the expectation that either volunteers or advertisements will support them. The lack of success for advertising on the Internet may lead to charges being levied on more Internet information sources.

connection—◡ **For definitions of bolded key terms, visit the online glossary available at http://connection.lww.com/go/thede.**

CONSIDERATIONS AND EXERCISES

1. Which type of search tool would you select to find information on:
   a. Diabetes
   b. Home Healthcare Classification (a standardized nursing terminology)
2. Access your favorite search tool and enter the appropriate terms to find information about:
   a. Cancer in children
   b. Diabetes in pregnancy
   c. Hepatitis C
   d. Cirrhosis but not alcoholism
   e. Epilepsy and epileptics
3. Studies looking at the accuracy of health information on the Web find a great deal of inaccuracies, even from supposedly reliable resources. What implications does this have for information for consumers and practitioners?
4. Create your own tool for evaluating a resource for use as a resource in a formal paper. Exchange lists with a peer and test the peer's list with several documents. Work with the peer to revise both sets of criteria as necessary.
5. Find an example of a true nursing online journal and a nursing e-zine.
6. How do the Internet networking entities differ in how messages are received and posted?
   a. In your opinion, which format would best meet the needs of a support group in your specialty area?
   b. Give reasons for this choice.

REFERENCES

About health on the net foundation (1998.) Retrieved February 9, 2002 from
   http://www.hon.ch/Global/about_HON.html.

eHealth Ethics Initiative, Internet Healthcare Coalition. *eHealth code of ethics.* Retrieved February 13,
   2002 from http://www.ihealthcoalition.org/ethics/code0523.pdf.

Fallis, D. & Frické, M. (2002). Indicators of accuracy of consumer health information on the Internet:
   A study of indicators relating to information for managing fever in children in the home. *Journal of
   American Medical Informatics Association, 9*(1), 73–77.

Fleishman, G. (1995), Looking for the right Internet connection. *Info World, 17*(5), 51–52, 56, 58.

HONcode Principles (1997). Retrieved February 9, 2002 from
   http://www.hon.ch/HONcode/Conduct.html.

Impicciatore, P., Pandolfini, C., Casella N., & Bonati, M. (1997). Reliability of health information for
   the public on the World Wide Web: Systematic survey of advice on managing fever in children at
   home [electronic version]. *British Medical Journal, Clinical Research Edition, 314,* 1875–1879.
   Retrieved June 18, 2002 from http://www.bmj.com/cgi/content/full/314/7098/1875.

McClung, H. J., Murray, R. D., & Heitlinger, L. A. (1998). The Internet as a source for current patient
   information [electronic version]. *Pediatrics, 101*(6), e2. Retrieved June 18, 2002 from
   http://www.pediatrics.org/cgi/content/full/101/6/e2.

Oliver, D. (1996). *Netscape 3 unleashed.* Indianapolis, IN: Sams Net.

Risk, A., & Dzenowagis, J. (2001, March). Review of Internet Health Information Quality Initiatives.
   Journal of Internet Medical Research, 4(3). Retrieved January 6, 2002 from
   http://www.jmir.org/2001/4/e28/index.htm.

Schloman, B. (August 19, 1999). Needle in a haystack? Finding health information on the Web. *Online
   Journal of Issues in Nursing.* Retrieved June 18, 2002 from
   http://www.nursingworld.org/ojin/infocol/info_2.htm.

Schloman, B. (2001). Nursing faculty and scholarly publishing: Survey of perceptions and journal use.
   Online Journal of Issues in Nursing, 5(1). Retrieved February 10, 2002 from
   http//www.nursingworld.org/ojin/topic11/tpc11_8.htm.

Sparks, S. M., & Rizzolo, M. M. (1998). World Wide Web search tools. *Image, 30*(2), 167–171.

Sullivan, D. (2001). *How search engines work.* Retrieved February 4, 2002 from
   http://searchenginewatch.com/webmasters/work.html.

Timeline: PBS life on the internet. (1997). Retrieved February 10, 2002 from
   http://www2.pbs.org/internet/timeline/index.html.

University of California. Berkeley Library WWW (2001). *Recommended search strategy.* Retrieved
   February 3, 2002 from http://www.lib.berkeley.edu/TeachingLib/Guides/Internet/Strategies.html.

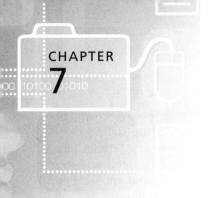
The Internet: The New Healthcare Paradigm

Objectives

After studying this chapter you will be able to:

1. *Describe consumer health informatics.*

2. *Identify uses of e-mail in healthcare.*

3. *Discuss the use of the Internet as support for clients.*

4. *List principles to be considered in a Web site.*

5. *Discuss principles that make a Web site accessible to those with disabilities.*

The growth of the use of computers in the United States is having an effect on how society manages information (CPS August 2000 Report, 2001). The percentage of U.S. homes that has a computer has gone from 8.2% in 1984 to 51% in 2000 (CPS August 2000 Report, 2001). With all likelihood, this number will continue to increase. The percentage of homes with access to the Internet grew from 18.8% in 1997 (the first year these statistics were collected) to 41% in the year 2000. Of homes with children, 65% have computers and 30% of the children in these homes use the Internet. Use does not differ by gender, but the group with the heaviest Internet use is in those aged 12 to 17 years, of whom 48% use the computer. The higher the education level, the higher the use levels are for the both the computer and the Internet. The figures for use of the computer by school children either at home or school is almost 90%. Nearly 25% of the U.S. population uses the Internet for information searches such as for health information.

Given the knowledge intensity of healthcare, it is not surprising to find that the computer and Internet have had a profound effect on healthcare. Changes are being seen in the roles and behaviors of both clients and healthcare professionals. Traditional healthcare relationships generally took place either face-to-face or by telephone. The provider had knowledge needed by the patient; the patient needed this knowledge and was expected to follow the orders issued by the provider. Today this relationship is being challenged both by patients, who now have access to information previously unavailable to them, and providers, who sense that there are benefits to be derived from a more collaborative relationship.

Consumer Health Informatics

In the push to reduce healthcare costs, many things have been tried: managed care, different types of insurance plans, reducing provider costs, and decreasing staffing. One group that has been consistently overlooked is the consumers themselves. Studies have found that consumers who have a better knowledge of their illness and treatment and support from others are able to use the healthcare system more effectively and are more apt to change their health-related behaviors (Gustafson, Hawkins, Boberg, Pingree, Serling, Graziano, et al. 2001).

Consumer health informatics is a new term that has been coined to describe patient-centered informatics. It is an applied science using concepts from health communication, education, social network theories, and behavioral sciences (Houston & Ehrenberger, 2001). The field encompasses consumers' participation in their healthcare using electronic technology, including viewing and entering information into their electronic medical records. One of its goals is to effect behavioral changes in clients as a result of information supplied to them using electronic means. Its origins can be found in the health communication literature that links patient education and self-help to better health outcomes.

Another aspect of consumer health informatics is the growing move to help consumers select healthcare the same way that they buy other goods; by seeking the best value. Driven by the need to curb costs and the desire of people to create their own health plans, several companies now provide this option. Consumers use the Web to view extensive information on doctors, hospitals, diseases, and treatments, including costs, and then create their own insurance plans. (Agovino, 2001). Employers who self-insure are also moving to make information of this kind available to their employees, as well as information about outcomes from various healthcare providers and agencies.

Empowered Client

A 1997 telephone survey found that 97% of adults who retrieve health information from the Internet believed that the Internet empowered them to make better choices (Miller & Reints as cited in Houston & Ehrenberger,2001). Empowerment in this context means an awareness of one's inherent abilities to be in control of one's healthcare. It has been found that consumers not only are willing to read scientific literature, but seek it out to learn about their conditions and various treatments. Sometimes consumers whose needs were not being met by their current providers have used these searches to find a provider whose specialty matched their needs.

As patients become empowered they expect more personal attention (Kaplan & Brennan, 2001). They desire the same services that the financial investment industry provides, namely personalized information that is targeted at them. Additionally, they expect to be full partners in their healthcare, not passive recipients.

These changes in patient expectations are creating further changes in the roles of healthcare providers. To meet these expectations, providers will need to relinquish the role of sole knowledge provider and accept the role of a partner in a collaborative relationship. Clients are coming to visits armed with information from the Web, sometimes information with which the provider may not be familiar. The provider must be ready to work with the client who has questionable information and be willing to discuss and, if need be, embrace alternative treatments from reputable sources.

ONLINE CLIENT HEALTHCARE RECORD

Until just recently, a person's healthcare record, whether in a hospital or clinic, was regarded as the property of the agency providing the care. Patients were not allowed to see their records; in fact, even providing patients with knowledge about their own body temperature was often regarded as improper. Today, however, patients are legally entitled to see their own medical records. Difficulties can arise because in most cases pieces of a person's life medical history are scattered in many different places. Unfortunately, the information in even one place may not be accurate or complete, as consumers who gain access to their healthcare records have found.

The Internet can provide a way to alleviate this situation. The first attempts at online health records involved the consumer's providing his or her own information (Bazzoli, 2000, May/June). Newer approaches are attempting to provide a collaboration between practitioners and consumers in creating and maintaining their health records. Some view this as a way to get consumers more involved in their healthcare and conscious of taking care of their health.

The practice of collaboration in a healthcare record, with both provider and consumer keeping copies, is still in its infancy, but as consumers take more control of their healthcare, it will grow. Whether it takes the form of a secure Internet record, or a smart card with pertinent information encoded in a magnetic strip, many advantages may be gained with a collaborative healthcare record. Having one's health information easily available will make it easier for patients who visit multiple providers to supply each one with an up-to-date record. This information will often be more than a referring provider currently sends (Landro, 2000). The presence of all an individual's health information in one easily accessible place will also provide safer care in the event of an emergency when regular records may not be available. Further, collaboration in the creation and maintenance of this online healthcare record between the provider and client will permit the provider to link information of interest to the client, thus providing more personalized care.

Currently, an online client healthcare record that delivers on its promises is still in its very formative stages. Kim & Johnson (2002) studied 11 online patient healthcare records identified through a Web search. They found that at a basic level these records provide Web-based access to personal medical information, but only a few provide the capacity for access to information in emergency situations, even though one of the benefits claimed for an online personal healthcare record is to provide this type of information. Many of these limitations directly derive from the data entry process, such as requiring clients to select entries from a list or type an entry with very little explanation. Overall, they found that in their current stage of development, patient healthcare records have limited functionality.

To make online healthcare records fully functional will require several things. If a record is to be useful, the information it contains must be correct. To ensure this, healthcare providers and clients will need to cooperate in creating these records. Few patients understand enough about medicine to be able to enter their own information correctly without some guidance. Additionally, fears about invasion of privacy must be addressed, both by the visibility of privacy policies and by penalties for violations of these policies.

E-MAIL COMMUNICATION WITH CLIENTS

The greatest use of the Internet is for e-mail, followed by a search for information. In a clinic survey, Kane and Sands (1998) found that 80% of primary care patients with access to the Internet wanted e-mail communication with their physician, and a growing number of clinicians and healthcare agencies are providing this service to their clients. Many reasons exist for using e-mail with clients. It is faster than regular mail, it requires less effort on the part of the sender, and it is asynchronous, freeing the individuals from a game of telephone tag (Pallen, 1995).

E-mail has been found useful in facilitating retention and clarification of information provided during visits (Kane & Sands, 1998). Patients who may be under stress during a visit often forget to ask important questions. Additionally, they often do not fully understand information provided about their self-care, or the need for further healthcare. When a patient is referred to other facilities, addresses and telephone numbers are easily included in e-mail, saving the patient from having to write them down or decipher someone else's handwriting. E-mail has also been found to increase compliance with immunizations. One study found that the use of computer program–generated e-mail or telephone messages to remind parents of the need for routine immunizations resulted in a higher rate of completion of the series of immunizations for children under 2 years (Dini, Linkins, & Sigafoos, 2001). Additionally, e-mail has been found to improve the visitation rates for well-child visits.

Kane & Sands (1998) believe that e-mail with clients should be characterized by a contractual relationship. They believe that before using e-mail with a client, clinicians should negotiate several issues such as how long the turnaround time will be, whether the e-mail will go through the office staff or be sent directly to the provider, what sort of content is permissible in the e-mail, and what compensation, if any, the provider will require for e-mail. Clients should also be instructed about any restrictions for e-mail, what content to place on a subject line, and to sign their full names to ensure accurate identification. Additionally, both patients and providers need to be aware that without encryption, their messages may be read by someone other than the intended recipients. Some consider that the discussion of these points with a client should be recorded in the health record and would even commit these points to writing, with one copy given to the patient and another placed in the record.

E-mail is not universally accepted by all providers. Concerns include privacy, time demands, liability, inappropriate use, and the continuing gulf between those patients who have access to e-mail and those who do not (Houston & Ehrenberger, 2001). One method of alleviating the time demands that e-mail can create is to develop a structured form that limits patient requests and facilitates a quick reply. Some healthcare agencies such as the Stanford Medical Group provide such a form on their Web site (Stanford Medical Group, 2002). It can be easily used for prescription renewals, referral requests, and follow up communication with the healthcare provider.

Use of the Internet for Support

Even in the earliest days of the Internet, clients sought online support to collect information and reach decisions (Houston & Ehrenberger, 2001). Today, using the interactivity of the Internet, healthcare providers can design consumer education that is tailored to the specific information needs of clients and their families. These same characteristics can also be used to provide support and education between and for professionals.

FORUMS

Forums are used by many Web sites to provide a place for an exchange of ideas. Forums are used by health-oriented Web sites to allow people to interact with others facing the same situation. One benefit of the environment of an online forum is that the discussions are **threaded**, allowing participants to read through the development of a topic in a linear manner. Some healthcare agencies provide Web sites that include tutorials and forums for their clients, with monitoring of the forums by a nurse or other healthcare professional. Examples include the well-researched CHESS (an acronym for Comprehensive Health Enhancement Support System) modules, which include private forums for consumers facing a common health crisis (https://chess.chsra.wisc.edu/Chess).

ELECTRONIC MAILING LISTS

Electronic mailing lists have also found several uses in healthcare: professionals supporting each other, professionals supporting clients, and clients supporting each other. Some of the benefits of professionals networking with other professionals are an exchange of care guidelines, formation of a different viewpoint on various aspects of care, finding new resources, and in general gaining new knowledge. When using this source of information, however, care must be taken in evaluating the message, both for content and the reputation of the poster. Some list posters do back up their statements with references; most do not. Never hesitate to ask a poster for textual references.

Electronic mailing lists are also used to provide support to clients. The Grief Net Support (http://griefnet.org/) organization that offers support to people who have endured the loss of a loved one maintains many lists, moderated by trained counselors. Their discussion groups are varied and oriented to the type of loss. They include, but are not limited to, support groups for those affected by terrorist attacks, widows or widowers, parents who have lost children, children who have suffered a loss, and those who are grieving the loss of a pet.

Electronic mailing lists to provide support when face-to-face contact in a group is unavailable, either because of time or distance constraints, has found many uses. One of the early support groups on the Internet was the Computerlink reported by Brennan (1994). This service not only provided networking among caregivers of patients with Alzheimer's disease but also allowed caregivers to leave questions for a nurse.

Electronic mailing lists have also been used in education, sometimes as part of a distance learning class and sometimes as an adjunct to a regular class. Gilbride, Breithaupt, and Hoehle (1996) used a listserv as an adjunct to the classroom. They found that students believed that the Internet helped them communicate with faculty and colleagues and that the discussions allowed them to connect classroom discussions to professional issues. Links to other support groups are included on the Web site for this book (http://connection.lww.com/go/thede).

SUPPORT GROUPS

One of the earliest uses of the Internet for support was the ComputerLink project (Brennan, 1996). This service provided support to those living at home with complex medical problems and their family caregivers. Users could access the service at a convenient time and select from a list of services. It was designed to link these people to each other and to a nurse moderator. Services were provided in three areas: communications, information, and decision support. Communication involved private e-mail, a forum where members could post and read messages, and a question-and-answer session. The information module provided an electronic encyclopedia and more than 200 indexed screens about selected illnesses, home care, and social services. In decision support, users were guided through an analysis process using their own words and preferences to make choices consistent with their values.

A similar service that provided computer-based support group for rural middle-aged women coping with a chronic disease was organized by a college of nursing (Cudney & Weinert, 2000). The program consisted of four components: conversation, direct access, health chat, and resources. Conversation permitted the participants to exchange feelings and ideas. Direct access to the other participants was provided in an e-mail format. The professionals in a health chat provided interactive discussions addressing women's health. The last component, the resource rack was a place for announcements and information such as telephone numbers for resources and information about additional sources of information.

Support groups may be a combination of a forum, e-mail, and a mailing list. Help given is similar to that received in face-to-face groups. Internet support has been used to work with those dealing with various conditions such as perinatal loss (DiMarco, Menke, & McNamara, 2001), disability issues (Finn 1999), menopause (Giordano, 1995), breast cancer (Sharf, 1997), alcoholism (Finfgeld, 2000), and chronic disease (Cudney & Weinert, 2000). An analysis of messages from one group found many positives for this type of support. Members of this group exchanged information, gave and sought encouragement and support, related personal experiences, gave thanks, and provided humor and prayer for each other (Klemm, Reppert, & Visich, 1998).

PROVIDING ACCESS TO RESOURCES

Another format for providing health information was adopted by a university medical center (Hern, Weitkamp, Haag, Trigg, & Guard, 1997). They created a site that provided access to many health-related resources, including the Arthritis Foundation and the National Stroke Foundation, as well as to full-text resources and literature databases. Then, working in partnership with many community groups including public libraries and other healthcare agencies, they provided public access points in the community. The site, NetWellness (http://www.netwellness.org/), is now sponsored by three university medical institutions.

Providing decision support as well as information is some of the aim of CHESS, the computer-based system developed by scientists from many specialties including decision sciences, information systems, and education that was mentioned earlier in this chapter (Gustafson, et al. 2001). This site contains, among many features, decision-support tools to assist clients to monitor their health status and risk behaviors. It also provides answers to questions, a library, information about relevant healthcare or community services, and personal stories of participants. Studies of this type of Web site have shown that they can help clients improve their quality of life and facilitate more efficient use of healthcare.

One hospital (Seper, 2002) provides online nurses 24 hours a day to dispense health tips, give medical referrals, and offer information about specific medications. Although nurses at this site will provide help to anyone, they are especially interested in working with teenagers who, they believe, will use anonymous online help instead of looking to chat rooms or other dubious sites for health-related information.

Not only is the Web being used to provide healthcare information, but organizations such as the American Medical Association and the Joint Commission on Accreditation of Healthcare Organizations are making sites available to allow consumers to comparison shop. Some of these sites offer comparisons of health plans; others help in finding a doctor. Still others provide comparison information about hospitals, nursing homes, and home care agencies. Information on disciplinary action against doctors is also available online. Access to most of these sites are free, but some charge a subscription fee.

CAUTIONS

When clients use the Internet for healthcare or information, they need to remember certain things. First, the information they get may be only an opinion; it may be an informed opinion, but it may not be. Unless they are very familiar with the reputation of the site sponsor and or the provider, clients should be careful giving their names, e-mail addresses, and especially their credit card numbers to Internet groups or Web sites. Additionally, clients should be advised that there are no overseers of Web content or policies. It may also be necessary to teach clients how to evaluate information they find on the Web (Martin & Youngren, 2000).

Other Uses of WWW Technology

The concept of hypertext in Web browsers has also been appropriated for use in private "Internets," or networks that are not available to the general public. There are two types—**intranets** and **extranets**.

INTRANETS

Intranets are networks that are accessed using a Web browser but are available only to users within a specific organization. They provide a cost-effective way to share information within agencies. Anyone in an organization who has struggled either to find the latest version of a procedure or to see that all who need updated information have it in their possession can appreciate an intranet. Intranets[1] can be extremely useful for storing documents that need frequent updating, such as procedures, clinical pathways, policies, and drug information. Because there is only one official copy of these items, all that is required to have current information accessible is to update the one document on the intranet.

An intranet may or may not be connected to the Internet. If it is connected, the contents of the intranet will be protected from the outside world by a firewall or encryption. Those within the institution, then, can access both the intranet and the Internet, but out-

---

[1] Internet, because it is a formal name, is always capitalized; intranet is not a formal name, thus should not be capitalized.

siders cannot access the information on the intranet. Intranets can also provide some of the same kinds of features provided on the Internet, such as e-mail, mailing lists, or news groups, although unless they are connected to the Internet, these features will be limited only to those on the intranet.

Like information on the Internet, information on an intranet is not limited to text. Graphics and multimedia files can also be made available this way. Digital video cameras can be used to record a procedure, then the file can be placed on the intranet giving users the ability to play it in slow motion, or to stop and start as necessary. This makes the intranet an ideal way to offer in-service continuing education programs and access to procedures. Preparing these documents does not need to be difficult. Although they often comprise a very large file, or one not really suited to the full Internet, all the major application programs (word processors, databases, spreadsheets, and presentation programs) convert documents to Web documents with a few mouse clicks. When preparing material for the intranet, thought should be given to adapting the material to take full advantage of browser capabilities.

Intranets of the future will provide more than a place to retrieve static information from HTML pages. Creating enterprise information systems that permit seamless transmission of highly important data throughout the entire agency requires powerful interfaces, which can be provided with standardized Web technology and standardized markup languages such as XML. Intranets will become interactive and permit not only the reporting of results and up-to-date information, but also the inputting of data for healthcare records.

EXTRANETS

An extranet is an extension of an intranet with added security features. It provides accessibility to the intranet to a specific group of outsiders. To access the extranet, a valid user name and password are needed. Besides offering the same services as an intranet, an extranet can be used by healthcare providers to access patient care information from outside of the institution. It can also be used to provide access to current patient data from patient monitors for authorized healthcare professionals who are not physically present in the hospital (Nenov & Klopp, 1996). As more and more information about clients finds its way into intranets and extranets, this will provide a venue for client access to their healthcare records as well as making it possible for clients to make appointments and perform other administrative tasks that now take up office staff time.

DIRECT CARE

In the early days of the Web, sites existed that allowed a provider to use information entered by a client to make a diagnosis and prescribe medicine. It was also possible to obtain a prescription drug by visiting one of these online physicians who theoretically evaluated the answers to a series of questions and made a decision without ever seeing a patient. Lawsuits and the threat of lawsuits have eliminated most of these, especially in the United States.

The Web is, however, being used to provide a second opinion. The patient first has his or her current physician send specified documents to the physicians at the site providing this service. An appropriate specialist is then identified, and a fee-based consultation over a secure server is arranged along with a follow-up consult a week later. The consulting physicians believe very strongly that one of the strengths of this program is involving the primary physician.

ONLINE PHARMACIES

If a person is going to use an online pharmacy to purchase drugs, there are some things he or she should know about the site. One of the most important is whether a registered pharmacist is available to answer questions. Users will also want to find out whether the site will accept their health insurance payments, whether the site runs on a secure server, and what the privacy policies of the site are.

World Wide Web Portals

A **portal** is by definition a Web site that offers a wide array of resources and services such as e-mail, forums, a search tool, and links to useful sites. It is the blending of all Internet tools into one useful service. Generally, a portal is targeted at a specific population such as professionals in a discipline, consumers with a particular condition, people looking for either general or specific health information, or shoppers looking for specific products, such as products needed to care for a baby. Currently many groups sponsor healthcare portals; some are commercial and some are nonprofit. Before recommending a site or portal to a client, it needs to be thoroughly evaluated. Because many portals depend on advertisements for support, special care needs to be taken to ensure that the information and links provided are complete and free from bias.

DEVELOPMENT OF A WEB SITE

Most healthcare agencies today have Web sites. The exact contents vary, but generally they provide information about the organization, often a map and directions to the physical agency, a list of the services offered, and other organizational information. Some healthcare agencies post healthcare information. Additionally, some hospitals with obstetric services feature a Web page that posts pictures of newborns that can be accessed by people the new parents specify.

Healthcare agencies may even develop a site specific to a given condition that functions more like an extranet; that is, access is restricted to only their clients. Organizations doing this need to develop very specific guidelines for their site (Prady, Norris, Lester, & Hoch, 2001), including that clients must have an understanding of the purpose of the site and its limitations. Privacy issues must be addressed for any data the site collects and any information that a client sends. Additionally, clients need to understand how to use the various parts of the site.

GENERAL DESIGN PRINCIPLES

There are two approaches to designing a Web page. The first uses an artistic approach, in which aesthetic sensibilities are primary. These are often designed by people schooled in print graphics, who often wish to emulate these effects on the Web. In the other, the Web designer sees the page as a way to assist a user to solve a problem (Nielsen, 1999). Although a pleasing design is helpful, sites that wish to successfully compete for viewers need to focus on users and their needs. Web users are an impatient lot; force them to cope with myriad decisions and much trial and error to find what they want and they will leave (Display 7-1).

Readability is another issue. A survey in 1992 by the U.S. Government revealed that about half of U.S. adults read at or below eighth-grade level (Smith, 2002). Providing information on the Web that is beyond the level of understanding of the intended readers is an expensive proposition. It not only discourages information seeking but damages self-efficacy. Several methods can be used to create a Web page, ranging from coding to use of an application program (Table 7-1).

ACCESSIBILITY FACTORS IN WEB DESIGN

The audience for healthcare Web sites includes not only people who are fully functional physically, but also those with disabilities. It is imperative, therefore, that healthcare Web sites be designed so that they are accessible by all. Worldwide, more than 750 million people are disabled in some way (Paciello, 2000). The 1997 U.S. Disability Census lists 52.6

Display 7-1 • THOUGHTS ON DESIGNING A WEB PAGE

A web page is an agency's front door to the world. Make it helpful.

Write down some answers to the following questions.

What is the purpose of the site?
Who is the intended audience?
What information should be shared? Is it copyrighted?
From a *user viewpoint*, what is the most intuitive organizational plan for the site? Try it out with someone outside the organization. Get feedback and change it.
Will it provide interactivity? If so:
    Who will respond to this?
    What features will be supported?
How will the site be publicized?

Use established Web conventions that are intuitive to users, such as blue underlined text for links.

The information
    Who will provide it?
    Who will approve it?
    Evaluate carefully for grammatical and spelling errors.
    Match the readability level to the audience.

Consider download time. Not everyone has unlimited Internet access.

Only use a graphic if it is small and/or contributes information necessary for understanding.
If graphics are used check to see how the page renders without them. Not all browsers have graphics capabilities, some users turn them off to shorten download time.
Keep file size as small as possible.

Think carefully before designing pages that require a user to have special plug-ins.

Is it necessary to make the content clear?
Is the user likely to have it?
Always include an URL that leads directly to a place for downloading the plug-in. Do not use the front page of the organization and leave users to hunt for it—they will not.

Consider maintenance of the site.

Who will maintain the site? Links are here today and gone tomorrow.
Who is responsible for what content?

Design a prototype and have outsiders test it without any input from anyone connected with designing the site to see whether its use is intuitive. Revise.

TABLE 7-1 ● *Comparison of Some Methods of Web Page Creation*		
Method	**Advantage**	**Disadvantage**
Office application program	Minimal knowledge required beyond use of the program itself.	Creates "dirty code" that is difficult to maintain outside the application program used to create it. Often creates a very large file. May not provide needed flexibility.
WYSIWYG (What You See Is What You Get) authoring tool	Fairly easy to use, but require some learning.	Some use non-standard code that requires special software on the server.
HTML editor	Provides good flexibility.	Steep learning curve
Coding HTML	Provides good flexibility.	Very steep learning curve

million people (19.7% of the population) as having one or more disabilities, with 33 million (12.3%) having severe disabilities (Americans With Disabilities, 1997). It is likely that the percentage of people with disabilities is even higher in the population of those who access healthcare Web sites.

Blindness and visual impairments are caused by many diseases and conditions including cataracts, cerebral palsy, diabetes, and glaucoma. Multiple sclerosis also often interferes with Web use. Many visually impaired users may use a screen reader, or a device that translates the screen text into voice. Screen readers read the text on each line of the screen from the far left to the far right regardless of any breaks. For example, if Table 7-1 were read by a screen reader, the following would be rendered when the first and second lines of that table are read:

> Office application program minimal knowledge required beyond creates dirty code that is difficult to use of the program itself maintain outside the application

Thus, users who employ a screen reader will find that a site using either a table or **frames** will have its text turned into gibberish. Because a screen reader does not "read" a **graphic**, when graphics are used, text alternatives (called *alt tags*) should be used. People who are colorblind may find it hard to distinguish between certain colors, whereas the hearing impaired may miss any audio. A dangerous feature is flickering items, which can cause seizures in people who are susceptible (Paciello, 2000).

Barriers to full use of the Web are experienced by those with physical or neurological disabilities who find it difficult to use a keyboard or mouse. Physical disabilities become more common as we age, making it imperative that healthcare Web sites be designed for all. The aim in Web design for people with some disability is, according to Demiris, Finkelstein, and Speedie (2001), to increase its functional accessibility. Those authors offer suggestions such as creating straightforward and clear Web pages and using icons and buttons that are simple, easy to understand, and large enough to not require precise dexterity for clicking. Other suggestions include the use of adequate contrast between text and background, intuitive navigation, avoidance of distracting features, and inclusion of users in the design phase. Additionally, and this should apply to all Web pages, the content should be written clearly and simply in language the users will understand.

The U.S. government has signaled its intention to encourage that Web sites be accessible by employees with disabilities with the passage of the Rehabilitation Act Amendments of 1998. Section 508 of that Act requires that when federal agencies develop or procure electronic and information technology, this technology be as accessible to Federal employees with disabilities as to those without disabilities (Electronic and Information Technology Accessibility Standards, 2000). It also requires that government sites that provide information to the public ensure this same accessibility.

Guides for making Web pages available to those with some disabilities are easily available on the Web. The World Wide Web organization and several other groups offer online information to make this job easier. Several of these sites provide a service that will check a Web page for accessibility errors and conditions. This book's Web page (http://connection.lww.com/go/thede) for this chapter contains the URLs of some of these groups.

Web design alone may not meet the needs of the disabled for Web access. There are also devices that can assist those with disabilities to use the Web. Providing clients with information about methods for overcoming limitations often becomes the nurse's responsibility. Specially designed keyboards can make Web and computer access easier for the physically disabled, whereas screen readers for those with visual difficulties will make computer use easier.

ELECTRONIC RÉSUMÉS

A growing number of agencies are using electronic databases to store, compare, and retrieve résumés of prospective employees (Puetz, 1997). These work much like bibliographic databases. The potential employer enters specific criteria and retrieves the résumés of those who meet the criteria. A résumé prepared for an electronic database needs to be prepared somewhat differently than a traditional résumé. The writer needs to include at the top a section for keywords and include terms that specify their discipline, credentials, specialties, and anything that makes the writer stand out such as special abilities with language or publications of articles and books. Format and style are also different. Because these résumés are stored electronically in a manner that eliminates many formatting options, bold facing and capital letters should be used for emphasis instead of different fonts and graphics.

 ## Summary

Consumer health informatics through the use of Internet technology is changing the role of both the consumers and providers of healthcare. Partnerships that take advantage of the ability to direct patients to pertinent information, information generated specific to a client's concerns, and the ability for a client to contact providers using e-mail or Web portals have the potential to improve the general health. The effectiveness of computer-generated health behavior interventions has been shown through many studies (Revere & Dunbar, 2001). The Internet and Web also provide the ability for professionals to offer support to various groups of clients and for clients to interact with one another.

These roles will require different skill sets, and for some, a willingness to give up older roles. Providers will find it helpful to be aware of the Internet activities in which their clients engage. They may want to monitor some of these, not as a traffic policeman, but to stay informed about the information that a client is receiving.

Many healthcare agencies already have and will continue to develop Web portals. The people responsible for the design of these pages need to become familiar with and employ design methods that promote accessibility to the information for those with disabilities. Nurses should become familiar with the devices that can make Web and computer access possible for those who need them.

connection—⁀ For definitions of bolded key terms, visit the online glossary available at http://connection.lww.com/go/thede.

CONSIDERATIONS AND EXERCISES

1. Given the statistics on computer and Internet use by the U.S. population, on which group would you concentrate the most effort in developing Web pages?

2. Describe an application of consumer health informatics.

3. List ways a nurse could use e-mail in working with clients.

4. Describe a use for an Internet support group in your practice (or in the area you might practice after you graduate).

5. Plan a Web site for a health topic.

6. Turn off the image loading in your browser. Look at some of the following pages as well as some of your favorite Web pages. At each site go down several levels. What recommendations would you make to the Web site builder for making the site more useful to those with visual disabilities? (Directions for turning off the image loading for a browser can be found at the Web site for this chapter (http://connection.lww.com/go/thede). Don't forget to turn it back on when you are through.)

   a. Welcome to the Internet Healthcare Coalitions: http://www.ihealthcoalition.org/
   b. Criteria for Assessing the Quality of Health Information on the Internet—Policy Paper: http://hitiweb.mitretek.org/docs/policy.html.
   c. Travel: http://www.orbitz.com/

7. Locate a Web page that offers health information. Copy the URL (see instructions on Web for chapter 6), access Bobby World Wide (http://www.cast.org/bobby/) and enter the URL to check for Web accessibility. Try this with several different health pages. What are the results?

REFERENCES

Agovino, T. (2001, December 10). New health plans leave decisions to consumers. *Cleveland Plain Dealer,* p. C4.

Americans with disabilities. (1997). Retrieved December 24, 2001 from http://www.census.gov/hhes/www/disable/sipp/disab97/asc97.html.

Bazzoli, F. (2000, May/June). Putting patients at the center. *Internet Health Care Magazine,* 42-43, 46–48, 50–51.

Brennan, P. F. (1996). The future of clinical communication in an electronic environment. *Holistic Nursing Practice, 11*(1), 97–104.

Brennan, P. F. (1994). Computerlink: An innovation in home care nursing. In S. Grobe & E. S. P. Pluyter-Wenting (Eds.) *Nursing informatics: An international overview for nursing in a technological era: Proceedings of the Fifth IMIA international conference on nursing use of computers and information science, San Antonio, TX, June 1994* (p. 407). Amsterdam: Elsevier.

Cudney, S. A., & Weinert, C. (2000). Computer-based support groups: Nursing in cyberspace. *Computers in Nursing, 18*(1), 35–43.

Demiris, G., Finkelstein, S. M., & Speedie, S. M. (2001). Considerations for the design of a web-based clinical monitoring and educational system for elderly patients. *Journal of the American Medical Informatics Association, 8*(5), 468–472.

DiMarco, M. A., Menke E. M., & McNamara T. (2001). Evaluating a support group for perinatal loss. *MCN: American Journal of Maternal/Child Nursing 26*(3), 135–40, 160–161.

Dini, E. F., Linkins, R. W., & Sigafoos, J. (2001). The impact of computer-generated messages on childhood immunization coverage. In R. Haux & C. Kulikowski (Eds.) *Yearbook of medical informatics: Digital libraries and medicine 2001* (pp. 210–217). International Medical Informatics Association.

Electronic and Information Technology Accessibility Standards. (2000). Retrieved February 14, 2002 from http://www.access-board.gov/sec508/508standards.htm.

Finfgeld, D. E. (2000). Resolving alcohol problems using an online self-help approach: Moderation management. *Journal of Psychosocial Nursing and Mental Health Services, 38*(2), 33–3, 48–49.

Finn, J. (1999). An exploration of helping processes in an online self-help group focusing on issues of disability. *Health and Social Work, 24*(3), 220–231.

Gilbride, D., Breithaupt, B. & Hoehle, R. (1996). The use of the Internet to support both on- and off-campus learners in rehabilitation education. *Rehabilitation Education, 10*(1), 47–62.

Giordano N. A. (1995). *An investigation of the health concerns of the menopause discussion group on Internet.* Columbia University Teachers College. Abstract obtained from CINAHL.

Gustafson, D. H., Hawkins, R., Boberg,E., Pingree, S., Serling, R. E., Graziano, F., & Chan, C. L. (2001). Impact of patient-centered, computer-based health information/support system. In R. Haux & C. Kulikowski (Eds.) *Yearbook of medical informatics: Digital libraries and medicine 2001* (pp. 224–232). International Medical Informatics Association.

Hern, M., Weitkamp, T., Haag, D., Trigg, J., & Guard J. R.(1997). Nursing the community in cyberspace. *Computers in Nursing, 15*(6), 316–321.

CPS August 2000 Report (2001). *Home computers and Internet use in the United States August 2000.* Retrieved February 13, 2002 from http://www.census.gov/population/www/socdemo/computer.html.

Houston, T. K., & Ehrenberger, H. E. (2001). The potential of consumer health informatics. *Seminars in Oncology Nursing, 17*(1), 41–47.

Kane, B., & Sands, D. Z. (1998). Guidelines for the clinical use of electronic mail with patients [Electronic Version]. *Journal of the American Medical Informatics Association, 5,* 104–111 (1998).

Kaplan, B., Brennan, P. F. (2001). Consumer informatics supporting patients as co-producers of quality. *Journal of the American Medical Informatics Association, 8*(4), 309–316.

Kim, M. J., & Johnson, K. B. (2002). Personal health records: Evaluation of functionality and utility. *Journal of the American Medical Association, 9*(2), 171–180.

Klemm, P., Reppert, K., & Visich, L. (1998). A nontraditional cancer support group. *Computers in Nursing, 16*(1), 31–36.

Landro, L. (2000, May 26). Tools that can help you keep your own accurate medical files. *Wall Street Journal,* B2.

Martin, S. D., & Youngren, K. B. (2000). The virtual community: Helping patients use Internet support groups. *Home Healthcare Nurse, 18*(5), 333–335.

May, S. (2002, February). *Healthcare Informatics, 44,* 48.

Miller, T. E. & Reints, S. (1998). *The health care industry in transition: The online mandate to change.* New York, NY: Cyber Dialogue, Inc.

Nenov, V. & Klopp, J. R. (1996). Remote access to neurosurgical ICU physiological data using the World Wide Web. In S. J. Weghorst, H. B. Sieburg, & K. Morgan (Eds.), *Studies in health technology and informatics* (pp. 242–249). Amsterdam: IOS Press in conjunction with Ohmsha, Ltd.

Nielsen, J. (1999). *Designing web usability.* Indianapolis, IN: New Riders Publishing.

Paciello, M.G. (2000). Web accessibility for people with disabilities. Berkeley, CA: Publishers Group West.

Pallen, M. (1995). Guide to the Internet: Electronic mail [electronic version]. *British Medical Journal 311,* 1487–1490.

Prady, S. L., Norris, D., Lester, J. E., & Hoch, D. B. (2001). Expanding the guidelines for electronic communication with patients: Application to a specific tool. *Journal of the American Medical Informatics Association, 8,* 44–348.

Puetz, B. E. (1997, February). Résumé writing in a wired age. *RN 60*(2), 28–31.

Revere, D., & Dunbar, P. J. (2001). Review of computer-generated outpatient health behavior. *Journal of the American Medical Informatics Association, 8*(1), 62–79.

Seper, C. (2002, February 2). Nurses online 24-7 at MetroHealth site. *Cleveland Plain Dealer,* C1;C3.

Sharf B. F. (1997). Communicating breast cancer on-line: support and empowerment on the Internet. *Women & Health, 26*(1), 65–84.

Smith, S. (2002). *Readability testing health information.* Retrieved March 17, 2002 from http://www.prenataled.com/story9.htm.

Stanford Medical Group. (2002). *Electronic mail services.* Retrieved February 13, 2002 from http://www-med.stanford.edu/shs/smg/email.html.

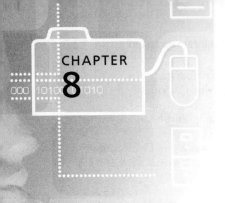

Telehealth:
Now and in the Future

Objectives

After studying this chapter you will be able to:

1. Define the two overall classifications of technology used in telehealth.

2. Discuss some ways that telehealth can deliver healthcare.

3. Illustrate opportunities for autonomous nursing practice in telehealth.

4. Discuss the main issues in implementing telehealth.

5. Analyze ways that telehealth could affect the present healthcare system.

During the 1998 Around the World Alone sailboat race, one of the racers, while in the South Atlantic, developed an abscess on his elbow that could have caused him to lose his arm. Using a wireless computer and satellite technology, he was put in touch with a doctor in Boston who directed his treatment thereby saving the arm. Not all **telehealth** applications are this dramatic, but this incident demonstrates the power of this new vehicle for delivering healthcare. Although much attention has been given to this aspect of telehealth (that is, the delivery of acute care or specialist consultations), telehealth has been shown to be far more versatile than previously thought. It can be used to provide home telenursing, electronic referrals to specialists and hospitals, teleconsulting between specialists and general practitioners or nurse practitioners, minor injury consulting, and as a call center (Wootton, 2001).

Terms such as telehealth or **telemedicine** have in the past have been used interchangeably to refer to health services delivered using electronic technology to patients at a distance. Given the wide breadth of services that can be provided for such clients, the term telehealth is more appropriate. The American Nurses Association (ANA) considers telehealth the umbrella term that encompasses telemedicine as well as telenursing and other applications. In its 1997 Report to Congress, the Office for the Advancement of Telehealth in concert with the Joint Working Group on Telemedicine defined telemedicine as the delivery of clinical services to patients in a geographical location separate from that of the provider and reserved the term telehealth to denote other applications for the use of telecommunications to promote healthcare

(Office for the Advancement of Telehealth & The Joint Working Group on Telemedicine, 2001). Officially, telehealth is defined as using electronic communications for transmitting healthcare information such as health promotion, disease prevention, professional or lay education, diagnosis, or actual treatments to people located at a different geographical location.

 ## Technology Classification

As the example of the sailor in the around-the-world race showed, the technology for delivering telemedicine does not have to be sophisticated. It would be hoped, however, that most cases would not involve self-treatment. Generally, there are two types of technology for delivering telehealth: store-and-forward technology and real-time technology that permits two-way communication. The boundary between these two modes is becoming less and less distinct, with many services using both types of communication

STORE-AND-FORWARD TECHNOLOGY

In store-and forward-technology, an image is captured electronically either by a digital camera, scanner, or other technology (e.g., x-ray machine) that generates electronic images which are then sent to a specialist for interpretation at a later time. The images may be still or have motion. Radiology, dermatology, and pathology are specialties that lend themselves very well to this technique, as does the interpretation of any test that creates an image that can be transmitted such as an electrocardiogram or MRI. Often this type of communication is from one practitioner to another. For remote communities such as those in Alaska, this method offers the only affordable way that medicine can be practiced (Puskin, 2001). This methodology is similar to having a mammogram that is read by a radiologist at a later date, except the patient has the radiograph done in a different location from where the radiologist is when he or she reads it.

REAL-TIME TECHNOLOGY

Real-time telehealth allows the patient and the provider to interact at the same time. Many telecommunications devices that permit two-way communication are used to provide real-time telehealth. The oldest of these is the telephone, but current telehealth technology generally includes two-way video and audio. Although this is possible with a modem and **plain old telephone service (POTS)**, often a higher quality of service is desired. The level of service that is needed depends on the type of services that will be offered. Often the service will require at least a T1 line or line on an integrated services digital network (**ISDN**), which must not only connect the sites but extend to the separate rooms where both the patient and the distant consultant are located. Large satellite systems that have a global audience are also used in telehealth. In short, any two-way communication technology offering both audio and video has, or will find, a use in telehealth.

Real-time telehealth also makes use of special instruments that can transmit an image to a clinician at a different location These include an ear-nose-throat scope, a camera that captures skin observations, and a special stethoscope. They can be used either in real-time or in store-and-forward mode. In addition, using a combination of robotics and virtual reality, a surgeon with special gloves and the appropriate audio and video technology is able to actually perform surgery by manipulating surgical instruments at the remote site. This procedure is known as **telepresence** and is another subset of telehealth. It is still in development and requires a 100% reliable system and a very high bandwidth but will eventually take its place in telehealth.

Some Telehealth Examples

As healthcare moves away from the hospital and into the home and community, and a much broader range of healthcare professionals (e.g., nutritionists, social workers, and home healthcare aides) is seen as a recognized part of healthcare, the therapeutic uses for telehealth will become greater. One problem about telehealth is that many third party insurance payers continue to focus primarily on acute medical care (Jones, 1997). The outcome is that many people remain underserved, with the result that illnesses that could be treated in their early stages progress to a stage at which they become very costly to treat.

HOME HEALTHCARE

One program in rural Kansas used interactive television to provide care for the elderly and disabled. This project used nurses to "visit" the patients at regularly scheduled times during the week (Lindberg, 1997). The system provided full interactive video and audio between the elderly clients in their home and the telehealth nurse. The nurse could view and enter patient data in an electronic record as well as monitor blood pressure, mental health status, diet, hygiene, and diabetic complications. When an intervention required the physical presence of a nurse, either the telehealth nurse or a home health nurse made the visit.

This project enjoyed many successes. In one case, the attention from the telehealth nurse stopped the recurrent hospitalizations of a 65-year-old with diabetes, high blood pressure, bipolar disorder, and manic-depressive disorder (Lindberg, 1997). In another, the nurse helped a 70-year-old with laryngeal cancer whose larynx had been removed and who postoperatively developed aggressive behavior problems. The "visits" by the nurse reminding him to take his medications allowed him to stay in his apartment and not be transferred to a nursing home. In still another case, a 71-year-old with multiple conditions had required a home health aide to dress and groom him before the televisits. When the television visits became regular, he started getting up every morning and dressing and grooming himself because he was going to be "on television." Projects such as this one demonstrate that telehealth has a great potential not only to improve the quality of life for many elderly people with chronic conditions, but to do so at far lower cost than providing only acute episodic care.

University Health System in Eastern North Carolina, which comprises the Brody School of Medicine at East Carolina University, a private hospital, Pitt Memorial, and University Home Care, offers a program called TeleHomecare. The program, which began in 1997 under a grant, is now part of the regular home care services provided to their clients (Personal communication, R. Saiid, 2002). Using **POTS**, telehome visits in this program include not only education but aspects of physical assessment including heart auscultation, pulse oximetry, and glucose monitoring (Figure 8-1). At the beginning of the service, a visit is made by a nurse who sets up the equipment and teaches the patient and a family member (if applicable) how to use it. From the beginning, this program has targeted its services to patients who had multiple hospital admissions for problems that

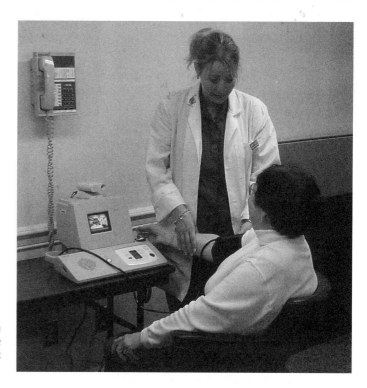

Figure 8-1 • Nurse instructing patient on use of home monitoring equipment. Picture courtesy of University Health System, East Carolina University.

could have been managed at home. Subsequent evaluations have shown that this program has decreased the need for hospital admissions and emergency department visits for these home care patients. Additionally, client acceptance has been high. The program enhances the care clients receive by providing interaction between client and nurse beyond regular clinic visits. Any client qualifies for this service as long as he or she does not need hands-on care. Nurses in this program treat those who have chronic conditions such as diabetes, hypertension, congestive heart failure, renal disease, infant apnea, and even preterm labor. It is sometimes used along with hospice care. The program has been recognized both nationally and internationally as a leader in telehome care.

A 4-year project funded by the Centers for Medicare and Medicaid Services (CMS) at Columbia University may again demonstrate the contributions of this cost-effective way of delivering healthcare. This project is evaluating the feasibility of using telemedicine to manage diabetes in the elderly (Shea, Starren, Weinstock, Knudsen, Teresi, Homes, et al., 2002). Participants in this project receive a home telemedicine unit for synchronous videoconferencing with a nurse and the electronic transmission of home finger-stick glucose readings and blood pressure data. They are also provided access to a project Web site. This project has a built-in research plan to evaluate not only cost-effectiveness but the acceptability of using telehealth in this capacity.

CLINIC VISITS

Other uses for telehealth are found in rural areas where residents traditionally have few options for healthcare, and few, if any, specialists. An example is the University Health System program which serves the rural area of eastern North Carolina (Balch & Tichenor, 1997). This program makes specialty medical consultations available to rural hospitals, clinics, and even prison clinics. A nurse in the distant location presents the patient to the specialist at the hub site, who interacts with the patient in much the same manner as he or she would in a face-to-face meeting. This group has also worked with school systems to offer not only consultations from nurses and other healthcare professionals but also health education classes regarding chronic diseases and other health topics (About telehealth project, 2002).

In another example, a nurse working in a tertiary-care hospital-based telemedicine center arranged specialty consultations for patients in smaller hospitals (Schlachta-Fairchild, 2001). In this system, patients did not have to travel to a large hospital but could go to the local hospital's telemedicine office and be connected with a specialist in a tertiary hospital. The nurse in this project served in a multitude of roles, including patient educator, staff educator, coordinator, and physician support resource.

TELENURSING

Telenursing as part of telehealth is not new. The project just described occurred more than 25 years ago and demonstrates well the use of nurses in telehealth. As can be seen in this and other examples, nurses play an important role in telehealth, often being managers of programs or lead coordinators (Puskin, 2001). Telehealth also offers a greater opportunity to provide preventive services, which are well within the purview of nursing. Examples of services that nurses have provided using telehealth include assistance in the bonding process of mothers and infants separated by distance, management of high-risk obstetrical patients, and rehabilitation of patients with spinal cord injury.

Telenursing offers nurses a chance to create more collaborative and autonomous roles and at the same time reduce the overall cost of healthcare. One example of this was demonstrated in a study in the United Kingdom that confirmed the potential value that telephone consultation with nurses had in reducing healthcare costs by reducing emergency admissions to the hospital (Lattimer, Sassi, George, Turnbull, Mullee, & Smith, 2000). Today, telenurses work in home care agencies, hospices, hospital-based telemedicine centers, managed care centers, disease management, rehabilitation centers, and all branches of the military (Schlachta-Fairchild, 2001).

EDUCATION

Most telehealth projects have a built-in educational component. In some, education is delivered during the "visits;" in others, through Web pages. Telehealth is also useful in the educational needs of healthcare professionals, not only for continuing education, but also for preparing practitioners. Clinical experiences for nurse practitioner and primary physician students, which often involves much driving time for instructors, have been shown to benefit from telehealth. One such application used both store-and-forward and real-time technology for providing clinical education. Store-and-forward methods were used to review student case presentations, whereas an ear-nose-throat scope, video camera, and high-quality stethoscope were incorporated into real-time use for evaluating student assessments, differential diagnoses, and management of some chronic problems (Chang & Trelease, 2001). Both faculty and student responses were generally positive, with over half of the students evaluating the technology as having enhanced their learning and retention a great deal. Faculty particularly expressed interest in using the technology for classroom presentations.

DISASTER HEALTHCARE

Telehealth has been used successfully in providing healthcare in disasters (Garshnek & Burkle, 1999). In 1985, the National Aeronautics and Space Administration (NASA) used satellite communication to furnish aid to people in Mexico City after the earthquake had devastated that area. Satellite communication was also used in 1988 after the Armenian earthquake to provide two-way interactive audio and unidirectional full-motion transmissions from several Armenian hospitals to four U.S. medical centers. This type of technology also provided consultations for casualties of small arms fire during the attempted Russian coup in 1993. These last two projects provided the groundwork for a project using a Web browser to create a relational database for consultation with Russia on clinical case records. As might be expected, the military has taken the lead in demonstrating many uses for telehealth including not only the war time disasters, but also delivery of humanitarian aide and hurricane relief.

 Issues

Telehealth in its various forms can provide many benefits such as enhanced patient care, reduced travel time, increased productivity, access to specialists, and enlarged educational opportunities for all. Many concerns, however, center on this mode of healthcare delivery. The 2001 Report to Congress on Telehealth by the Office for the Advancement of Telehealth and The Joint Working Group on Telemedicine listed five: lack of third-party reimbursement, legal issues, safety standards, data security, and the telecommunications infrastructure (The Office for the Advancement of Telehealth & The Joint Working Group on Telemedicine, 2001).

REIMBURSEMENT

Reimbursement remains a large barrier to the widespread adoption of telehealth. Most of the examples in this chapter were supported with grants and, despite successes, were discontinued when the grant expired. Our healthcare system today is shaped by third-party payers, both government and private. Any service for which Medicare does not pay will lag in development. Before passage of the 1997 Balanced Budget Act (BBA), Medicare recognized only very limited aspects of telehealth. This act shifted the debate from the question of whether payment ought be made at all to how it ought be paid (Puskin, 2001). Before passage of this act, telehealth reimbursement services were limited by very restricted eligibility criteria that did not reflect actual telehealth practice.

Although this act was an important first step, the policies under the BBA as interpreted by Center for Medicare and Medicaid Services (CMS), formerly the Health Care Financing Administration (HCFA), were still very limited. They required the patient to be present during a consultation, thus greatly limiting the use of store-and-forward technology. Reimbursement was limited to those practitioners who were eligible for payment under Medicare. Most cases also required the referring practitioner to be present during the consultation. In practice, however, nurses usually present the patient. Fee splitting was another issue that limited the practice. Under the prior rules, the referring practitioner received 25% of the fee and the consultant 75%, a fee that was unacceptable to the consultant. Additionally, services were limited to federally designated rural areas known as Health Professional Shortage Areas (HPSAs). Many rural areas have a sufficient number of primary care providers but lack specialists. Additionally, despite adequate healthcare services, many inner city residents often lack access to healthcare resources as a result of poverty, poor public transportation, and personal debility.

Some of these issues have been addressed with the passage of the Medicare, Medicaid, and State Children's Health Insurance Program (SCHIP) Benefits Improvement Act of 2000 (BIPA), which became effective October 1, 2001 (Puskin, 2001). The services that are eligible have been enlarged and fee-sharing has been eliminated, as has the requirement that the referring practitioner be present during a consultation. The new act clarified that home healthcare agencies, which are paid under a prospective payment system in which the agencies are paid a fixed amount per provision of home health services, may use their prospective payment money for telehealth visits. However, under this act, telehealth encounters still do not meet the definition for a Medicare home visit. (Office for the Advancement of Telehealth & The Joint Working Group on Telemedicine, 2001). This act requires that within 2 years after enactment of this legislation, the Secretary of the Department of Health and Human Services (DHHS) conduct a study to identify additional services and locations for which reimbursement should be permitted, and additional practitioners who should be reimbursed (Puskin, 2001).

Although it seems obvious that telehome visits save money, the current Federal policies may not be enough to encourage greater use of telehealth. Sadly, there have been few statistically significant studies demonstrating a cost savings (Office for the Advancement of Telehealth & The Joint Working Group on Telemedicine, 2001). This may be due to the small number of telehealth consultations in a specialty or the lack of a standard evaluation for studying telehealth efficacy. Also affecting the spread of telehealth is that any savings in money accrue to the payer, not the agency providing the care. Unless the treating agency is part of a managed-care plan, there is no great motivation for expanding these services. Still, the few studies do indicate cost savings, and some evidence indicates that private insurers are recognizing this and providing more coverage than was previously documented (Puskin, 2001).

LEGAL ISSUES

The Tenth Amendment to the U.S. Constitution guarantees to the states those powers not delegated to the United States nor prohibited by it to the states. Under this amendment, states have assumed the power to regulate healthcare practitioners for the protection of their citizens. No state, however, has authority over practice in another state. Transport nursing and telehealth both create problems with these assumptions. If a nurse practicing and licensed in State A provides nursing care to a client in State B in which the nurse is not licensed, which state has the responsibility and authority to regulate the practice? Given the litigious nature of U.S. society today, it is interesting that at this point there have been no reported lawsuits in which interstate telehealth practice was a critical factor (Hutcherson, 2001). This may be due to the fact that present and past telehealth practices have been high-quality programs that carefully monitored intervention outcomes and resulted in a high degree of patient satisfaction.

The various state boards involved in regulating healthcare practitioners have all been wrestling with the various questions in this issue. Is the care provided at the location of the provider or the patient? Should the healthcare provider be licensed in both the state where the patient resides *and* where the provider is located? The medical community appears split on this issue, with the Federation of State Medical Boards adopting a model act based on where the patient resides and the American Medical Association wanting to continue the present system in which a practitioner must be licensed in all states in which he or she practices (Gaffney, 1999). This latter view is shared by the American College of Radiology and the American Physical Therapy Association.

The National Council of State Boards of Nursing (NCSBN) in 1997 proposed a mutual recognition model referred to as the Nurse Licensure Compact that would be implemented through interstate compacts. Under this concept, nurses holding a valid license in one state could practice in another state that had implemented the compact, provided the nurse followed the laws and regulations of the state nurse practice act in the locality in which the patient was located. This is similar to a driving license in which one is licensed in one's state of residence but may drive in another state. While driving in the second state, however, the driver must follow the laws of that state. As of October, 2002, 18 states have approved this compact, although North Dakota's law will not be implemented until sometime in 2003 or 2004 (NCSBN, 2001). The Nurse Licensure Compact also calls for a Coordinated Licensure Information System that contains personal, licensure, and disciplinary information. Currently, the NCSBN maintains a disciplinary database to which a number of states contribute (Gaffney, 1999). The compact at this time applies only to registered nurses, although the NCSBN has developed a model for advanced practice nurses.

One question that has not been settled is whether telehealth practiced over state lines is actually interstate commerce and thus able to be regulated by federal statutes. Under the U.S. Constitution, the provision of services across state lines is interstate commerce and within the jurisdiction of the federal government. There is a precedent for federal involvement when it is determined that the best interests of the patient are threatened by disparity in state standards for healthcare. For example, the Clinical Laboratories Improvement Act (CLIA) authorizes CMS to regulate all clinical laboratories across the country and the Mammography Quality Standards Act (MQSA) requires all mammography facilities in the United States to meet stringent quality standards and to be inspected annually by an Food and Drug Administration–approved accreditation body (Hutcherson, 2001). It is likely that in the future this approach will be applied to some type of national licensing for healthcare providers. Given the many stakeholders and legitimate issues on both sides, expect to this to be a lengthy debate.

SAFETY STANDARDS

A concern with all new applications of technology in healthcare is the safety of the patient. All the projects discussed thus far in this chapter have been of a very high quality with no compromise in patient safety. A persistent question in this area is whether there is a need for certification or additional credentialing for those engaged in telehealth practice. If there is a need, is it for validation of competencies related only to the equipment or also to the clinical care delivered through this new medium (Certification in Telehealth: Should We Do It?, 1999). Whether these questions stem from financial, quality, or safety concerns is problematical. A task force from the Office for the Advancement of Telehealth (OAT) issued a report in 1999 that raised a number of issues that needed to be considered before establishing any certification process. Hutcherson (1999) points out that healthcare workers are quite adept at adapting to new technology and tools, having experienced the introduction of many in the past century, and that there is consensus among the healthcare community that current professional licensure is adequate for telehealth (Hutcherson, 2001).

Concerned with safety and standards of practice in telehealth, the ANA has published three monographs on telehealth. The *Core principles on telehealth,* published in 1998, addresses telehealth as a whole (Chaffee, 1999). Many of these principles focus on standards that ensure patient safety and legal practice. They also call for development of clinical telehealth guidelines. In 1999, nurses representing many associations, federal agencies, universities, and the armed services collaborated to develop 11 competencies for nurses involved in telehealth, which the ANA published as *Competencies for telehealth* (ANA, 1999). The specific performance criteria for each competency statement were left to nursing organizations and individual facilities to develop. The third publication, *Developing telehealth protocols: A blueprint for success*, is a checklist for use in the design of effective telehealth systems. It was published in 2001 and is a collaboration between the ANA, the Office for the Advancement of Telehealth, and the Joint Working Group on Telemedicine.

In an endeavor to set standards in telenursing, the American Academy of Ambulatory Care Nursing in 2001 published *Telehealth nursing practice administration and practice standards,* which addresses nine standards for telenursing including staffing, competency, ethics, patient rights, and the use of the nursing process in telehealth (American Academy of Ambulatory Care Nursing, 2001). They followed this with publication of the *Telephone nursing practice core course manual.* Additionally, the American Telemedicine Association and the American Psychological Association have created clinical guidelines (Office for the Advancement of Telehealth and The Joint Working Group on Telemedicine, 2001).

DATA SECURITY

Telehealth requires electronic health records, which leaves telehealth susceptible to all the privacy, confidentiality, and security issues surrounding electronic health records. Additionally, there are other considerations in telehealth. The OAT together with the DHHS Office of the Assistant Secretary for Planning and Evaluation are studying the privacy concerns unique to telehealth (Kumekawa, 2001). These issues include the presence of nonclinical technical personnel during a consultation and observation of the teleconsultation by clinical personnel not visible to the patient. There is also a need to provide security during transmission of data. Any of these issues can present problems complying with the Health Insurance Portability and Accountability Act.

TELECOMMUNICATIONS INFRASTRUCTURE

Telecommunications infrastructure costs represent a large percentage of the overall costs in many telemedicine budgets. This is especially true in rural areas where transmission costs are higher than in urban areas and most access is by POTS. To help reduce the costs, the Telecommunications Act of 1996 directed that rural healthcare providers be given discounts in data transmission to equal the costs in urban centers (Office for the Advancement of Telehealth & The Joint Working Group on Telemedicine, 2001). However, POTS is very slow, and for many purposes, the two-way audio and video provided are not of high enough quality. Additionally, transmission is very slow as it is in most present-day wireless devices.

To see the full scope of features that telehealth can offer, such as telepresence, requires very high data transmission speeds. The development of Internet2 many help to overcome this barrier. Internet2 is a 13,000-mile network with a transmission rate of 2.3 **gigabytes** per second, which is a result of collaboration between the federal government, academia, and industry (Issues: Future Technology Trends, 1999). At present, however, this backbone is mostly a research network connecting a few businesses and many universities. Although short of these speeds, DSL and ISDN offer some improvements over POTS. The cost of providing these lines to all rural areas, combined with the need for speed, may eventually make satellite telemedicine networks the medium of choice, especially in rural areas. At present, satellite transmissions are still prohibitively expensive, but when they are affordable they do offer data transmission speeds three times faster than an ISDN connection and 30 times faster than a T1 line

Another issue is equipment interfacing. It will be difficult to achieve telemedicine's potential without interoperability and interconnection of equipment (Office for the Advancement of Telehealth & The Joint Working Group on Telemedicine, 2001). This lack makes networking between, and sometimes within, projects a frustrating and expensive task. Telecommunications standards also need to include technical standards for image quality in video transmissions for the various specialties. For example, the level of clarity and color needed to correctly diagnose skin conditions in dermatology may differ from that needed for radiology. Clinical protocols and guidelines will also need to be developed. It must be remembered that telehealth has not only national implications, but global ones, as well; thus, standards will need to be developed internationally.

OTHER ISSUES

As telehealth becomes more developed, issues dealing with patient and provider acceptance and satisfaction will become more evident. In all the telehealth projects that have been reported, satisfaction by both patients and providers was high. Most such, however, have been pilot projects supported by grants. Some people involved in healthcare fear that in the rush to reduce healthcare expenses, technology will replace face-to-face consultation. The ANA has taken the position that telehealth should augment rather than replace traditional healthcare (ANA, 1996). They see a potential for "abuse" of the technology by replacing professionals in patient care in homes, schools, and other settings where healthcare is given.

The East Carolina University project showed the need to attend to the sociocultural aspect of telehealth (Balch & Tichenor, 1997). To address this issue, frequent demonstrations with all involved healthcare personnel are needed, as well as a phased introduction to the telemedicine infrastructure. The project also found that staffing needs were higher than anticipated both to meet needs inherent in both technology and client care. With multiple sites and limited resources, scheduling telehealth activities needs a very organized and systematic approach. Additionally, telehealth requires a high level of teamwork.

Information management in telehealth presents many challenges to informatics, not only technically but also in terms of strategies needed to manage information from more than one site. Agencies involved in telehealth will need an overall strategic information plan that considers not only the data needs at the agency but those at the distant sites. If both the agency and practitioners at the distant location are to function fully, they will both need to be able to access all the information about a patient and to enter data.

 ## Summary

As technology improves, the possibilities for telehealth are endless. Telehealth technologies can be classified as either store-and-forward or real-time. Store-and-forward is an asynchronous method in which images are sent to a distant location and examined at the convenience of the specialist. Real-time telehealth, a synchronous mode, involves having the patient and the consultant interact at the same time. Although telehealth is starting to expand, many of the projects reported in the literature were supported by grants. Telehealth offers many opportunities to nurses. Telehealth has also proved valuable in education, both professionally and for patient care and for disaster care.

Before telehealth becomes more widespread, certain issues need to be resolved. Reimbursement is probably the largest concern, with Medicare still reluctant to offer payment for telehealth except in rural areas. The licensure problem needs to be resolved to allow telehealth practice across state lines; this may even need to be resolved internationally. As with any innovation affecting healthcare, the need for attention to patient safety is also paramount. The telecommunications infrastructure also presents problems in some cases. Perhaps one of the most important issues is the acceptance of this technology by patients and healthcare providers. The financial issues are not solely in the reimbursement area. As with many innovations, the way healthcare is delivered will change. These changes will create opportunities for many, but if more preventive care does reduce the number of visits to emergency departments and hospital admissions, they also have the potential to upset the financial base of the present day acute care system.

connection— For definitions of bolded key terms, visit the online glossary available at http://connection.lww.com/go/thede.

CONSIDERATIONS AND EXERCISES

1. Define the two overall classifications of technology used in telehealth.
2. Discuss some ways that telehealth can deliver healthcare.
3. Write two or three paragraphs illustrating how nurses can operate autonomously in telehealth.
4. Select one of the issues in implementing telehealth and discuss the different approaches to resolving the issue.
5. Explore the ways that telehealth could have an impact on the healthcare system in your country.

REFERENCES

About telehealth project. (2002). Retrieved April 13, 2002 from http://eahec.ecu.edu/telehealth/abth.html#purp.

American Academy of Ambulatory Care Nursing. (2001). *Telehealth nursing practice administration and practice standards.* Retrieved April 16, 2002 from http://www.aaacn.org/resource/telephon.htm.

American Nurses Association (n.d.) *Telehealth monograph.* Retrieved April 16, 2002 from http://www.nursingworld.org/tan/99sptoct/products.htm.

American Nurses Association (1996). *Telehealth—issues for nursing.* Retrieved April 17, 2002 from http://www.ana.org/readroom/tele2.htm.

American Nurses Association (1998). *Core Principles on Telehealth.* Pub#9901TH. Washington, DC: American Nurses Publications.

American Nurses Association (1999). *Competencies for Telehealth Technologies in Nursing.* Pub#9907TH. Washington, DC: American Nurses Publications.

American Nurses Association (2001). *Developing Telehealth Protocols: A Blueprint for Success.* Pub#DTP20CM2. Washington, DC: American Nurses Publications.

Balch, D. C., & Tichenor, J. M. (1997). Telemedicine expanding the scope of health care information. *Journal of the American Medical Association, 4*(1), 1–5.

Certification in telehealth: Should we do it? Retrieved April 16, 2002 from http://telehealth.hrsa.gov/jwgt/certdraft.htm.

Chaffee, M. (1999). A telehealth odyssey. *American Journal of Nursing, 99*(7), 27–32.

Chang, B. & Trelease, R. (2001). Can telehealth technology be used for the education of health professionals? *Western Journal of Nursing Research, 23*(1), 107–114.

Gaffney, T. (May 31, 1999): The regulatory dilemma surrounding interstate practice. *Online Journal of Issues in Nursing.* Retrieved April 16, 2002 from http://www.nursingworld.org/ojin/topic9/topic9_1.htm.

Garshnek, V., & Burkle, F. M. Jr. (1999). Applications of telemedicine and telecommunications to disaster medicine historical and future perspectives. Journal of the American Medical Association, 6(1), 26–37.

Hutcherson, C. M. (September 30, 2001). Legal Considerations for Nurses Practicing in a Telehealth Setting. *Online Journal of Issues in Nursing, 6*(3). Retrieved April 16, 2002 from http://www.nursingworld.org/ojin/topic16/tpc16_3.htm.

Issues, future technology trends. (1999). Retrieved April 17, 2002 from http://telehealth.hrsa.gov/pubs/future.htm.

Jones, M. G. (1997). Telemedicine and the national information infrastructure: Are the realities of health care being ignored? [electronic version] *Journal of the American Medical Association, 4,* 399–412.

Kumekawa, J. K. (September 30, 2001) Health information privacy protection: Crisis or common sense?" *Online Journal of Issues in Nursing, 6*(3). Retrieved April 16, 2002 from http://www.nursingworld.org/ojin/topic16/tpc16_2.htm.

Lattimer, V. Sassi, F., George, S., Turnbull, J., Mullee, M., & Smith, H. (2000). Cost analysis of nurse telephone consultation in out of hours primary care: Evidence from a randomised controlled trial. [electronic version] *British Medical Journal, 1320,* 1053–1057.

Lindberg, C. C. S. (1997). Implementation of in-home telemedicine in rural Kansas: Answering an elderly patient's needs. *Journal of the American Medical Association, 4*(1), 14–17.

National Council of State Boards of Nursing (2001). *State compact bill status.* Retrieved October 16, 2002 from http://www.ncsbn.org/public/regulation/mutual_recognition_state.htm.

Office for the Advancement of Telehealth and The Joint Working Group on Telemedicine 2001. *Report to congress on telemedicine (2001). Executive summary.* Retrieved April 12, 2002 from http://telehealth.hrsa.gov/pubs/report2001/exec.htm.

Puskin, D. S. (September 30, 2001) Telemedicine: Follow the money. *Online Journal of Issues in Nursing, 6*(3) Retrieved April 16, 2002 from http://www.nursingworld.org/ojin/topic16/tpc16_1.htm.

Schlachta-Fairchild, L. (2001).Telehealth: A new venue for health care delivery. *Seminars in Oncology Nursing, 17,*(1), 34–40.

Shea, S., Starren, J., Weinstock, R. S., Knudson, P.E., Teresi, J., Homes, D., et al. (2002). Columbia University's Informatics for Diabetes Education and Telemedicine (IDEATel) Project Rationale and Design. *Journal of the American Medical Association, 9*(1), 49–62.

Telehealth: A new venue for health care delivery. *Seminars in Oncology Nursing, 17*(1), 34–40.

Wooton, R. (2001). Recent advances telemedicine. [electronic version] *British Medical Journal, 323,* 557–560.

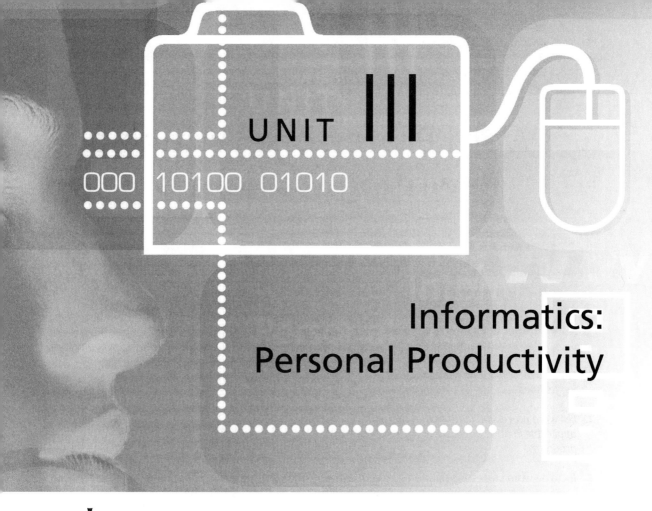

UNIT **III**

000 10100 01010

Informatics:
Personal Productivity

LEARNING to use the productivity tools bundled in office software suites effectively not only improves output but saves time. Few of us use many of the features of these products, preferring instead to limp along manually doing things that are done much more effectively using the feature designed for that purpose. We excuse ourselves by saying that we don't have time to learn to do it when in reality the time it would take to learn the feature is often less than the time we spend doing it manually. These are the challenges that the tools in an office software suite present to users. The opportunities they provide when mastered are improved abilities in communication.

In the three chapters in this unit, when any instructions are given they have been tested in the Windows versions of both the Corel and Microsoft Office Suites. Chapter 5 introduced the concept that many of the application programs behave similarly, in these three chapters that explore word processing, presentation programs, and spreadsheets, more of these similarities are considered. Approaching these programs with an idea about their similarities allows one to increase one's computer fluency, because skills learned in one program transfer to others, both current and future.

CHAPTER 9

Word Processors: Writing and Rewriting Without a Hassle

Objectives

After studying this chapter you will be able to:

1. *Experiment with many word processing features.*

2. *List word processing features that are applicable in other application programs.*

3. *Increase word processing skills.*

Software programs that are designed to help a user manipulate text, edit, rearrange, and retype documents on a personal computer are called *word processors*. The popularity of word processing attests to the fact that written communication is still the primary means of spreading information and knowledge. Effectively using a word processor is part of computer fluency and has become a necessity to advance in nursing. One of the benefits of mastering basic word processing skills is the transferability of these skills to other application programs, most of which use the basic editing features of word processors when any text editing is required.

Word processing software packages do vary in some of the features they offer. All packages, even the text editing software that comes with an operating system, offer the ability to insert, delete, cut, and paste text; search and replace words; store and retrieve documents; and **word wrap** (the automatic insertion of line breaks when text exceeds the width of the page). Even e-mail software offers many of these features. Full-featured word processors such as Corel WordPerfect, Lotus WordPro, and Microsoft Word, however, offer the writer many more features.

 The Document

Open a word processor and a blank document appears, in some ways resembling a blank piece of paper. The top of the screen has menus and icons that provide access to the features of the word processor. The bottom of the screen usually has what is called a *status line*, or a line that provides information about the document, such as the number of the current page, the distance of the insertion point from the left margin, and whether the Caps lock is on or off. In Windows word processors, the very bottom line of the screen will contain icons for any open programs, and for some programs, a separate icon for every open document.

In the blank section of the screen, the user types a document, which often will be printed when finished. Although typing skills are a great help in entering text, that is the only resemblance that a word processor has to a typewriter. In fact, thinking in terms of the printed page, as one does with a typewriter, interferes with maximizing word processing features. In word processing, a user should separate the tasks of writing from those of formatting the page. Concentrate first on writing, then format later is a good rule for word processing.

Separation of formatting from writing is evident in the views of a document that a user can access. The draft or normal view shows just the text and is ideal for writing. In this view, when a new page becomes necessary a dotted line appears (solid line, in some word processing packages) to indicate a page break. The top and bottom page margins are not visible and do not interfere with one's thinking, nor is one tempted to paginate (create artificial page breaks) before editing is completed. The Print text command shows how the text will look when printed. In print view, one sees items that will appear on the printed page, such as page numbers. Some word processors also have a Web view, and most can be used to create Web pages. When used for this purpose, they may create files that are very large or have hypertext codes that are not compatible with all Web browsers.

ENTERING TEXT

Two modes are available for entering (inputting) text in a word processing program: insert and overtype. Users can toggle between these two modes by tapping the Insert key. The default mode is the insert setting. In this mode, when the user enters new characters, the original text automatically makes room for it. In typeover (may be called overtype or strikeover) mode, any new characters will replace those already in the document. Sometimes, as a result of an accidental tapping of the insert key, a user may be in overtype mode when this is not desired. To remedy this, tap the insert key again. If in doubt about which mode a user currently is in, the status line usually provides this information.

When entering text into a word processor, users do not have to be concerned about where a new line should start. A feature called **word wrap** flows the text over to the next line when the computer finds that the word added to the line will cause it to exceed its allowable length. This line break is flexible and will change when necessary if text is added or deleted, or if the length of the line is altered by a user changing margins, **font**, font size, or font attributes When the user adds a line break by tapping the enter key, the line break is inflexible; that is, it is permanent (unless deleted). This type of line break, called a hard return, is used when the user wants to start a new paragraph, or in situations in which the user knows that the text should always start on a new line (e.g., when creating a list).

CHANGING THE APPEARANCE OF THE TEXT

The appearance of text can be changed in many ways. Attributes can be applied to selected text, or applied before the text is entered. The font (typeface) and size of the font can also be changed. As with many functions in application programs there are several ways to apply text appearance changes.

Attributes

An **attribute** is a characteristic that changes the appearance of a printable symbol, such as a color. Attributes that can be applied to characters in most word processors include **boldfacing**, *italicizing*, and <u>underlining</u>. Attributes can be turned on before or after characters are typed. To select an attribute before typing, choose the appropriate symbol from the tool bar, or click on Format>Font. To make the change after typing, select the text and apply the attribute in the same manner.

Fonts (Typefaces) and Font Size (in Points)

A **font** is the name given to the typeface style that is used for the characters in the document. The font and its size can be changed for the entire document, or for just a small section. Like attributes, changes can be made before or after text is entered. A dropdown box for both fonts and size is generally found on the toolbox near the top of the screen, or they are available in the font menu under Format on the menu line. Some programs use the term **point size** to refer to the size of the print. The fonts and sizes available are a function of the printer in use as much as the application program (Figure 9-1). Fonts should be chosen carefully. Using too many different fonts together is confusing to readers.

Editing Text (Basic)

Basic editing involves "navigating" around a document and using the editing keys. Navigation entails using the arrow keys or the mouse to move the insertion point. These actions allow the user to move the insertion point without disturbing any text. To insert new text, the user places the insertion point where he or she wishes the new words to be and then starts typing. Characters can be erased with either the Delete or the Backspace key (Table 9-1). Spaces and hard returns (forced line breaks) as well as forced page breaks are deleted as if they were text characters.

Different Fonts and Sizes		
8 point	**12 point**	**20 point**
Arial	Arial	Arial
Courier	Courier	Courier
Times New Roman	Times New Roman	Times New Roman
Kaufmann	Kaufmann	Kaufmann
Franklin Gothic	Franklin Gothic	Franklin Gothic

Figure 9-1 • Font and point size.

TABLE 9-1 • *Delete Versus Backspace Key*	
Deleting a Small Amount of Text	
Using the Delete Key	*Using the Backspace Key*
Removes the character that is to the *right* of the insertion point.	Removes the character that is to the *left* of the insertion point.

DELETING TEXT

Although the delete and backspace keys work well for deleting a few characters, they are cumbersome when it is necessary to delete a large amount of text. To delete a large block of text, place the mouse pointer at the beginning or end of the unwanted text, hold down the left mouse button, and drag the pointer to the other end, or hold down the shift key and use the arrow keys to select the text. The text will change color (called **highlighting**) to show it has been "selected." Release the mouse button when the text is highlighted. With the text selected, tap the delete key or depress the right mouse button and choose "delete" from the pop-up menu.

CUTTING, MOVING, AND PASTING TEXT

With word processing, as in all application programs, the user has the ability to copy and/or move sentences, paragraphs, pages, and the entire document. When text is to be moved from one location to another, it is "cut" from that location and "pasted" into the new location. When text is copied, it is left in its original place and a copy is pasted in another location.

To move text, first select it and then cut it out by clicking on the scissors icon on the toolbar. This removes the text from its current location and places it in the computer's memory on what is called a **clipboard**. The user then moves the insertion point to the new location for the text by using arrow keys or the mouse pointer. Then he or she pastes the contents of the clipboard to the new location by clicking on the paste icon (a dark clipboard with a light object in the bottom right corner) on the tool bar. All these options are also available from the edit menu.

To copy text, after selecting the area intended, the user clicks on the copy icon on the tool bar (to the right of the scissors) then moves the insertion point to the new location and pastes the text. Once it is on the clipboard, text or any object remains until replaced by another object or text. Hence, the user can paste the same item multiple times. Originally, the clipboard only held one item, but some newer application programs allow multiple items to be placed in different parts of the clipboard.

 ## Saving

It is a good idea to save frequently when creating a document in a word processor. To facilitate finding the file again, use a file name that is descriptive of the file and place it in a folder that pertains to the subject of the document. Back up all important documents, such as term papers, on a diskette that is separate from the computer. If the document is vital, have two back-up copies and keep one in a different location.

Files saved by a word processor are in a proprietary format, or one that is specific to the brand of the word processor that created it. Sometimes it is necessary to give a file to someone who uses a different type of word processor. To do this, you can save the file in an rtf format that usually maintains all the font attributes when transferred from one application to another (see Figure 5-6 in Chapter 5). Note that the extension in the file name will change when you do this.

Retrieving

To retrieve a document, the user needs to know the location and name of the file. If a file was saved to a diskette in Drive A, to retrieve the file, place the diskette in the A drive, type the file name (including the "a:\") and tap enter. For example, if a file was named "mypaper" and saved to a diskette in the "a" drive, to open the file, enter a:\mypaper in the appropriate box. If the file is in the current working folder, or the user knows its location and how to change working folders, it is usually much easier to retrieve it by selecting from the list of that folder (See Chapter 5 for a discussion of folders).

Paragraphs

A *paragraph* as defined by a word processor is any text separated by hard returns (created by tapping the enter key). It may be one word or many pages, but in formal papers a paragraph is generally at least three sentences long. Paragraphs can be aligned or formatted different ways.

JUSTIFICATION (ALIGNMENT)

Justification or text alignment refers to how the left and right margins of the paragraph appear. Different justification can be applied to a paragraph, paragraphs, a page, or an entire document. Text can be justified in four ways (Figure 9-2). Unless a very good printer and font are available, the easiest documents to read are justified flush left, so called because of the straight left margin and the even spacing between words.

PARAGRAPH FORMATTING

The default formatting for a paragraph is often with the first line indented 1/2 inch to the right. Paragraphs, however, may also be formatted as **outdented** or **hanging paragraphs**, as required by fifth edition of the American Psychological Association's (APA) format for references (Figure 9-3). All these styles are easily created by a word processor by placing the insertion point anywhere in the paragraph and accessing the paragraph menu, which is found under Format on the main menu line.

Page Properties

The printed page is the ultimate focus of a word processed document. A page has many properties that are used to change its printed appearance. Most are accessible from the page setup menu, which is usually found under File on the menu line.

Left Justification (Left Margin Straight)

Learning to use a word processor is not so much a factor of learning the commands, but of knowing what is possible. Once you know what is possible and can ask, "How do you do x?" instead of being oblivious to the fact that it is possible to do x, you are 75% of the way to using a function effectively.

Right Justification (Right Margin Straight)

Few writers, even professionals, get it right the first time. Rewriting is as germane to writing as breathing is to staying alive. A word processor makes rewriting relatively painless thus allowing a writer to appear at his/her best. Editing, however, leads to unintended results when one formats manually.

Center Justification (Text centered horizontally)

When an individual first moves from a typewriter to a word processor, and before one has learned to think "let the computer do it," some features in word processing can cause confusion, and yes, frustration! Much of the frustration new word processor users experience comes from ideas ingrained by the use of typewriters and a fixed page.

Full Justification (Both Margins Straight)

Those reared in the printed page world sometimes find it very anti-intuitive that they do not have to, indeed should not, use the enter key to paginate. The problems that manually creating new pages causes become evident when they try to edit the text. Unintended results occur when users use the enter key to create a new page. New pages created in this manner are fluid and will change as the text above is added or deleted. The result is that the "new page" will not be a new page.

Figure 9-2 • Justification (alignment) examples.

LAYOUT: PORTRAIT OR LANDSCAPE

The amount of text that can be printed on a page of any given size is limited. The limits are determined by the margins, font, and font size of the type used. Sometimes, especially with tables, it becomes desirable to change the page layout (called page size by some word processors) so that the long side is horizontal instead of vertical. This creates a **landscape** page layout. The most common page layout is with the long side horizontal, which is termed a **portrait** layout.

CENTERING VERTICALLY

Sometimes it is desirable to center the text on a page not only left to right, but also vertically, or top to bottom. This can be useful in creating a title page.

MARGINS

Both layout and centering a page vertically must be applied to an entire page. Left and right margin changes, however, can be applied to one paragraph, to a page, or to the en-

Hanging Paragraph

Manually creating a hanging paragraph instead of using this feature not only wastes time, but creates problems when one needs to edit the text.

Indenting of Both Margins

Create page breaks only when it is imperative that the new text be on a fresh page and then use the forced page break (Ctrl+Enter). If it is necessary for all of a given set of text to always be on the same page, use the "Keep Text Together" Feature found under format (Paragraph in some word processors.)

Figure 9-3 • Examples of paragraph formatting.

tire document. The usual margin for apiece of 8-1/2 ×11 inch paper is 1 inch on all four sides. This may or may not be the default setting for the word processor. If this is not the case, the left and right margins should be changed to 1 inch. When this is done, it is also possible to make 1-inch margins the default for any future documents. Top and bottom margins and defaults may also be changed.

 ## Printing

In Windows-compliant programs, tapping Ctrl-P automatically prints the document or starts the printing process. The File menu also contains a print function. Using this option, a block of text, one page, a range of pages, or the entire document can be selected for printing. Although many features that improved the appearance of a printed page such as a header or page numbering can be applied at any time, others, such as entering page breaks to improve the pagination for looks, should not be introduced until all editing is finished and the document is ready to be printed.

PAGE BREAKS AND KEEPING TEXT TOGETHER

Page breaks work the same way as word wrap; the computer starts a new page when it finds enough new type has been set to fill a printed page. Like a line break caused by word wrap, this page break is fluid and will change as needed when the document is edited. For this reason, page breaks should not be entered as the document is written, unless it is known that subsequent text must start on a new page, such as when creating the first page in the References section. Writing in normal (i.e., draft) mode helps one resist the temptation to enter page breaks too soon.

To force a page break, tap Ctrl + Enter. This is analogous to a hard return; that is, no matter what editing is done before the forced page break, the text that starts after it will always be on a separate page. Page breaks created by repeated tapping of the Enter key create fluid page breaks that will change as the document above and below it changes, which produces inappropriate page breaks. Using the appropriate line and page break feature preserves the ability to edit one's writing, which is the key to effective communication.

Sometimes, although one does not necessarily need a new page, one wants to be sure that a given block of text when printed will always be on the same page. This can be done by using the "keep text together" feature. Use the help feature to learn how this is done.

HEADERS, FOOTERS, AND PAGE NUMBERS

A header is text that is printed on the top of each page, and a footer is text that is printed on the bottom of every page (Figure 9-4). Some formal documents require headers on all pages. On others, the user may want to use a header as clarification for the reader. Manually entering headers and footers results in their moving to a location other than the top of a page when there is any editing of the document that either adds or deletes a line. For this reason, headers and footers should be inserted using the word processor header/footer function. Headers and footers may have any attributes that can be applied to text, and can be left, center, or right justified. Some word processors print a header above the margin, thus creating a smaller top margin. This can be reset. A header or footer can include page numbers, or page numbers may be inserted without using headers or footers. If both a header and a page number are needed, include the page number as part of the header. The page number will then not try to print in the same location as the header. Check the application's help function for header, footer, or page numbers to learn to use these functions.

 ## Some Common Word Processor Features

Most people use only a very small portion of their word processor's capability, ignoring features that can make a document more professional looking as well as saving time in creating the document. The online help feature provides instructions in how to use many other features.

Header

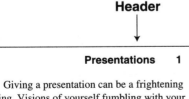

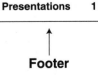

Footer

Figure 9-4 • Headers and footers.

SPELL CHECK

Many misconceptions exist about how spell check works. A computer does not think; it only makes comparisons (Figure 9-5). When spell check is used, the computer compares each set of characters between spaces with the words that are in its dictionary. If it finds a set of matching letters, it assumes that the word is spelled correctly.

Most word processors use a wavy red line to underline any words that are considered misspelled at the point of data entry. When this line appears, to find out how the word processor thinks the word should be spelled, place the mouse pointer over the word and right click. A list of suggestions will appear. If one of those words is the correct one, select it, and the speller will replace the misspelled word. If "No Suggestions" appears, and the user knows the word is spelled correctly, the user can add that word to the dictionary. If one is engaged in writing for a specialty field for which many of the words are not part of the default dictionary, additional dictionaries, such as a medical dictionary, can be added.

One function related to the speller is the ability of word processors to automatically change what is seen as a misspelled—or more usually mistyped—word to what it considers the correct format. This function is often referred to as *auto correct* or *quick correct*. To provide for this function, the word processor stores a list of common misspellings together with the correctly spelled word. If a word is typed in a way that matches the misspelling, the correct word is automatically substituted for the misspelled one. New words can be added to this function, and words that may not be a misspelling in a certain context can be deleted.

THESAURUS

Although not as large, the thesaurus is set up much like a printed one and is much quicker to use. Like spell check, the thesaurus is located in the Tools (sometimes under language) menu. To use the thesaurus, place the insertion point on the word for which a substitute is desired, and access the thesaurus. A window pops up that lists some possible synonyms. Some word processors also provide antonyms. Select the proper word, and click on the box that tells the computer to replace it.

GRAMMAR CHECKERS

Perfect functionality has not yet been reached with grammar checkers. Still, using one will not hurt anything. They are excellent at picking up syntactical errors such as subject-verb disagreement and run-on sentences. Grammar checkers may also be located under Tools.

I have a spelling checker
I disk covered four my PC.
It plane lee marks four my revue
Miss steaks aye can knot see.

Eye ran this poem threw it.
Your sure real glad two no.
Its very polished in its weigh,
My checker tolled me sew.

Figure 9-5 • Speller peccadilloes.

FIND AND REPLACE

Find and replace is another very useful tool. Find will locate every instance of a set of characters, which is usually a word or phrase. This feature is available in most application programs including Web browsers and e-mail packages. The find-and-replace feature can replace one set of characters with another. Perhaps a user types the word "nurse" when he or she really wants to write "Registered Nurse." By accessing find and/or replace on the Edit menu, the word processor can be told to find every instance of "nurse" and replace it with "Registered Nurse." The replacement can be automatic, or the user can decide which occurrences to replace.

FOOTNOTES AND ENDNOTES

Footnotes and endnotes are different features, but each is accessed and entered the same way. A footnote is a piece of text printed at the bottom of a page. It is usually additional information that may add to a reader's knowledge. An endnote is a piece of text that is printed at the end of a document, for instance, a list of references. Word processors automatically place these notes in the proper position and number them accordingly. The drop-down box to access this feature is found on the Insert menu.

GRAPHICS

The term *graphic* (or *graphical*) in the computer environment refers to any item that is not text or a table. Graphics can be inserted in a document, or in some word processors actually drawn in the word processor as well in the presentation package that is part of all the office software suites. Usually this item is an image, but text can also be placed in a frame known as a *text box* and then treated as a graphic. Most suites also come with **clip art**, or small pictures or symbols that can be used in a document or presentation package.

COLUMNS

Column creation is accessed from the Format menu. Users are then asked to designate the number of columns and can either accept the default spacing between the columns or change it. Using a forced page break in a column forces the text to the top of the next column.

TABLES

Tables can be created by clicking on the table icon on the tool bar and dragging to create the number of rows and columns wanted. Extra columns can be added or deleted at any time. If the default column size does not match a need, columns can be resized by placing the mouse pointer on the grid line between columns until it changes shape, depressing the left mouse button, and dragging the line. To enter text into a table, simply type. The rectangle, or cell, will enlarge as needed.

Many options for formatting a table are available. Although some word processors have more detailed features, all provide the following functions:

▼ Adding a row to the bottom of the table by placing the insertion point in the right-most cell on the bottom row and tapping the tab key.

▼ Navigating the table, by tapping the tab key to go to the cell on the right, shift-tab to go the cell on the left, or using the arrow keys to move the insertion point up or down a row.

▼ Changing the appearance or style of a table. This includes removing all the borders, or changing their attributes. Several ready-made formats are part of each word processor package. Table attributes can be accessed either by right clicking on the table or by clicking on table on the menu line.

▼ The ability to calculate using elementary formulas.

▼ The ability to change cell sizes, either by a menu, or dragging row or column borders.

▼ The ability to both join and split cells either vertically or horizontally.

SORTING

When typing a list of names, it is not always convenient to enter them in alphabetical order. The sort function, however, automatically alphabetizes them based on the word (e.g., first, second) in the line that the user designates. Sort can be applied to a list, column in a table, or paragraphs. The sorting function is useful in organizing references for a paper. Use the help function to learn how to sort.

MAIL MERGE

Mail merge takes a set of data and places the different pieces into a desired form. In using names and addresses to write a form letter, the user creates a set of data that includes **fields** such as title, first name, middle name, last name, address, and so forth. A letter, or form, is then planned in which these items are placed appropriately (Figure 9-6).

AUTOMATIC NUMBERING

Most word processors automatically assume that whenever a number is entered at the beginning of a line followed by a punctuation mark and some text, the next paragraph should be numbered with the next number. Additionally, some word processors then indent each paragraph regardless of the wishes of the user. Overriding this indent can be done by right clicking on the paragraph and changing the indent. The maneuver to stop the numbering varies with the word processor, but tapping the enter key twice will stop it in one program and delete the unwanted number in another. The advantages to automatic numbering are that it saves having to enter the numbers when a list is what is wanted, but even more valuable, if the items in the list are reordered, the numbers automatically change so they remain in sequence. That is, if item 4 is moved to the line after item 1, it becomes number 2 and the former number 2 becomes 3, and so on.

The automatic numbering feature is not an outline feature because the default generally has only one level. To create an outline with various levels, it is necessary to change the format of the numbering feature. This can be done either before one enters any numbers and text or afterward. This feature is on the Insert menu in some word processors and the Format menu in others. This function is very useful for creating an outline for a paper or a multiple choice test.

```
(Title)Ms.
(First Name)Lucy
(Middle Name)X.
(Last Name)Caro
(Address)25 East Southwick Drive
(City)Anywhere
(State)Any State
(Zip)42424-1001
```

Sample of one record in a data set

```
(Title) (First Name) (Middle Name) (Last Name)
(Address)
(City), (State) (Zip)

Dear (Title) (Last Name):

        You have been selected from many people to
enjoy a special vacation at our new resort at the
beautiful sea shore. (First Name), we know that you will
not object to paying a small fee of $2000 for this
privilege. You need to contact us by Friday at the latest
to take part in this great opportunity. Call us anytime at
1-800-BELIEVE.

Sincerely,


Joe Barnum
A sucker is born every minute
```

Sample of a form letter

```
Ms. Lucy X. Caro
25 East Southwick Drive
Anywhere, Any State 42424-1001

Dear Ms. Caro:

        You have been selected from many people to enjoy a special vacation at our new resort
at the beautiful sea shore. Lucy, we know that you will not object to paying a small fee of
$2000 for this privilege. You need to contact us by Friday at the latest to take part in this great
opportunity. Call us anytime at 1-800-BELIEVE.

Sincerely,


Joe Barnum
A sucker is born every minute
```

Form letter after it has been merged

Figure 9-6 • Data set, form letter, and result of merge.

When the outline function is on, tap the enter key to create the next numbered item. To move to the next level below, tap the tab key, and the symbol reverts to the next lower level. To change to a level above, tap shift-tab. Figure 9-7 illustrates an outline format. The labels for each level (e.g., number 1, a.) can be changed by the user. A regular out-

1. This is level one of an outline
   a. This level two accessed by tapping the tab key after the number 2 appeared.
   b. The "b." appeared automatically when the enter key was tapped.
2. Shift-tab moved back to the first level.
   a. Level two again
      i. Level three
         (1) Level four
            (a) Level five
3. After tapping Shift-Tab 4 times, we are back at level one again.

Figure 9-7 • Example of an outline.

line format with Roman numerals as the top level and uppercase letters for the second level can be selected, or the user can create any desired style.

CROSS REFERENCING

With the popularity of the Web, publishers of word processing software have added the ability to insert a Web link into a document. Clicking on the link, if the user is online, will retrieve the page in the link just as it does in a regular Web page. Links within the document, known as cross referencing, are also possible (e.g., *"see page X-23"*). The page number then is "generated" before printing to ensure its accuracy. It is also possible to use referencing or to mark items to be included in a table of contents.

MACROS

A **macro** is a small program that automates a function. If the same functions are continually accessed, such as creating a superscript, a macro can be created to perform this function automatically. Although complex macros are programmed, it is also possible to create a macro by recording keystrokes as a function is performed. After creating a macro, it

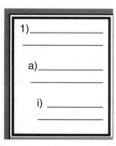

Figure 9-8 • Outline format.

can be placed on the tool bar or assigned to a key. To place a macro on the tool bar, place the mouse pointer on the tool bar and click with the right mouse button, then follow the directions. To record keystrokes to create a macro, click on "tools/macro/record," enter a name for the macro, implement the keystrokes, and stop the recording by clicking on the square on the small window that is present when a macro is being created.

Increasing Word Processing Skills

Most users of word processing software avail themselves of only a small fraction of the features that their word processors offer. This limits output and results in time wasted as they manually do what the word processor would do more quickly. Online help gets better with every version of the office software suites and is a great source of assistance in increasing one's word processing skills. Classes can help too, but they only open a door to the intricacies of the program; one must enter that door and try the features not only in class but in all settings. Becoming aware of what a word processor can do, then learning the features in a "just in time" manner, can keep the learning to a manageable level.

When experimenting with a new feature, save the document before experimenting. Then, if the result is unacceptable, you can always close the document without saving and retrieve the original document. The undo feature is also often a ticket back to square one. When learning new features, expect some frustration, but remember that you will be rewarded by saving time the next time this feature is needed.

As one becomes more expert in word processing, one often wants to access features quickly. To meet this need, many features have shortcut keys. Additionally, most of these shortcuts perform the same functions in other programs, including Web browsers (Table 9-2).

Summary

Word processors have become very popular. The basic editing skills pioneered in word processors are used in most application programs including e-mail programs. Once text is entered into a word processor it can be altered in many ways. Attributes can be added; the font or font (point) size can be changed; text can be deleted, copied, or moved. Learning to let the word processor perform such functions as line breaks and page breaks involves reconceptualizing the idea of a document from a fixed-page entity to a document that changes while it is being edited. Time spent learning to let the computer perform features such as centering a page vertically, formatting a paragraph, and entering headers and footers plus learning to cope with automatic numbering is returned many times over in creating future documents.

Word processors have many other features that not only make tasks easier but also make them economically feasible, such as sorting, mail merge for personalizing notes, and cross-referencing to make it easier for a reader to locate information on another page of a document. The short-cut keys in Table 9-2 provide an excellent way to access features not only in word processing programs, but also in other application programs.

connection⟶   **For definitions of bolded key terms, visit the online glossary available at http://connection.lww.com/go/thede, as are directions for using many of the features discussed in this chapter.**

TABLE 9-2 • *Universal Commands in Word Processors and Other Applications*

Common Word Processing Shortcuts

Want to:	Use:
Navigate a document	
Move the insertion point without changing any of the text?	Arrow keys or the mouse
Move from beginning of a word to beginning of the next?	Ctrl + right or left arrow key
Move from paragraph to paragraph?	Ctrl + up or down arrow keys
Delete and insert characters	
Delete a character that is to the left of your insertion point?	Backspace
Delete a character that is to the right of your insertion point?	Delete key
Select a word?	Click twice with mouse pointer.
Select text?	Place mouse pointer at beginning or end of the text, depress and hold left mouse button and drag to opposite end of the text.
Select text slowly?	Place insertion point at beginning or end of the text, depress and hold the shift key, and use arrow keys to enlarge selection.
Enter text over selected text?	Just type, first key press will delete selected text.
Select the entire document?	Ctrl + A
Type over the existing text? *	Insert key (use this key to toggle back to the regular insert mode too.)
Force line and page breaks	
Force a new line?	Enter key.
Force a new page? *	Ctrl + Enter
Format a paragraph	
Indent the first line of a paragraph? *	Tab key
Create a hanging paragraph? *	Format/Paragraph
Miscellaneous	
Find a phrase in the document?	Ctrl + F
Print?	Ctrl + P
Undo the last entry?	Ctrl + Z
Move from cell to cell or input box to input box?	Tab
Move back to prior cell or input box?	Shift + Tab
Cut, copy, and move text	
Copy a selected portion of text to the clipboard?	Ctrl + C
Cut out a selected portion of text and place on the clipboard?	Ctrl + X or Shift + Delete
Paste anything on the clipboard to new location?	Ctrl + V or Shift + Insert
Saving and retrieving a document	
Save a document?	Ctrl + S
Retrieve a document?	Ctrl + O

* Indicates those functions that are not universally applicable. All others apply in Windows application programs and often in Web browsers as well.

CONSIDERATIONS AND EXERCISES

1. Enter a paragraph into a word processor and:
   a. Select the paragraph and change the font and font (point) size.
   b. Place the insertion point at the beginning of a word, tap the Insert key, and enter the letters "abc" and see what happens. Tap the Insert key again to stop this mode of entering text.
   c. Click on the Undo icon (or tap Ctrl + Z) to undo this change.
   d. Boldface one sentence.
   e. Create a hard page break at the end of the paragraph.
   f. Make a hanging paragraph by clicking on Format > Paragraph on the menu line (will be under Special on the Indents and Spacing tab in Microsoft Word.)
2. Experiment with automatic numbering.
   a. Enter the number 1, a period, and tap the Tab key.
      i. Enter the word HOUSE.
      ii. Tap the Enter key.
      iii. What happened?
   b. Enter the word CAR after the "2." and tap the Enter key.
   c. Type the word BOAT and tap the Enter key.
   d. Stop the automatic numbering.
   e. Select all the text on this page by using Ctrl + A and then delete it.
3. Experiment with outlining.
   a. Find Bullets and Numbering on either the Insert or Format menu.
   b. Select Outline Numbered.
   c. Select the format that looks like Figure 9-8.
   d. After the 1 that appears on the screen after you click "OK,"
      i. Enter the word HOUSE.
      ii. Tap the Enter key.
      iii. Tab the Tab key.
      iv. Enter the word KITCHEN.
      v. Tap Enter.
      vi. Enter the words FAMILY, ROOM.
      vii. Tap Enter.
      viii. Tap Shift + Tab.
      ix. Enter the word CAR.
      x. Turn off the outline feature the same way that the automatic numbering was turned off.
4. Copy the entire document to another document.
   a. Tap Ctrl + A to select the entire document.
   b. There are four ways to place the selected text on the clipboard. Select one and perform the activity.
      • Tap Ctrl + C
      • Tap Shift + Delete
      • On the tool bar click on the Copy icon.
      • On the menu line click on Edit > Copy.

   c. Paste the text on the clipboard into a new document.
      i. Leave the current document open.
      ii. On the menu line click on File > New.
      iii. Select one of the following four ways to paste the text on the clipboard in the new document.
- Tap Ctrl + V.
- Tap Shift + Insert.
- Click on the paste icon on the tool bar.
- On the menu line click on Edit > Paste.

   d. Return to the original document by clicking on the icon on the bottom of the screen. (If a line of icons is not seen there, place the mouse pointer there until one appears, or click on Window on the menu line and select the appropriate document from that list.)

5. On the page-setup screen (on the menu line click on File > Page Setup.):
   a. Change the page orientation to landscape (Size or paper size).
   b. Change the margins to .75 inches (7 cm).

6. Insert a header that is right justified and contains a running head, five spaces, and a page number. Use the help feature to discover how to do this. You may have to experiment a little.

7. Change the view of the document from print (page) to normal (draft) mode or the other way around if you are already looking at the document in the normal (draft) mode. What happens to the header?

8. Create a table of three columns and three rows. Enter the following text:
   a. In the first cell in the first row enter DATE.
   b. Tap the Tab key.
   c. Enter the word TIME and tap Tab.
   d. Enter the word PROJECT and tap Tab.
   e. Enter today's date and tap Tab.
   f. Enter the present time and tap Tab.
   g. Enter "Creating a table" and tap Tab.
   h. Using Help, ask how to create a header row in a table then follow the instructions and make the top row a header row. (When the top row is a header row, if the table rows span more than one page, a header row or rows will print at the top of each page—just as a page header automatically prints on the top of each page.)
   i. Play with the table formatting function. (Right click over the table for a list of some options.)

9. Use the information for this chapter on the Web page (http://connection.lww.com/go/thede) and center the text on a page vertically.

Presentation Software: Looking Professional in the Spotlight

Objectives
After studying this chapter you will be able to:

1. *State and define the features that presentation software packages provide.*

2. *Describe some uses of presentation programs.*

3. *Apply principles of good design in creating visuals.*

Nurses and students give many presentations, sometimes informally to one another, but often before a group. Feeling confident in this endeavor is something that comes with practice. Having good visuals to facilitate delivery of the presentation helps provide this confidence. Using visuals not only adds interest to a presentation but also improves the listeners' retention rate. Only 38% of what an audience learns comes from the audio messages—55% comes from the visual messages (Visual Presentation Issues, 2001). Today, presentation software can help produce high-quality visuals and make the user look more professional.

One very effective and easy way of adding visuals to a presentation is to create projected visuals, or those in which the image is broadcast onto a screen. A lighted screen has the ability to rivet the attention of an audience, making it easier for them to receive the message. Projected visuals include overhead transparencies, 35-mm slides, and computer-projected slides. When using a projected image, speakers are perceived as better prepared, groups are more likely to reach consensus, and people are more likely to act on recommendations they learn about during the presentation.

Presentation software simplifies the creation of visuals by presenting the user with templates that facilitate building various types of projected visuals, such as a title slide or one where the important reference points are highlighted by adding bullets. If one creates slides for use with computer projection equipment, then film clips, sound, movie-like transitions between slides, and animation can be added to the presentation. These shows can be used for a presentation or to create a show that runs unattended. Some of the more common presentation packages are Corel's Presentations, Harvard Graphics, Lotus' Freelance, and Microsoft's Power Point.

 ## Basics of Slide Creation

Each brand of presentation software, as well as specific versions within that brand, vary in how features are implemented, but all packages have more similarities than dissimilarities. Each of these packages provides drawing tools that allow one to create a sketch and then to copy and paste it into a word processor. If one desires to place an entire slide into a text program tapping Ctrl + A will select all the objects on the screen. These objects can then be placed on the clipboard by clicking on the copy icon and from there pasted into the text. The drawing can also be saved, although in some presentation programs it will be saved as a slide. Despite naming the visuals slides, presentation programs are not limited to producing only computer slides. It is possible to develop many types of visuals including 35-mm slides, transparencies, or even a booklet with text and pictures.

Although when creating an individual visual one does not need to be concerned with consistency in backgrounds, when creating a series of slides it is important. To facilitate this consistency, presentation program screens consist of three layers that the user manipulates independently. This concept differs from other application programs in which the user works with only one layer. The three layers are a background layer, a layout layer, and the editing layer to which text or images are added (Figure 10-1).

THE BACKGROUND LAYER

One of the first choices a user makes when creating a slide show is the background. This layer is often referred to as the *master*. Presentation programs all come with various background choices that the user can either accept as they are or modify. Some backgrounds may have images on them that, although interesting, may get in the way of the message to be communicated. There is usually a way to eliminate objects in the background or the entire background for either one slide or all the slides in a show.

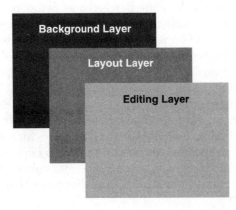

Figure 10-1 • Three layers of a slide.

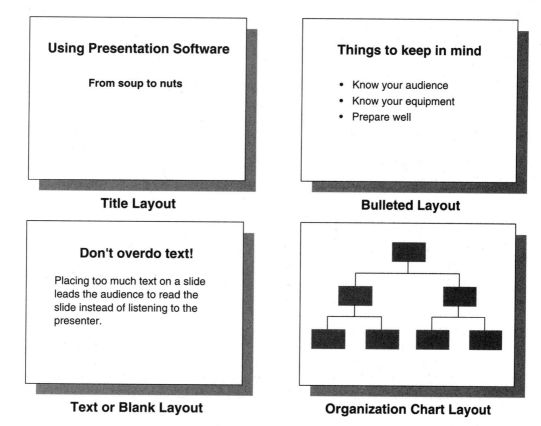

Figure 10-2 • Some slide layouts.

THE LAYOUT LAYER

Although in a visual production the background should be constant, the message the user wishes to convey on each individual slide often necessitates a different positioning of the objects (pieces of text and images) that make up the slide. For example, the first slide in a visual presentation is often a title slide. Obviously, the title should predominate, although one's name and credentials may also be included. A slide with bullet points pertaining to the information to be delivered may be next. To facilitate the construction of such slides, presentation software provides a set of ready-made templates, or layouts, from which the user selects. The array of layouts varies from program to program, but there are generally preformatted layouts for a title slide, bulleted slide, text slide, organizational chart slide, and a blank (Figure 10-2).

Once a layout is chosen, directions for entering text appear on the screen. Text is usually entered into rectangles (*text boxes*). Although these rectangles remain visible to help in creating the slide, one may leave any of them blank; these rectangles will not be visible when the slide is shown or printed (Figure 10-3). Each layout has a pre-selected text **font** and size, but these features are modifiable.

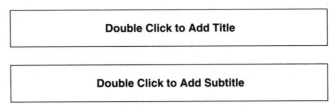

If left empty, the rectangles will NOT print or be seen when the slide is shown.

Figure 10-3 • Title slide layout as it appears when creating a slide.

THE EDITING LAYER

As with word processing, several different views can be used in editing. Entering text is done in either the slide view that focuses on the slide, the outline view that focuses on the text being entered, or a combination view (may be called *normal*) that allows users to enter both notes and information on the slide. There is also a slide sorter view that depicts 12 slides at once. This view allows a user to move, insert, copy, edit, or delete *complete slides*. The play or slide-show view projects the slide on the monitor as it will appear during a presentation. One can switch between views by clicking on View on the menu line and selecting the appropriate view, or by using icons on the screen.

Creating a slide may be done in any but the slide sorter or slide projection views. In either the combination or slide view, the user can enter text directly onto the slide. In both modes, text may also be entered on the outline panel. In any slide creation view, moving between levels on bulleted slides follows the same principles as using the outline function in a word processing program. Tapping the enter key allows the user to enter the next point, tapping the tab key will create the appropriate bullet for the next lower level, and tapping shift-tab creates the correct bullet for the next highest level.

In the outline view, moving to the next slide can be done by using shift-tab to move to the top or title level. In any of the editing views, a new slide may always be made by clicking on the appropriate icon. A new slide may also be started by clicking on Insert on the menu line and selecting new slide. The vertical scroll bar provides the opportunity to move between slides that have already been created.

IMAGES

Images on a slide may be custom drawn, inserted from **clip art**, pasted from the clipboard, scanned and imported, or downloaded from the Web. Most images may also be resized and moved on the slide. If an image consists of many parts, sometimes it is necessary to select the entire image by tapping Ctrl + A, then holding down the shift key and deselecting other objects. Once selected, the objects may be grouped into one object or may be moved or resized as a unit.

The **clip art**, or a small drawing that has already been created and is in a computer file that comes with a presentation program, is often the preferred source of images. Other images are also usually available from the vendor's Web Site. These generally are royalty free, but other images found on the Internet may not be. Many types of clip art have limitations on how they can be used. If one is buying a package of clip art, be sure to read the fine print before you purchase the software.

Occasionally an image may not project well when one is using visuals. To prevent this from marring a presentation, check the appearance of the slide in the Play or Show view before committing to using the visual in the presentation. Generally, if an image looks good in playback mode, it will project well, but if possible check the image with the projection equipment, and the version of the presentation software that will be used in the presentation.

Although using a scanned image, clip art, or images from the Internet makes it possible to include very detailed pictures, these images can sometimes confuse the learner. For example, in presenting information about circulation through the heart, a detailed picture would probably not aid understanding as much as a schematic drawing that only depicted the four chambers and the veins and arteries leading into and out of the heart.

When adding images, remember that the point of visuals is to communicate a message to the audience. Clip art can be appropriate if it emphasizes that message; when it is only used to enliven a slide, it seldom adds much to the presentation. A little variety, especially when it pertains to the message, can be helpful, but be careful not to distract the audience.

CHARTS AND TABLES

A table or chart is often clearer in communicating meaning than text. When using a table, one is limited in the size that can be created. Presentation software provides the ability to import a graph or data directly from a spreadsheet as well as the ability to copy and paste the graph.

SPECIAL EFFECTS

Although one can add special effects independent of the visuals, those that are made possible by presentation software are generally available only when the computer itself is used for the presentation. When doing a computer slide show, especially when using special effects such as sound and video clips, the complete presentation should be tested on the equipment that will actually be used during the presentation itself. It is also important to use moderation with any special effects. Like images, special effects can be helpful to some messages, but they become distracting when used inappropriately.

Sound
Sound can be added by recording it using a microphone attached to the computer and special software, or through a sound file. Some sound files can be found on the Internet, whereas others can be purchased as software. After the file is selected, follow the directions prescribed by the presentation package you are using to attach the sound to a slide. The steps for doing this can be found by searching for "add sound" in the help feature.

Video

Video clips are equally easy to insert. The video, however, must be in digital format instead of the analog mode used for ordinary video tape. Conversions from analog tape can be made, or cameras that record directly to the computer can be used. If one is planning to add video, limit its length to 45 to 60 seconds; any length beyond that often distracts the audience. As with sound, before using video in a presentation, check the equipment. Have a copy of the presentation without video available in case the video portion of the presentation equipment fails on the day of the presentation.

Transitions

A transition is the way a slide makes its entrance. There are many different types of transitions. Some cause a slide to fade in, some cause the slide to appear first at the center, then expand the view, and others cause the slide to sweep across the screen. These transitions and more are available in presentation software. Transitions can be dramatic, enhance your message, or distract the audience. The best rule is to use them sparingly.

Animation

Often referred to as custom animation, this term is used somewhat optimistically in the more well-known presentation software. Generally, animation takes the form of progressive disclosure, although newer versions of presentation software offer others. Progressive disclosure is a technique in which one item at a time is revealed until all the items are displayed. When revealing bulleted points, for instance, those that have been discussed can be dimmed or converted to a different color while the current point has center stage. Custom animation can also be used with images.

There are also many options for how bulleted items will be revealed. Some of these options are for the item to slide in from any direction, bounce in, fade in, or even curve in. Like all options, this feature should be used judiciously. Progressive disclosure can be used with 35-mm slides and transparencies but requires a different slide for each point.

Animated gifs (a type of image files from the Web that show movement) can be used in some versions of some presentation program presentations. Unless it is known for sure that this will work on the computer you will use for presentation, do not plan a presentation around the movement in the image.

SPEAKER NOTES

Speaker notes are entered as text while designing the slide. Although the notes are not seen on the slide, they are connected to the slide in a way that allows them to be printed for use either as notes during the presentation, when rehearsing, or for handouts. Some presentation programs allow the slides and notes to be sent to a word processor as a table. Once in the word processor, the table, notes, and visuals can be edited. This can be used to produce an instructional booklet or to print slides and notes for use in rehearsing the show and to use as Plan B in case the technology fails.

 ## Presentation

There are two options for showing the slides with a computer. First, open the program and play the slides, second, compile the show so it will play on a computer that does not have the program that was used to create the show. If one is planning to present the slide show on a different computer, be certain that the file does not get too big to move. The size of the file varies with the number of slides, but it varies even more with their contents. Adding images of any size increases the size of a slide. Additionally, if one is compiling a show, the resulting file can be two or three times the size of the original file. The size of the file a user can transport depends on the mode of transfer. If using a Zip or Jaz drive, flash memory, or CD-ROM, the problem is not likely to occur, but the computer used to present the show must have the capability of reading the storage device that is used. If a 3-1/2-inch disk is the only alternative, it is possible to use the slide sorter to break the show into several parts that can be reassembled when on the new computer. E-mailing the file as an attachment to someone at the site of the show is another possibility.

NONLINEAR PRESENTATION

When giving a presentation, you should be somewhat flexible. Some audiences may ask questions, others do not. A presenter can also misjudge the time needed for the presentation. If using the computer for the presentation, these eventualities can be handled easily. Depending on the program, the presenter can prepare a hidden slide to show if a specific question is asked or if time permits. One popular presentation program will advance (or retreat) to a specific slide when that number is typed and followed by tapping the Enter key. With this program, keeping a list of slide numbers while presenting will allow a presenter to easily show any slide in the show.

CREATING 35-MM SLIDES OR TRANSPARENCIES

Creating 35-mm slides using the slides from a presentation program is also possible. Some institutions provide an in-house slide development service that uses the file to create the slides. Commercial slide services are also available. Many services accept the file by modem transmission. Transparencies may also be created with a presentation program, but because a transparency is generally in **portrait** orientation and slides are in **landscape**, translating a slide show to a transparency requires editing the slides (see Figure 5-5).

TRANSFERRING TO THE WEB

Presentation programs contain an option to create a Web based show from the slides. Use of this feature requires special considerations. Few slide shows have much meaning in an independent mode. Most depend on the presenter to interpret the points on each slide. Therefore, if creating a Web-based slide show, create the slides so that each one presents a complete message and together they form a whole. Additionally, slides created with a presentation program are graphic objects and create large files. To view the show a user must download each slide individually. The result may be that downloading is a very slow process for those using **plain old telephone service** (**POTS**) with the result that few will watch the entire show. There are usually much better alternatives for creating a Web presentation.

Designing the Slides

The overall design principles that one uses often depend on how and where the slide will be used.[1] Backgrounds should be selected with this in mind. There are many backgrounds from which to select, some of which may detract from the message. For best visibility select a dark background and light text if the slides will be presented in a dark room, and a light background and dark text if a light room will be the site of the presentation.

Transparencies present their own design requirements. Before starting to enter any content, select the portrait page orientation to match the way transparencies are shown. The use of a background should be limited to just an object with no background color. This can be accomplished by changing the color schemes of the selected master or by not using any background. Unless a color printer will be used to print the transparencies, use black text, but in any case use dark-colored text. If colored images are used, check the slides in black and white before printing.

If, after creating slides, the background is not suitable, it can be changed for all the slides without changing any of the slide contents. Changing the background may, however, affect how the various layouts and text are positioned; therefore, it is necessary to check all slides after changing a background.

TEXT

When placing text on visuals, include only the essential elements of concepts. State ideas as though they were headlines. A visual is not meant to give the entire idea but rather to serve as a focus to assist the audience in following your presentation. Visuals are also helpful to the presenter as a guide to the oral presentation.

Audiences should be able to get the point of the visual within the first 5 seconds after it appears. It is argued that a presenter should be quiet for those 5 seconds to allow the audience to grasp the point (Radel, 1997). To accomplish this, it is necessary to limit the text. One way to determine whether you have too much information on a visual image is to place the information on a 4×6-inch card and try to read it from a distance of about 5 to 6 feet.

Never write the presentation on a series of slides that are intended to be read to the audience. Audiences can read faster than a speaker can talk and may become torn between reading ahead and listening (Radel, 1997). This practice also leads the speaker to pay more attention to the slides than to the audience.

A facet of presentation packages that can be both advantage and disadvantage is the number of fonts available, many of which are unsuitable for text in a projected visual. Even though it is always tempting to select a "jazzy" font in the hope that it will enliven a presentation, too often this choice creates readability problems. When making a selection, remember that fonts can elicit an emotional response from the audience; thus, choose one that is not only visually appealing but that elicits the desired response. If it is a factual presentation, keep the font simple. In a small group, a font that appears more personal may be more appropriate.

[1] Although a presentation program can be used to create many types of visuals, the term *slides* will be used here to denote any visuals created with a presentation program.

Font	Comparison
Kaufmann at 12 points Times New Roman at 12 points Arial at 12 points	*Presentation Skills* Presentation Skills Presentation Skills
Kaufmann at 16 points Times New Roman at 16 points Arial at 16 points	*Presentation Skills* Presentation Skills Presentation Skills

Figure 10-4 • Different fonts in the same point size.

The background templates for presentation programs have preselected fonts that are generally suitable for presentation. It is possible to change these font styles either for an individual slide or the entire presentation. Changing a font may disturb the layout on some slides due to the difference in size of the text in different fonts (Figure 10-4). The measurement unit for text size is points. **Point size**, however, is not always an accurate guide. Some fonts at 12 points, despite being one-sixth of an inch in height, are very difficult to read.[2] This is due to what is called the x factor, or the height of lower case letters. In making transparencies, do not use any font that makes the printed text smaller than 1/4 inch. Thus, the smallest font that should be used in making transparencies is 18 points. For computer or 35-mm slides, the smallest easily readable text size is 24 points.

Some fonts (e.g., Garamond, and to a lesser degree, Times Roman) have projections from the type-body called *serifs* that are fine strokes across the ends of the main strokes of a character. Serifs create softer edges to the characters, which adds to readability on paper. When they are projected, however, they may have a tendency to look fuzzy. For projected visuals use a sans serif (i.e., without serifs) font such as Arial (Figure 10-5). This font follows the basic rule in choosing a display font—that the letters appear crisp and clean.

The appearance of text can be altered with attributes other than the type of font. Adding boldface text is one way to emphasize a point, as are underlining and italicizing. Italicizing, however, tends to make text more difficult to read; if it is used, give the audience more time to read the slide. If a point or points are emphasized with any of the above-mentioned attributes, be consistent throughout the presentation—that is, use the same attribute for the same type of information throughout.

COLOR

Although color can be used to draw attention to a feature, it should never be used as the only distinguishing characteristic. As with fonts, it is important to be consistent in using color. After an audience grasps the implications of a given color, the visuals are more easily comprehended. Although the eye can perceive millions of colors, screen colors should

---

[2] Most printed documents from computers are set in either 10 or 12 point.

Sans-serif font: Arial	Generally easier to read online
Serif font: Times New Roman	Easier to read in a print format

Figure 10-5 • Comparison of sans-serif and serif font.

be limited to about six, which number is all that the eye can track at one glance (Faioloa & DeBloois, 1988).

Color, like text fonts, also has an emotional appeal. Red can be seen as exciting or as the color of fire and blood, whereas green is usually seen as calming. The meaning of colors varies with cultures. Purple may indicate spirituality, mystery, aristocracy and passion in some cultures; in others it may symbolize mourning, death, nausea, conceit, and pomposity (Morton, 1998).

Color combinations should be selected that are compatible but offer a contrast. When placed on top of one another, some colors, such as red on black, give a three-dimensional appearance that may make an object appear closer than the background. Additionally, objects sometimes appear larger on one color than another. Reading accuracy is best when the colors used for background and text are on the opposite sides of the color wheel that is found in the Font specifications of many programs. Keep in mind that 9% of the population has some kind of color perception problem, usually a deficiency in discriminating red from green. When using a gradient background (Figure 10-6), it is imperative to use a very readable text and to test the slide for readability. Many of the backgrounds that are provided with presentation programs are gradient backgrounds.

It is important to test color combinations. If using a presentation program to make 35-mm slides, if possible make a test slide and check to see how well the slide projects using a slide projector. It can also be helpful, if using a computer presentation, to test the slides with the projector. If this is impossible, find out the resolution and number of colors supported by the projection unit. If it is lower than the computer monitor itself, set the video output to a lower resolution when creating the visuals.

Figure 10-6 • A gradient background.

ORGANIZING A PRESENTATION

Creating good visuals does not alone ensure a good presentation. The visuals and the presentation must reinforce each other. This requires good planning, preparation, and rehearsal. The first step in preparation is to understand what message the presentation will be trying to communicate. In making this decision, take the characteristics of your audience into consideration. An approach for an audience of laypeople will differ from one given to an audience of professional peers. Similarly, an approach needs to take into account whether the audience agrees with the conclusions in your topic or has not yet made a decision.

One rule of thumb in presentations is to first provide an overall introductory view of what will be said, follow with the material, and then summarize what has been said. When planning a presentation, keep in mind that most people attending a presentation will remember no more than five key points (Feierman, n.d.). To ensure that important points are remembered, start planning for the presentation by stating the five key points that the audience should retain. Build an outline around these points.

Creating the Visual Presentation

After the overall planning is done and the slides are in the desired order, a background can be added, images finished, the text smoothed out, and any desired progressive disclosure or slide transitions added. In deciding which features of a presentation program to use, keep the objective of getting a message across to the audience as the primary goal. After finishing the preparation of the visuals, rehearse the presentation by using them in computer format. Make any necessary changes, and then, if using 35-mm slides or transparencies, prepare to make the conversion. Make any necessary handouts or notes, and rehearse before the actual presentation.

Creating Handouts

It is very easy to print the slides in a handout mode with room for notes next to them. This type of handout has drawbacks, however. With your entire presentation in hand, the audience may decide to not stay for the presentation. Or, as in the case of converting slides to a Web-based presentation, the slides may not contain the information you wish the audience to retain. Create handouts that are as well-thought out as the presentation itself. When the handouts do not mimic what is onscreen but are designed to allow the audience to follow the handout, the attention of your audience will likely increase (Chronister, 2002). Leaving some blanks for pieces of information that will be added during the presentation can transform the audience from passive to active as it listens to fill in the blanks.

 ## Copyright

Although most issues about copyright in presentations or Web pages center around images, the unauthorized use of text can also violate copyright laws. Copyright is protection given to creators of artistic work including text, film, music, and images, whether published or unpublished, to decide how and where their work may be used. Since April 1, 1989, almost everything created privately and originally is copyrighted whether it

TABLE 10-1 ● *Highlights of Fair Use*		
Factors	**More Likely to Be**	
	Fair Use	*Unfair Use*
Use made of object	Educational, non-profit	Commercial
Nature of work used	Fact	Imaginative
How much is used	Small amount	Large amount
Effect on future value of the work	Original is out of print or otherwise unobtainable	Competes with sales of original publication
		Avoids required royalty payment

carries a notice or not. This includes e-mail. Assume that anything you see published or on a Web site is copyrighted. Exceptions are any work created by the United States Government.

Fair use is a limitation placed on exclusive use of a work that applies in some circumstances. Unfortunately, no undisputed definition of fair use exists; rather, it is an area with increasingly contested boundaries, and some have said that those boundaries should be crossed at one's own risk. There are, however, some guidelines based on four factors: the character of the use, the nature of the work used, the amount of the work that was used, and the effect that the use will have on the market for the original work. Table 10-1 addresses some factors that may impinge on a decision about whether a use is fair or not. Perhaps the best rule is, when in doubt, ask permission.

Images and cartoons are probably the most frequently used items in presentations or Web pages that violate copyright laws. The rules about images state that unless you created the image, you do not own it. Unless an image is stated to be in the public domain, assume that it is copyrighted. Many Web sites that feature images are rather vague about who owns the rights to the image. Clipart that comes with most presentation programs can be freely used for any use, educational or commercial.

Summary

Even a small presentation given to a group of colleagues will be better received if the appropriate visuals are used. As a nurse progresses up the career ladder, knowing how to make impressive presentations is an aid to advancement. Professional effective communication is the key to a successful career. Although several vendors make presentation packages, they all have similarities. Basically, these packages facilitate the job of creating good visuals by providing a constant background for the visual and tailored layouts. It is possible to modify any of these things at any time. Although there are many options available, such as adding images or special effects such as sound, video clips, animation, and progressive disclosure, they should be used only to enhance the message. In the same vein, select colors, fonts, backgrounds, and layouts to enrich a message (Table 10-2). All presentations need planning and organizing. Handouts

TABLE 10-2 • *Basic Rules for Creating Visuals*	
Designing Visuals	
Text	Limit to 6 or 7 words in a line and 6 lines on a slide
Fonts	Choose a sans-serif font for projected visuals. Limit number of different fonts used.
Font Size	Transparencies $\geq$ 18 points
	Sides $\geq$ 24 points
Colors	
Text and background	Contrasting—opposite sides of color wheel
For emphasis	Be consistent
Number used	Total of no more than 5 or 6

should reflect what the audience needs to take away from the presentation, and not just the slides.

There are several issues involved in creating a presentation. A word processed file created from the presentation program is helpful in rehearsing the presentation when the computer is not available. Additionally, it provides an excellent back-up if the technology fails. Ensuring that there are no copyright infringements is also important in preparing a presentation.

connection—⌐ **For definitions of bolded key terms, visit the online glossary available at http://connection.lww.com/go/thede.**

CONSIDERATIONS AND EXERCISES

1. Describe the purpose for each of the three layers in a presentation program.

2. Experiment with different backgrounds and decide whether they would be desirable in a specific type of presentation, such as a research report, a class project, or a welcoming speech. If they are not appropriate, how could they be modified to be more useful for your purpose?

3. Experiment with adding text and images to the different slide layouts in the presentation program you have on your computer.

4. Using the Help feature, search for the term "animation" and animate some text in a bulleted slide.

5. You have found a cartoon on the Internet and wish to use it in a presentation. Under what conditions should it be used?

6. Create a three- or four-slide presentation on a topic of your choosing. Add a background and use more than the title and bullet layouts. Add an image. Use the principles of good design found in Table 10-2.

REFERENCES

Chronister, T. (2002, May). Technology should not keep audiences in the dark. *Presentations*, 62.

Faioloa, T., & DeBloois, M. L. (1988). Designing a visual factors-based screen display interface: The new role of the graphic technologist. *Educational Technology, 28*(8), 12–21.

Feierman, A. (n.d.). *The art of communicating effectively.* Retrieved May 18, 2002 from http://www.presentingsolutions.com/effectivepresentations.html.

Morton, J. (1998). *Color, the chameleon of the web.* Retrieved May 18, 2002 from http://www.colormatters.com/chameleon.html.

Radel, J. (1997). *Effective presentations.* Retrieved May 16, 2002 from http://www.kumc.edu/SAH/OTEd/jradel/effective.html.

Visual Presentation Issues. (2001). Retrieved October 15, 2002 from http://www.agocg.ac.uk/reports/mmedia/video3/app3.htm

Working With Numbers: Letting the Software Do the Hard Part

Objectives
After studying this chapter you will be able to:

1. *Identify similarities between word processing and spreadsheet software.*

2. *Use computer conventions to create mathematical formulas for computer applications.*

3. *Explore functions specific to spreadsheets.*

4. *Select the appropriate chart to communicate a specific point.*

Numbers are often part of the information nurses need to manage. Computers, together with specialized software, provide freedom from the drudgery of manual calculations and make managing numerical information much easier. The first spreadsheet program, developed in 1979, greatly accelerated the acceptance of computers in the business world. What is most remarkable about the first spreadsheet is that the design is so functional that few changes have been made to it over the years. Instead, many more features have been added, such as graphs and components, which make it easier to enter formulas. Because the design is so intuitive, there is probably the least variation in performing functions in different vendors' spreadsheets than in any other application type.

Spreadsheets are not the only type of application program that simplify managing numerical data. There are programs, called financial managers, that allow checkbooks to be balanced and the management of a personal budget, including providing help in categorizing items to facilitate tax preparation. There are also programs that use data from a financial manager or spreadsheet to create and print tax returns. Another type of numbers manager is statistical packages.

 Spreadsheets

A spreadsheet is a table with rectangles, or cells, which are capable of containing data or a formula to produce information or knowledge from the data in other cells. In Figure 11-1, notice the top row above the cells consists of letters in alphabetical order and the first column contains

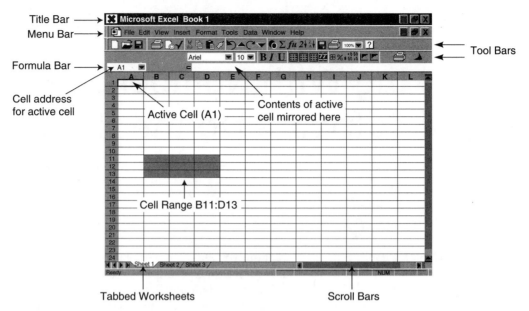

Figure labels:
- Title Bar
- Menu Bar
- Formula Bar
- Cell address for active cell
- Active Cell (A1)
- Contents of active cell mirrored here
- Cell Range B11:D13
- Tool Bars
- Tabbed Worksheets
- Scroll Bars

Figure 11-1 • Spreadsheet screen.

numbers that increase in increments of one. The cells are named by the letter at the top of the column and the number of the row, hence the cell in the upper left corner is named A1. In some spreadsheets, the **insertion point**, or **cursor**, changes shape depending on what activity it is prepared to do. When moving around the cells, the insertion point may be a cross, but it may switch to an I bar when entering or editing text.

The Screen

The spreadsheet screen is similar to all application programs associated with a **graphical user interface** (GUI). At first glance, the main difference between a spreadsheet and a word processor seems to be that the document screen in a spreadsheet is a table. Many of the familiar icons used in word processing are in their usual places, such as the title bar (Figure 11-1). There are, however, some differences. For instance, there is a formula bar under the toolbar. At the bottom of the screen there are tabs.[1] For behavioral similarities between word processors and spreadsheets, see Table 11-1.

VOCABULARY

The vocabulary of spreadsheets is not very complex. A *cell* is the name given to the rectangles in the table. A *row* is a horizontal group of cells, and a *column* is a vertical group of cells. **Cell address** is the name given to a cell, and it is derived from the letter of the column and the number of the row where it is located. The **active cell** (*A1* in Figure 11-1) is

---

[1] In a GUI, a tab is a *bump* shaped like the protrusion on manila folders on which a label is placed. Clicking on a tab gives access to the screen (worksheet) represented by that tab.

TABLE 11-1 ● *Functions That Spreadsheets Share With Word Processing Programs*	
Function	**Characteristics Special to Spreadsheet**
Resizing and moving windows and graphics	No differences. Select object or window and drag to resize.
Toolbars	Like most application products, can be edited to suit working preferences.
Drop-down boxes and dialog boxes	Identical to word processors.
Editing	Delete will delete the contents of the entire cell unless you are entering or editing data. Backspace works identically to other programs when cursor is an I-bar type. Data can be entered with the numeric keypad.
Enter key	Moves the active cell to the one beneath the current active cell.
Selecting	Can select, cut copy and paste pieces of text, a cell, group of contiguous cells known as a range, or graphic objects.
Cut, copy, and paste	Identical to word processors.
Click and drag	Identical to word processors.
Undo and redo	Can only undo the last change.
Create files	Files are workbooks. Workbooks can contain many worksheets.
Automatic backups	Identical to those in word processors.
More than one document open at the same time.	Can have several workbooks and worksheets within a workbook open at one time. (Like all programs, if you open more than the RAM in your computer will support, you will notice that all actions are slowed.)
Navigation	Similar to tables in word processing, except for enter key. Enter key moves down one row. Tab key moves active cell to the right, Shift-Tab moves active cell to the left. Arrow keys and page up and down work identically. Ctrl-Home goes to the beginning of worksheet and Ctrl-End to the end.
Horizontal Scroll Bar	Is on the right side of the bottom of the screen to make room for the tabs for the different work sheets in a workbook.
Formatting Attributes including changing the appearance, size or type of font. Text justification	Can also format the contents of the cell, i.e., specify that numbers in selected cells should contain decimals, dollar signs, and the like.
Graphics	Graphics, besides clip art or drawings can consist of charts. Spreadsheets are excellent at creating charts (graphs).
Printing	If the table will not fit horizontally on one page, the columns will be printed on another page. This may break up the continuity of the table. The best results occur when a range of cells is designated to be printed. Keeping the size of a worksheet to a printable size is another option. The print option will print selected cells, the current worksheet, or the whole workbook.
Speller	Works almost identically to that in a word processor.
Templates	Same principles.
Web access	As in word processing, you can link to the Web or publish a table, chart, graphic, or any combination to the Web.
Record macros	Same principles. Be careful if you receive a macro from another source; macros may harbor viruses. Scan the file with an up-to-date virus checker before using it.

analogous to the insertion point in other programs and is the location where any information entered will be placed. Besides being visible in the table by bold lines, the contents of the active cell are mirrored on the formula bar line. A **range of cells** is a group of contiguous cells, for example, cells B11:D13. The range of B11 to D13 in Figure 11-1 would be expressed as B11:D13 or B11..D13, depending on the spreadsheet application's publisher. Users can name ranges of cells and use this name in commands instead of the cell location.

Two terms that may at first seem a little confusing are **worksheet** and **workbook**. A worksheet refers to one table, whereas a workbook consists of one or more worksheets. On a worksheet, there is room for 256 columns and 65,536 rows. When working on a project, however, it is advisable to keep the size of a worksheet smaller than this. A spreadsheet that is using 256 columns, unless it is used for research data, may be more manageable if it is broken down into several worksheets. The worksheets are indicated by the tabs on the bottom of the screen. A user moves between the worksheets by clicking on the tab. To name a worksheet, double-click on the tab and enter a name. When they are saved, worksheets create a workbook.[2] Spreadsheets also allow users to have several workbooks, each containing many worksheets, open at the same time.

The contents of a spreadsheet are not confined to a table. It is possible to add pictures or charts to any worksheet.[3] These items can be positioned next to the data in the table to which they apply, or they can be placed on a separate worksheet. Worksheets do not need to remain in the order in which they were created. They can be placed in any order in the workbook by dragging the tab for that worksheet to the desired location.

There are times when a spreadsheet is used as a template for others to use. In these cases, it is an excellent idea to use a separate worksheet to document what has been done and what is expected of the user. Any spreadsheet that will be used repeatedly should also have documentation. Documentation helps the user remember the assumptions on which various items are based.

USES FOR SPREADSHEETS

Although spreadsheets are used extensively for budgets and the management of financial records, they are useful whenever calculations are needed. For example, a nursing information system could link to a spreadsheet that had ready-made drug calculation formulas available. Before formulas are used in this fashion, however, they should be triple-checked for accuracy. Additionally, the numbers that will be entered into the formula should be very visible on the screen for the user to check the accuracy of the numbers that he or she entered.

The real power of a spreadsheet is derived not only from its ability to organize and edit data but from its ability to recalculate when a number in a referenced cell is changed. A **referenced cell** is one that is included in a formula in another cell. For example, in Figure 11-2, the cell D1 contains a formula. It references the cells B1 and C1. Any changes made to the contents of either of these cells will cause the number in cell D1 to change. Notice that the formula is seen on the formula bar.

[2] The name *notebook* is used by some spreadsheets to denote this same concept.

[3] *Chart* is the name computer programs give to a graph, such as a bar or line graph.

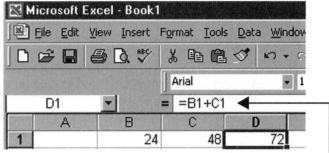

Figure 11-2 • Referenced cells.

Referenced Cells

FORMULAS

A spreadsheet formula is a mathematical equation that provides instructions to the computer for processing the data. Formulas can be either relative or absolute (Figure 11-3). A relative formula, which is the default, when copied to another cell, adjusts to the move by changing the referenced cells. An absolute formula retains the original cells when moved.

Errors can creep into a spreadsheet when entering cell addresses in a formula. To prevent this, spreadsheets provide a point-and-click method of entering cell addresses. After entering the symbol indicating that a formula is about to be entered, (e.g., an equal sign or the "@") put the mouse pointer on the first cell the address of which will be in the formula and click once with the left mouse button. The cell address appears in the formula. Enter the necessary mathematical symbol, then point and click at the next cell needed. When the formula is complete, tap the enter key.

	A	B	C	D
1				
2		24	48	B2 + C2
3		64	36	B3 + C3
4				

	A	B	C	D
1				
2		24	48	B2 + C2
3		64	36	B2 + C2
4				

A. Relative Formula

B. Absolute Formula

In A, the formula in cell D2 was copied to cell D3. Because it was a relative formula it automatically changed its contents from B2 + C2 to B3 + C3. In B, the formula in cell D2 was designated an absolute formula. When copied to cell D3 the contents did not change.

Figure 11-3 • Relative and referenced formulas.

To simplify the use of some common formulas, spreadsheets provide many that are already constructed, called functions.[4] They include a wide variety for many purposes, some of which are statistical. The statistical functions beyond simple descriptive statistics are not as easy to use as those in a statistical package. When reading about functions, the word **argument** may be used. Argument, in computer instructions, means the data the user furnishes on which the program will perform the stated function. While setting up formulas to average some numbers, for instance, instructions in the help menu might read AVERAGE (argument1, argument2, . . .). This means that the user substitutes the numbers that need to be averaged for argument 1, enters a comma, then enters the number for argument 2, and so on. The number in the argument can be a number, a cell, or even a range. The parentheses are an integral part of the formula, and must not be omitted.

Creating Formulas

The principles and symbols of formula calculation are identical in all computer programs. The characters used to communicate that the computer should perform a specific calculation, such as multiplying or dividing, are not, however, always the same as the ones used on paper. An asterisk (*) is used to denote multiplication. If the familiar X were used, the computer would be unable to distinguish whether the keystroke refers to the character "x" or a symbol for multiplication. A computer formula for the multiplication of 5 times 50 becomes 5*50. Assuming the numbers were in cells C3 and C5, the command becomes (C3*C5). To write this formula in a spreadsheet, enter the formula, preceded by either an equal sign (=), or the (@), depending on the publisher of the spreadsheet program, for example, (=C3*C5) or (@C3*C5).

There is no divide key on the computer. To signal division, the computer uses the forward slash (/) (located under the question mark). To instruct the computer to divide 10 by 5, the formula is 10/5. A formula entered for division looks like (=C3/B2) or (@C3/B2).

The results of division are not always an integer or whole number (Table 11-2). In a formula, specify whether the result is to be the integer (whole number with any decimals truncated) or to be rounded to a specified decimal place. Asking for just the integer or rounding to a given decimal place are two different operations. This occurs because, the integer truncates or cuts off the fractional part of the answer and shows the largest whole number that is the result of dividing the two cells. Rounding produces accuracy to the decimal point specified.

To raise a number to another power, called exponentiation, use the caret (^), which is located over the 6. In telling the computer to raise 2 to the power of 4, the formula looks like (=2^4) or to raise the number in cell C3 to the power of 4, (=C3^4).

Priority of Mathematical Operations

In performing arithmetical computations, computers do not follow a strict left-to-right order. Three factors determine the order in which mathematical procedures will be performed:

---

[4] Be careful when entering functions. If a space is not placed after the function name and before the open parentheses in the function, it may not calculate.

TABLE 11-2 ● *Different Types of Arithmetic Division in Computer Programs*

Divide the Number	By	Answer		
		As an integer	*Round to 2 decimal places*	*Round to 0 decimal places*
29	5	5	5.80	6
32	6	5	5.33	5
Formula		INT(29/5)	ROUND (29/5,2)	ROUND (29/5,0)
Spreadsheet example		INT(B3/B5)	ROUND ((B3/B5),2)	ROUND((B3/B5),0)

▼ The kind of computation required.
▼ Nesting, or the placing of an expression within parentheses.
▼ Left-to-right placement of the expressions in the command.

The computer arbitrarily performs mathematical operations in the following order:

▼ Anything in parentheses is performed first.
▼ Exponentiation is done next.
▼ Multiplication and division follow in a left-to-right manner.
▼ Addition and subtraction are performed last.

If there are ties (two commands to multiply, or one to multiply and one to divide), a left-to-right order prevails (Table 11-3). For example, in the expression "15/3 * 5" the 15 is divided by 3 and then multiplied by 10 for an answer of 25. If, however, the formula were written with a parentheses as 15/(3*5) the first operation would be to multiply the 3 by 5, hence the answer would be 1. In the command 5 + 4 * 3, the multiplication of 4 by 3 would precede the addition of the 5. The result of this statement would be 17, not 27.

For some formulas, it is necessary that the calculations not be done in the order just specified. In these cases, the formulas are nested. For example, if it were necessary to add the contents of two cells before dividing by another cell, the addition operation would be enclosed in parentheses. To illustrate the formula would be written "(6 + 8)/2." If the parentheses are omitted, the 8 would be divided by 2 and then added to the 6 for an answer of 10. When written with the parentheses the answer is 14. Parentheses can also be nested. In this case, the calculation in the innermost set of parentheses will be performed first. In the expression (3*(4+6))/2, the first thing the computer will do is add the 4 and 6, then multiply the resulting sum of 10 by 3, divide the resulting 30 by 2, for an answer of 15. Many spreadsheet users follow the principle of nesting any operation. Instead of

TABLE 11-3 ● *Acronym to Remember the Order in Which Computers Perform Calculations*

Please	Excuse	My	Dear	Aunt	Sally
		Equal (left to right)		*Equal (left to right)*	
Parentheses	Exponentiation	Multiplication	Division	Addition	Subtraction

writing 5*3 + 6*4 the formula would be written (5*3) + (6*4). The answer will be the same in either case, but when parentheses are used it is easier to find mistakes in a formula. These rules, which follow algebraic protocols, are used in all application packages that allow calculations such as spreadsheets, statistical packages, and databases. When using the acronym (or mnemonic) in Table 11-3, remember that when two mathematical operations are equal, such as multiplication and division, the calculations will be left to right.

OTHER SPREADSHEET FEATURES

Besides the normal functions that can be applied across the board in most application programs, such as changing the font, point size, or changing the color of the background or text, spreadsheets possess some unique characteristics that require specialized functions.

Formatting Cells with Type of Contents

There are generally two different types of contents in a spreadsheet cell: text or numbers. Numbers, depending on what they reference, can be formatted in different ways. If a number represents a dollar amount, the cell may be formatted to automatically add a dollar sign ($) to any number entered into that cell. If the number is the result of division, the cell may be formatted to only show a given number of decimals. Alternatively, the number may automatically be represented as a percentage (%). How cells are formatted varies with the specific spreadsheet, but all require that the cells to be formatted be selected, then the attribute applied. Search the help menu with the word "format" to discover how to perform this task.

Freezing Headings

When the rows in a spreadsheet become too numerous to be viewed on one screen, it becomes difficult to know what the numbers in each cell represent. Spreadsheets provide a way to freeze the headings, so they are always on the top or the left side of the screen. To learn how to accomplish this task, use the help menu and search under the term "windows," then depending on the program's publisher, select "freeze windows" or "split window panes."

Automatic Entry of Data

In constructing a spreadsheet, there are times a user needs to have column headings that are used sequentially, such as the days of the week. Spreadsheets have a feature that allows the user to make a few entries and then have the computer complete the series. This function also works with numbers. The spreadsheet will even enter numbers that are not next to each other if the sequence increases or decreases by the same number (e.g., 2,4,6). It is also possible to create one's own list of data for automatic data entry. This function is indexed in the help menu under "automatic fill."

Database Functions

Spreadsheets are capable of some database functions. A user can re-sort the order of a range of cells or the entire spreadsheet, ask questions of the data, filter out unwanted items, and find specific items. As would be expected, none of the database functions are as robust as those in a true database, but they are functional for many simple operations.

A spreadsheet, or any range of cells, is also easily exported to the companion database (program that is part of the same office suite) for more extensive data manipulation. Any data that are structured in a table format, whether in a spreadsheet, a table in a word processor, a statistical package, or a database, can be easily passed from program to program.

Linking Cells From Other Sources

There are times when a value a user wants to include as part of a spreadsheet is in another workbook or another worksheet within the same workbook. It is very easy to use a cell as a value in another sheet or workbook, and this method is much less prone to error than trying to check the other sheet, copying the value, and entering it into a formula. When cells are linked, if the value in the linked cell changes, the change will be visible in the worksheet containing a reference to that cell. To use information from other worksheets or workbooks, check the help menu for "linking."

Other Features

There are many other spreadsheet functions, such as data entry forms. When data need to be entered onto a spreadsheet, a user can create a simple data entry form that will show only one row, called a record, at a time. When compared with database forms, spreadsheet forms are minimally functional.[5] Like word processing, printouts can be dressed up with headers, page numbers, and page breaks.

SPREADSHEETS AS DECISION MODELS

A natural tendency with spreadsheets is to regard them as an elaborate calculator and forget that the power of having all referenced cells recalculate after a change permits one to test different theories. Spreadsheets also provide other features to allow testing theories or solving problems. A cell with a formula, for instance, can be set so that the value in a referenced cell will change to produce a given value. This is useful when the answer needed is known but requires working backward to find it. Different spreadsheets give different names to these features. As in any other computer program, when using a spreadsheet for decision making, it is imperative to know the assumptions upon which the spreadsheet is based.

TIPS FOR BETTER SPREADSHEETS

Designing a spreadsheet that effectively communicates does not happen by adopting a casual approach. If spreadsheets are to be useful, they need to be well organized. If one is designing a complex sheet, a table of contents should be included. Explanations of any logic or assumptions should also be included on the first worksheet. If others will be using the spreadsheet, clear instructions and labels are imperative. Users of computer items rarely have the same viewpoint as the creator. For complex formulas, especially those that reference the results of formulas, test the formula with simple numbers, particularly if the spreadsheet will be used with many different values.

---

[5] If both the spreadsheet and database from the same office suites are available on the computer, it is possible to create a form in the database for use in entering data in the spreadsheet.

Another helpful organizing trick is to always start different blocks or sections on a worksheet at the right lower corner of the previous block or place it on another worksheet. This allows rows and columns to be inserted within a block without changing any other block. Above all, keep the spreadsheet as simple as possible. Organize work by using different worksheets in a workbook instead of placing everything on the same sheet. Probably the most helpful tool is to spend time planning a spreadsheet before the computer is even turned on. It is easier to make changes before any data have been entered than after a user has laboriously worked something through.

Statistical Packages

A statistical package takes data and performs the calculations required for a statistical test in a fraction of the time that it would take a user to even write down the formula. Statistical packages allow users to manipulate data, such as reversing the data for a variable—for example, taking all fives and changing them to ones while changing all ones into fives. It is also possible to write formulas that make other data changes.

STATISTICAL PACKAGE SCREENS

There are three screens in statistical software: a screen for entering variables, the data screen, and the output screen. When the variables are entered, their type is designated, for example whether the variable is scale, nominal, or ordinal. The screen where data are entered resembles a spreadsheet with a case occupying one row. When a statistical test is performed, a document is created that is visible on the output screen (Figure 11-4). The document is cumulative, or, in other words, the results of each statistical test are added to the document. The document in the output file can be printed, or it can be saved to a file. It is also possible to edit this file by selecting and deleting items. In some packages, although the file itself is in a proprietary format, it can be exported to an ASCII format, in which case it can be opened and edited by any word processor or text editor.

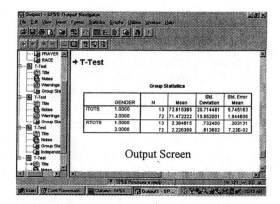

Figure 11-4 • Data and output screens for SPSS. Used with permission of SPSS, Inc.

VOCABULARY

The vocabulary of statistical packages is identical to that used for research. Before doing statistics, whether manually or with a computer, the user must be clear about the difference between independent and dependent variables. The user also must know which statistical tests are appropriate for which level of data, as well as the probability level that will satisfy the hypothesis.

TIPS FOR BEST USE

A statistical package will perform a given test when it believes that it has the appropriate information regardless of whether that test is valid for the hypothesis the user is testing. For example, if asked, a statistical test will provide an average, standard deviation, and variance for identification numbers, as well as test for differences or correlation if the user gives it another variable that meets the conditions of the test. The results, however, will be meaningless. There is no substitute for understanding the requirements of the statistical test needed and the assumptions.

Charts

A **chart** is a graphical presentation of a set of numbers, or what is sometimes called a graph. Charts are used to communicate meaning that can be difficult to understand from a raw set of numbers. Creating charts with a computer is relatively easy. Like statistical packages, a computer will produce any type of chart, whether it communicates anything meaningful or not. Using charts appropriately involves knowing the message that needs to be communicated and selecting the type of chart that best accomplishes this aim. Although word processors, databases, presentation packages, and spreadsheets all facilitate the creation of charts, spreadsheets in many cases have the most powerful chart-creating tools. Perhaps the biggest plus for creating charts in a spreadsheet is that if the numbers in the cells used to create the chart change, the chart automatically reflects this change.

VOCABULARY

To construct a meaningful chart, it is necessary to understand the vocabulary. Table 11-4 and Figure 11-5 can assist in this task.

TYPES OF CHARTS

Spreadsheets take the drudgery out of creating charts as well as present the option for creating not only many different types of charts, but of making them three dimensional, changing the orientation of the x axis to that of a vertical position, and combinations of all these factors. Each of these features can emphasize objects in the chart that may misconstrue the true meaning of the base numbers. Compare the two- and three-dimensional charts in Figure 11-5. In which does the figure for April stand out more? Most of these variations can be used in all charts. When using these variations, be certain that they reflect the point that needs to be communicated. As a user of charts, be aware that these distortions exist.

TABLE 11-4 • *Chart Vocabulary*	
Term	**Meaning**
X axis	The horizontal axis (line) of a bar, line or scatter graph, generally represents time values, categories, or divisions.
Y axis	The vertical axis (line) of a bar, line or scatter graph, most often used to represent amounts.
Data	Numbers without meaning, those that are unprocessed.
Data series or set	A set of numbers that will be represented in the chart, usually on the Y axis, or a group of items that will be represented on the X axis.
Axis title	The title for the information displayed on an axis.
Graph title	A description of the graph used to title the graph.
Legend	The visual representation of each item in the data series. May be a color, shape, or both.
Data point	The point where a number is plotted. It is the intersection of its value on the X and Y axis.
Data labels	Labels that show the actual value of a specific data, or the data points.
Two-dimensional charts	A chart that represents data on the X and Y axis.
Three-dimensional charts	A chart that adds a third axis, referred to as the Z axis. Can be very misleading, use only when there is a need to communicate an added dimension.

Pie Graphs

Pie graphs are used to communicate the proportion of various items in relation to the whole. They are designed to show percentages, not amounts. A pie chart may also be used to show a proportional relationship between a slice and the whole. Figure 11-6 illustrates different types of pie charts.

XY Charts

Bar and line charts are sometimes referred to as XY charts because they are constructed with X and Y axes. No matter which type is used, there are conventions that, when they are adhered to, create the most easily comprehensible charts. Placing amounts on the Y axis meets the common expectation that an upward movement is associated with an increase in amount, whereas downward movement indicates a decrease. When the X axis is used for the passage of time, the most effective form of communication is achieved when

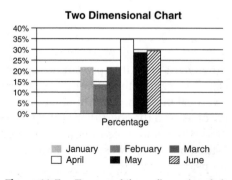
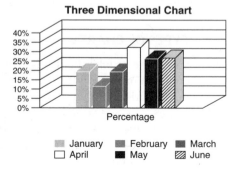

Figure 11-5 • Two- and three-dimensional charts.

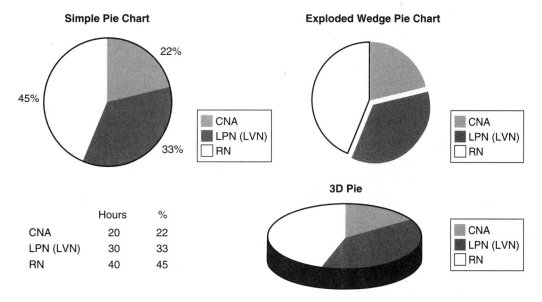

	Hours	%
CNA	20	22
LPN (LVN)	30	33
RN	40	45

Figure 11-6 • Pie charts. These pie charts all represent the same data. Notice how the exploded wedge looks almost as large as the piece at 7 o'clock to 12 o'clock. The same distortion occurs in the 3D pie. Without the percents it is difficult to determine which slice is largest in both the exploded wedge and the 3D pie.

the earliest time is placed on the left and time elapses to the right. To prevent a distortion of value, it is best if the Y axis starts with a zero. If this approach is not followed, include an explanation with the chart.

In an XY chart, data can be added to other data in two different ways: they can be stacked or they can be made cumulative. In a stacked chart, each data set uses as its baseline the previous data set. A stacked chart can also be a 100% chart where each data set is a percentage of the whole. In a cumulative chart, the data accumulate for each series. Figure 11-7 is a cumulative graph.

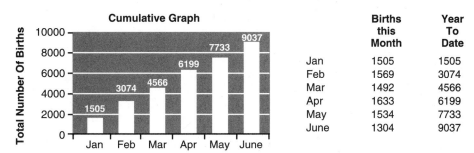

	Births this Month	Year To Date
Jan	1505	1505
Feb	1569	3074
Mar	1492	4566
Apr	1633	6199
May	1534	7733
June	1304	9037

Figure 11-7 • A cumulative graph. Each bar in this graph adds the births for each month to the total for the month before. Thus each bar represents the total number of births year to date.

Bar Charts. Bar charts are generally associated with comparisons of amounts. Figure 11-8 depicts several types of bar charts that compare the number of births for the months of January to June. The simple bar chart shows the total number of births each month, whereas the cluster, stacked, and 100% formats, allow comparisons of the number of vaginal and cesarean births each month.

Line Charts. Line charts also show amounts, but their emphasis is on communicating changes in data over a time period elapsed, as opposed to the comparisons represented by a bar chart. Figure 11-9 uses three different types of line charts to depict the change in blood pressure during the first year of life

CREATING THE CHART

Computer application programs allow the creation of many different types of charts. The first task in creating any chart is to select the cells that represent the data to be charted. After the appropriate cells have been selected, click on the chart tool and select the type of chart that will best represent those data. It is often possible to preview how the chart will look before the final selection is made. One can also edit the title and legend, as well as change the fonts, for any of the data. Once you have clicked on the icon to indicate that you have finished, the chart appears on the spreadsheet. At that point, it can be resized,

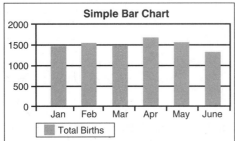

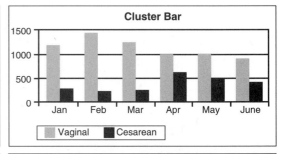

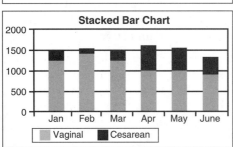

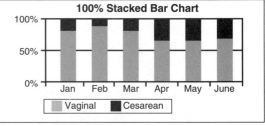

Data For Charts			
	Vaginal	Cesarean	Total Births
Jan	1223	282	1505
Feb	1372	197	1569
Mar	1205	287	1492
Apr	1010	623	1633
May	1032	502	1534
June	902	402	1304

Figure 11-8 • Bar charts. The simple bar chart represents the number of births each month for January to June. The cluster bar compares the number of each type of birth by placing each on the zero line, while the stacked bar chart shows the total births, but starts the cesarean birth numbers at the end of the bar for vaginal births. The 100% stacked bar allows the comparison of percentages for each type of birth for each month.

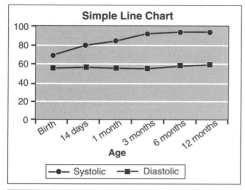

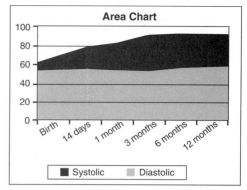

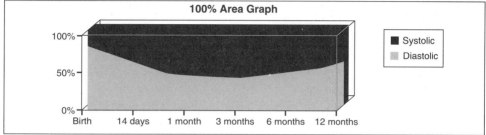

Age	Data Systolic	Diastolic
Birth	69	55
14 days	77	54
1 month	85	52
3 months	90	50
6 months	91	53
12 months	91	55

Figure 11-9 • Line charts. The simple line graph depicts the changes in the average systolic and diastolic blood pressures during the first year of life. In the area chart, both the systolic and diastolic start at zero. In the 100% area graph the diastolic is seen as a percentage of the systolic. The area and 100% area charts show clearly the changes in pulse pressure.

moved, or edited. To edit a chart, right click on the object that needs editing to obtain a drop-down menu of choices.

 ## Summary

Spreadsheet programs have taken much of the drudgery out of calculations and deserve a place on any manager's desktop. Spreadsheets have much in common with other application programs, especially word processing. Their basic structure is a table, with a column of numbers on the left side and a row of letters at the top, which are used to give names to each cell. The keys used as mathematical operators in spreadsheets are the same as in any other computer program that calculates, as is the order in which calculations are performed.

Statistical packages can be used in performing statistical tests and as a learning tool in grasping the true meaning behind a statistical test. When they are done well, charts can communicate more effectively than raw numbers. The type of chart should be selected based on the information that needs to be communicated. When making a chart selection, keep in mind that some types of charts distort the true figures behind the chart.

Although the programs discussed in this chapter make managing numbers easier, if they are not used carefully, they can create great misinformation. As with all computer use, nurses and other healthcare professionals should use common sense when interpreting computer numerical output. This includes understanding the assumptions that various models use. Given thoughtful use, software that calculates numbers can assist all healthcare professionals in managing information.

connection—⌐   **For definitions of bolded key terms, visit the online glossary available at http://connection.lww.com/go/thede.**

CONSIDERATIONS AND EXERCISES

1. List some of the similarities between a word processor and a spreadsheet.
2. Calculate the answer as a computer would to the following:
   a. 5*3+3
   b. 12−6/3
   c. (5+15)/5
   d. (6+4)*3)/15
   e. 10/2*3 (When operators are equal use the left right rule.)
3. Using nesting , write formulas for the following. Nesting means placing a subordinate mathematical operation in parentheses within another set of parentheses e.g. (30/(14−4) in which 4 will be subtracted from 14 BEFORE this sum is used to divide 30. (Ans. is 3.)
   a. Multiply 4 times the sum of 8 + 4.
   b. Raise 2 to the power of 5, then multiply by 5 and divide by 10.
   c. Multiply the sum of 4 + 5 times the sum of 3 + 6.
   d. Return the highest whole number (this is an integer with a decimals truncated) possible if 2020 is divided by 23.
   e. Round 25 divided by 3 to two decimals.
4. In a spreadsheet, create a formula to calculate the number of intravenous (IV) drops per minute when the IV tubing calibration rate is 20 drops per minute, the time for the infusion is 8 hours, and the total volume to be infused is 1000 cc.
5. Experiment with some features of a spreadsheet. Use the help feature when necessary.
   a. Using fill series, create columns with the months of the year.
   b. Using the freeze headings (locked titles), lock these headings.
   c. Enter two of the formulas in Question 2 or 3.
6. You have data that represent the number of pressure ulcers for each of three different types of mattresses that are used in your unit. You wish to communicate that one of these mattresses is far superior to the others. What would be the best type of chart to show this?
7. You want to show what percentage of all admissions to your emergency department occur during each shift. Which type of graph will show this best?
8. You wish to show the changes in the number of pounds gained each month of a pregnancy from month 3 to delivery of a healthy infant. You have the average number of pounds gained each month (i.e., 2 pounds in month 3, 5 pounds in month 5) for 300 pregnant women from the third month of pregnancy to delivery. What type of chart will you select to show changes over time?

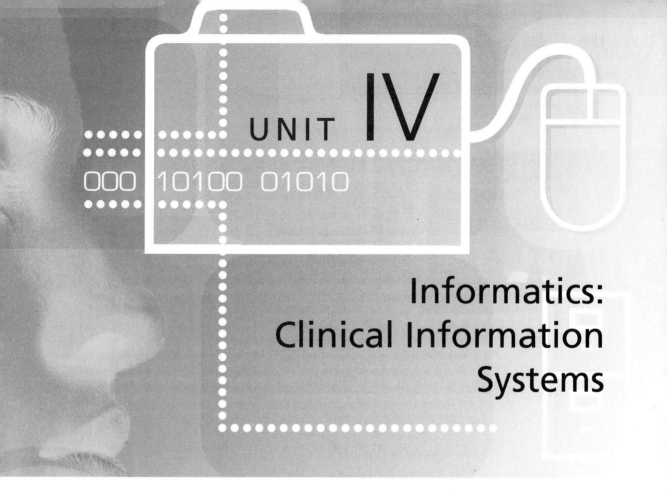

UNIT **IV**

OOO 10100 01010

Informatics:
Clinical Information
Systems

As this decade unfolds, more changes in healthcare are bound to occur. Informatics is becoming more and more important in the quest for patient safety, a factor put into focus by the Institute of Medicine's reports. Other demands on this relatively new field are created by requirements by third-party payers for data that provide outcomes for healthcare. These demands illustrate the reality of the interdisciplinary nature of healthcare; no single specialty can provide the needed data if these goals are to be met.

This unit starts with an exploration of the subspecialty of nursing informatics and proceeds to look at the entire field of direct clinical informatics. Chapter 12 looks at nursing informatics as a specialty and explores the roles and standards of the role. Chapter 13 examines the development of standardized terminologies and their role in nursing and healthcare. This task presents both the greatest challenges and opportunities for nursing, the challenge to gain the cooperation of all nurses and the opportunity to make nursing care visible not only to patients, but to third-party payers and health policy planners. Chapter 14 explores healthcare information systems as an enterprise-wide system using this as a background to emphasize the informatics tasks of all nurses.

Informatics Nurse Specialist: A Specialty in Two Disciplines

Objectives
After studying this chapter you will be able to:

1. List the four main areas of patient information.

2. Review the role of the American Nurses Association in developing nursing informatics as a specialty.

3. Describe the roles available for an informatics nurse specialist.

4. Examine the research needs in nursing informatics.

5. Interpret the informatics skills needed by all nurses.

6. Identify professional informatics organizations.

7. Discuss the benefits that nursing informatics can bring to nursing.

One might say that the first informatics nurse specialist was Florence Nightingale. Recognizing the value of data in affecting healthcare, during her service in the nineteenth century in the war in the area of Russia called the Crimea, she collected data and systematized record-keeping practices (Audain, 1998). Using these data, she developed the pie graph to dramatize the need for reform to stop the needless deaths caused by the unsanitary conditions in military hospitals.

With the advent of the computer, the use of data is far more widespread than it was in Nightingale's time. When decisions are based on the data available, the need for the collection and analysis of nursing data become very important. Without nursing data, the value of nursing will continue to be hidden to many people in policy-making positions. Through nursing informatics, the healthcare information systems that are being developed will include the nursing data needed to show the value that nurses add to healthcare.

The overall focus of nursing informatics in the clinical area is to integrate information from all areas into a usable whole that provides the clinical nurse with easy access to pertinent data and information so the nurse can provide high-quality care. The many sources of information needed for patient care were broadly classified into four areas by studying the information needs of practicing cardiovascular nurses (Corcoran-Perry & Graves, 1990). These areas are: information about the patient, institutional information, domain knowledge, and procedural knowledge.

The information needed in each category goes beyond immediate needs. Patient data include not only data pertinent to immediate physical care, such as results of the history and physical, medications, and laboratory reports, but also demographic information and information about the patient's support system. Institutional information includes data of immediate concern, such as tracking a piece of equipment or a person, as well as agency policies concerning admission criteria, release of information, and confidentiality of patient data. Information needed for external bodies, such as that needed for reporting to third-party payers, regulatory agencies, and policy-making bodies, can also be included in this category. Domain knowledge pertains to nursing knowledge as well as to knowledge from related disciplines. It includes knowledge from literature and clinical experiences. Procedural knowledge focuses on the procedure for performing tasks such as starting an intravenous line. Nursing informatics adds value to nursing by providing systems that integrate information from all these sources and presenting it in ways that are useful to the practicing nurse.

As healthcare information systems evolve, they are going to focus not only on a way to capture, analyze, and present data for individual patient care and policy making, but also on ways to provide evidence-based practice. Bakken (2001) states that this evidence needs to include randomized clinical trials, systematic reviews, practice guidelines, and clinician-client encounters. Informatics is the specialty charged with synthesizing these different data sources into a workable whole useful to healthcare practitioners.

Like many specialties, nursing informatics is a broad field. A report from the National Center for Nursing Research (Pillar & Golumbic, 1993) proposed seven areas for nursing informatics:

1. Using data, information, and knowledge for patient care
2. Defining data in patient care
3. Acquiring and delivering knowledge about patient care
4. Creating new tools for patient care from new technologies
5. Applying ergonomics for nurses who use computers
6. Integrating systems
7. Evaluating the effects of nursing systems

Practice in each of these requires different knowledge and skills on the part of the informatics nurse specialist. There are also informatics skills that all nurses need. To understand the role and value that nursing informatics adds to nursing, it is necessary to recognize that nursing is not confined to tasks, but that it is a cognitive profession. Providing the data to support this is a joint function of nursing informatics and clinicians.

Nursing Informatics Specialty

The American Nurses Association (ANA) has been one of the leaders in recognizing the value of informatics to nursing. They supported the formation of the Council on Computer Applications in Nursing, which was first convened in 1984 under the chairmanship of Harriet Werley. A resolution to promote the development of computerized nursing systems in nursing practice was passed in 1986, followed in 1989 by the creation of the Steering Committee on Databases to Support Clinical Nursing Practice (Elfrink, Bakken, Coenen, McNeil, & Bickford, 2001), renamed in 1998 the Committee for Nursing Practice Information Infrastructure (CNPII).

In 1992, the ANA recognized nursing informatics as a specialty, with the first certification examination being given in 1995. The prerequisites for taking the examination for certification include an active registered nurse license; 2 years of practice as a registered nurse; 2,000 hours of practice in the field of nursing informatics in the past 3 years or 12 semester hours of academic informatics credits or the completion of a graduate program in informatics; and 30 hours of continuing education within the past 3 years that are applicable to the field (ANCC Certification, 2001). Passing the examination provides certification for 5 years, at which time the certification may be renewed if specified educational and practice requirements are fulfilled.

The ANA has released several publications focusing on nursing informatics. Among their topics are the standards and scope of nursing informatics practice. The standards of practice are organized in a problem-solving way that is similar to the nursing process itself (Scope and Standards of Nursing Informatics Practice, 2001). Informatics nurses are charged with identifying and clarifying issues and selecting, developing, implementing, evaluating, and adjusting informatics solutions to nursing practice issues.

 ## Roles for Informatics Nurse Specialists

As can be seen from the broad areas included under the heading of nursing informatics, as well as the evolving nature of nursing informatics, the roles of informatics in nursing practice are diverse (Table 12-1). Informatics nurse specialists may be involved in developing, implementing, and evaluating information systems or facilitating the creation of nursing knowledge. Their positions include project managers, consultants, educators, researchers, and product developers (Scope and Standards of Nursing Informatics Practice, 2001).

All nursing informatics specialists interact with various people on many different organizational levels (Heller & Romano, 1988). These interactions are important in collaborating, interpreting data, and gaining support for new practices. Such meetings are also needed to assist the informatics nurse specialist in identifying how information flows through an organization, assessing for real and potential communication problems and, when necessary, devising alternative methods of communication. To fulfill these functions, nursing informatics specialists need a knowledge of nursing, information science, systems theory as it applies to clinical and managerial decision making, change theory, cognitive theory, and the impact of organizational and group dynamics on healthcare systems (Romano & Heller, 1990).

User liaison is an important service performed by nursing informatics specialists. In this role, the nurse acts as the communications link between nurses and others involved in computer-related matters (Anderson, 1992; Hersher, 1985; Hersher, 1995). Nursing information systems specialist is another role that nursing informatics specialists may fill. In this job she or he manages all nursing applications and may head the nursing computer coordinating committee. Nurse informaticists may also act as data systems managers for a specialty such as Oncology.

Nursing informatics specialists working for either a healthcare agency or a vendor may find themselves part of a team installing an information system or training new users. They may also be involved in product management or product definition. In this position, the nurse may also be responsible for seeing that the product is updated. This involves be-

TABLE 12-1 ● *Possible Roles for Informatics Nurse Specialists*	
Possible Roles	**Responsibilities**
Project manager	Planning and implementing of an informatics project. Project managers must be able to communicate effectively with all levels of management, users, and system developers. They must also be familiar with all factors involved in the project including, but not limited to, managing change, assessing the need for the new project, and planning for its implementation.
System specialist	May work at many different levels from the unit to the full agency. Acts as a link between nursing and information services being both a nursing resource and representative.
Consultant	Provides expert advice, opinions, and recommendations from consultant's area of expertise. Must be able to analyze what the client wants, as well as what is needed, and integrate these to create what is possible, technologically and politically. May be employed within an organization, by a vendor, or self-employed.
Systems educator	Provide training for use of information systems. Includes new systems as well as orientation for new employees. If employed by a vendor, may be responsible for documenting a new system and providing "train the trainer" education for healthcare agency personnel.
Researcher	Using informatics to create new knowledge. Encompasses research in any area of nursing informatics. May involve basic research on the symbolic representation of nursing phenomena, clinical decision making, or applied research of information systems. Could be involved in developing decision support tools for nursing.
Product developer	Participates in the development of new information systems including the designing, developing, and marketing of informatics solutions for nursing problems. Must understand the needs of both business and nursing.
Policy developer	Contributes to healthcare policy development by identifying nursing data, their availability, structure, and content that are used to determine health policy. These policies encompass not only information management, but health infrastructure development and economics.
Entrepreneur	Analyzes nursing information needs in clinical areas, education, administration, and research; develops, and markets solutions.
Other	Any role that involves assisting in the process of managing information. May be performed by a clinician whose primary responsibilities are clinical, or one whose primary responsibilities involve informatics.

ing aware of new developments in the field as well as the current and future needs of clients.[1] Some nurse informatics specialists working for vendors are involved in marketing. For marketing, skills in listening and anticipating needs, as well as the ability to identify the real decision maker, are necessary.

Many nurses in nursing informatics are involved as consultants, either working independently or working for an organization (Display 12-1). Consulting is a high-pressure field in which people often must make instant decisions based on an analysis of only the known facts and personal knowledge. This role involves both that of a liaison and an expert. Many consulting jobs require heavy travel. Nurses in academia who are involved in nursing informatics are also usually involved in associated research.

[1] When working in a role that involves working with system users, a client is not necessarily a person outside the agency, but any individual who needs the services that an informaticist can provide.

My mother introduces me these days as "my daughter who used to be a nurse." But that's not true-I am and always will be a nurse. I'm just practicing in a *different* area. Advances in technology have improved our ability to care for patients. What nurses (or others, like my mother) don't often think about is that these technological advances also include computer systems. Nurses need to have the skills to be able to use a PC, a monitor, or other piece of equipment, just like they need the skills to be able to do a physical assessment. You cannot keep up with the information or reports needed in today's world unless you have some system (besides paper) to help you.

I got into the field of nursing informatics several years ago when I was manager of a hospital ambulatory services department. Being responsible for the business aspects of the department as well as the clinical aspects, I was on the project team for implementation of the new computer systems. I found that my innate curiosity and need to always ask "Why?" proved very helpful in this endeavor. I also discovered that a computer is only a tool; it takes humans to analyze information needs and to plan how to best meet them—discovery that led me to the field of nursing informatics.

I have never regretted the move! Just as in clinical nursing, you never know what to expect on a given day. Although you anticipate what you need to do each day, anything can happen to interrupt those plans and change your priorities. The next thing you know, it's 5:30 PM and you haven't been able to do one thing on your to-do list.

I start out each day by turning on my PC. Then I open my e-mail system. I read my new messages and respond when necessary. This usually takes an hour or two. Sometimes an e-mail I receive will require a telephone contact for follow-up, or users may contact me by telephone. Much of the time spent in my office I'm either answering a question, providing clarification, explaining how a function works, or troubleshooting. When I am troubleshooting, I often access the software system with which the caller is having difficulty. This allows me to try to do what the user has done or attempted to do, so I can assess whether the caller is using the right function or routine, and using it correctly. If the function is being used appropriately, I try to recreate what the user has done to see whether I can elicit the same response or responses that she or he did. This method gives me a better picture of the difficulty and allows me either to solve the problem or to pinpoint a software problem. One day, I logged 6 hours and 45 minutes of telephone time; most of which was nonstop.

Sometimes I need to contact one of the vendors to get a problem resolved. Talking with vendors may also include discussing product enhancements, a new product or fea-ture that they are developing and releasing to clients, or an upcoming class or meeting. Software testing is another function of the job. There may be new features or updates released that need to be tested. This process involves creating different situations in which you enter data and print reports to make sure the software does what it's supposed to do. This can take hours, days, or even weeks to complete.

Reports are the end result of information processing. When you buy software, you sometimes get *standard* reports (those that most users need) but you usually have to write *custom* reports. That is another role of the nurse informaticist: users give me requests for reports that they would like to have. To create them I may be able to modify an existing report, or I may need to create a new one. This involves determining which file or files the information resides in, how the output of the report should look, what fields the report needs to include, what to name it so that the users will know which report to run, and perhaps which menu to put it on. Writing reports can take anywhere from a few minutes to several days, depending on the complexity, as well as the amount of time you can devote. (Remember all those interruptions!) Testing a report is also part of modifying or creating one. As the creator, I need to test it to be certain that it produces what the user wants. Then, I need to have the user test it to see whether the data and design meet his or her needs.

Another role of the nurse informatics specialist is that of teacher. I develop the lesson plans and teaching materials to train the staff on the use of the computer systems. Training is done formally or informally, depending on the situation, and can last a few minutes or several days. In addition, I attend meetings, both in my department and with other departments. Many times, I am the leader of the meeting, which also involves putting together the agenda and handouts, and doing minutes. There are also user group and informatics organizations to which I belong.

A key element in this role is communication. When you are working in nursing informatics, you are providing help and support to end users: staff, managers, directors, and vice-presidents, as well as the programmers/developers. (Very often, the programmer or developer is at your vendor's location and not in-house.) Nursing informatics is extremely dynamic, and I love the challenge. It offers me the opportunity to work with many different people, do many different things, and to be creative. This role is never boring!

Judith Hornback, RN, BSN, MHSA
Informatics Nurse Specialist
Senior Consultant, RHI, Inc.
Highland, Indiana

Educational Preparation

One characteristic that stands out in informatics nurses is the commitment to life-long learning. Most nurses today who are practicing in the field of nursing informatics have gained their knowledge through self-learning and continuing education. Before commencing on a career in nursing informatics, it is helpful to have a thorough, in-depth understanding of clinical practice in nursing. This type of knowledge comes with experience that goes beyond a degree. Computer competency alone, although helpful, is insufficient for a career as a nurse informatics specialist. Computers are only a tool in informatics; information management is the focus.

Preparation for being a nurse informatics specialist can be acquired in many different ways: through a formal academic degree, formal education leading to a certificate, formal educational courses, continuing education courses, professional conferences, and on-the-job learning. Many of the specialty and professional societies provide seminars and workshops for informatics. The American Medical Informatics Association (IMIA) and the Healthcare Information Management Systems Society (HIMSS) have large educational and research meetings, including tutorials for novice practitioners (Educational paths, 1996). Additionally, some universities sponsor 1- or 2-week intensive informatics courses.

The nursing working group of the American Medical Informatics Association (AMIA) classifies nursing informatics programs into four categories: online courses, graduate programs with a specialty in nursing informatics, graduate and undergraduate programs, and courses in nursing informatics and individual courses in nursing informatics (Lange, 2001). The online courses may be stand-alones, lead to a certificate in nursing informatics, or belong to a formal degree granting program, which may or may not be 100% online. Degree granting programs may offer just a concentration in nursing informatics, or they may make nursing informatics the main focus of the degree.

Many educational institutions have begun informatics programs. Some focus on nursing informatics, others encompass the entire healthcare informatics field. Given the many areas of nursing informatics, it follows that each educational program will have a different focus. Some focus on applied informatics, others on informatics research. At present, no accrediting bodies examine informatics education. Thus, there are many questions that prospective students need to ask of any program (Display 12-2).

Research in Nursing Informatics

There are many areas for research in nursing informatics that can guide nursing practice as well as improve nursing information systems. One such is **decision support**. Before decision support systems for nursing can be developed, research is needed to identify how, when, and why nurses make decisions. Many factors affect this, including ethics and institutional and social factors. It is necessary to uncover not only the actual decisions nurses make, many of which may be traditionally thought of as medical decisions, but to provide support for the fact that nurses actually make these decisions (Pillar & Golumbic, 1993). Research to identify the tacit knowledge of expert nurses is also needed to provide

---

Display 12-2 • QUESTIONS TO ASK REGARDING FORMAL EDUCATIONAL INFORMATICS PROGRAMS

Questions specific to an informatics program (in addition to those normally asked of any educational program)

What is the focus of the informatics program?
    Clinical systems
    Knowledge generation
What types of jobs do graduates of the program obtain?
Who are the faculty in informatics?
    What are their qualifications to teach informatics?
        Clinical
        Academic
    What are their interests in informatics?
How long has the program been operating?
What courses are currently available versus those still in the planning stages?

---

high-quality decision support systems.[2] Other areas in nursing informatics open for research include the study of methods to design systems that support or automate the structuring and processing of nursing information to produce clinical decisions, the identification and establishment of standardized nursing languages, and the development and building of clinical databases to manage information for administration and add nursing knowledge for patient care (Romano, Heller, & Mills, 1996).

Informatics Missions for All Nurses

Informatics nurse specialists cannot work in a vacuum. The best systems are developed by collaboration between informatics nurse specialists and practicing clinicians. This avoids one of the common reasons for system failure: neglecting the expertise of end-users. To make this a productive relationship, practicing clinicians need to have a basic understanding of the role data play in providing not only individual patient care, but also in tracking and trending patient care. As data are synthesized and converted to information, all nurses will need to learn to use this information/knowledge wisely. Everyone needs to realize that a computer can work only with those data that it has. The principle "garbage in, garbage out" (GIGO) should be accompanied by the corollary "data lacking, output defective" (DLOD). When evaluating output, look at the data categories (fields) on which it was based.

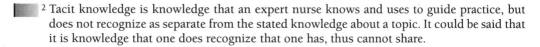

[2] Tacit knowledge is knowledge that an expert nurse knows and uses to guide practice, but does not recognize as separate from the stated knowledge about a topic. It could be said that it is knowledge that one does recognize that one has, thus cannot share.

Informatics Organizations

The major professional organizations in informatics are multidisciplinary. The Healthcare Information and Management Systems Society (HIMSS) and International Medical Informatics Association (IMIA) are two examples. These organizations publish journals and sponsor meetings, and are a source of up-to-date information in the field. Their annual meetings allow members to establish a network of people with whom ideas can be shared. In addition, they provide a place to share information about specific problems.

HIMSS, which was founded in 1961, is a not-for-profit organization dedicated to promoting a better understanding of healthcare information and management systems. At present, HIMSS represents more than 12,000 healthcare professionals in over 35 chapters (About HIMSS, 2002). Many nurses are involved in this organization, which meets annually. The organization publishes a quarterly journal and several guides to the field. They offer accreditation as a Certified Professional in Healthcare Information and Management Systems (CPHIMS).

The IMIA is a nonpolitical, international, scientific organization. IMIA's goals include promoting informatics in healthcare and biomedical research and advancing international cooperation (International Medical Informatics Association, 2002). IMIA sponsors many working groups on various topics; two of these topics are specifically nursing oriented: nursing informatics and nursing informatics education. The IMIA nursing working group sponsors an international nursing informatics conference every three years. A glance at the titles of these conferences shows the progression of themes in nursing informatics (Table 12-2).

The American Medical Informatics Association (AMIA) is the organization that represents the United States at IMIA. The nursing working group within AMIA (AMIA-NW) is responsible for promoting the integration of nursing informatics into the broader context of healthcare with activities such as, facilitating the education of professionals, influencing policy makers regarding the use of nursing information and fostering innovation and scientific exchange (AMIA-NW, 2001). AMIA-NW sponsors a nursing informatics electronic mailing list, nrsing-l.

There are also professional informatics organizations that focus on nursing, although most are local. One that is national is the American Nursing Informatics Association (ANIA). Founded in 1992, ANIA is a nonprofit organization formed to support nurses

TABLE 12-2 ● Titles of International Nursing Informatics Conferences	
1982	*The Impact of Computers on Nursing*
1985	*Building Bridges to the Future*
1988	*Where Caring and Technology Meet*
1991	*Nurses Managing Information in Health Care*
1994	*An International Overview of Nursing in a Technological Era*
1997	*The Impact of Nursing Knowledge on Healthcare Informatics*
2000	*One Step Beyond: The Evolution of Technology and Nursing*
2003	*E-health for All: Designing a Nursing Agenda for the Future*

who design, implement and manage information systems for education, practice and research (ANIA, 2001).

A local group with many members nationwide, as well as internationally, is the Capital Area Roundtable in Nursing Informatics Group (CARING). It was organized in 1982 to provide educational experiences and articles, act as a clearinghouse for speakers and programs, and provide a professional network for those involved in informatics in the Washington, DC area, as well as for those who can be reached electronically (Caring, 2001). In 2001, the group had over 650 members from 43 states and 11 countries. They have monthly meetings and produce a newsletter.

Nursing informatics groups are not confined to the United States. One very active group is the British Computer Society Nursing Specialist Group. They are one of five Health Informatics Specialist Groups of the British Computer Society. One of their aims is to contribute to information and technology debates about information management both nationally and internationally (About the NSG, 2001). This is accomplished by using focus groups and interacting with other groups such as the Royal College of Nursing and the Nursing Informatics Working Group of IMIA. In addition to these activities, they publish a quarterly journal.

Nursing Benefits From Nursing Informatics

When properly used, nursing informatics has the potential to improve patient care as well as to make the value that nursing adds to healthcare visible. Patient care can be improved in several ways. Technology, wisely used, can reduce the burden of paperwork on clinicians, as well as improve the communications that take up so much of a nurse's time. Unfortunately, many systems today lack the input from both experienced clinicians and informaticists that is needed to accomplish these aims.

Information systems can assist nurses in many tasks by providing **decision support tools**. A decision support tool correlates information from sources such as patient data and literature and offers advice based on this integration (Kohn, Corrigan, & Donaldson, 2000a). A well-designed decision support system is able to synthesize information that the clinician may not remember or even may never have known. For example, in giving a medication, a decision-support tool would examine not only the recent literature about the drug, but the patient's record for any allergies, drug incompatibilities, or other contraindications. Then it would report any inconsistencies to the nurse, along with any information needed to correctly administer the drug. If the system were to be combined with a bar coding system in which the nurse ran a scanner over the medication packet and the patient's identification bracelet, it would also assist in preventing a medication from being administered to the wrong patient.

Information systems provide other methods for improving patient safety. The Washington, DC based Institute of Medicine's (IOM) 1999 report "To Err is human" found that errors occur for one of two reasons: either a plan is not carried out correctly, or the plan is incorrect (Kohn, Corrigan, & Donaldson, 2000b). Informatics is now able to facilitate the prevention of many errors by not only using decision-support tools but by tracking functions that are implemented improperly. Electronic tracking will allow clinicians to determine the source of the problem. The results may indicate a need for more education, or find that organizational policies need to be revised or that a combination of both are needed.

Additionally, situations that require the ability to obtain and analyze data quickly will always occur in healthcare. Well-designed clinical systems will provide data that can be analyzed to aid in addressing these situations, replacing the present paper-based system that makes obtaining data costly and time-consuming. Thus, solutions will be provided in a more timely manner and major consequences will be avoided.

Perhaps the biggest benefit that informatics can add to nursing is to assist in the process of identifying the value that nursing adds to healthcare (Display 12-3). Given the GIGO and DLOD principles, the value of identifying data that describes nursing practice becomes apparent. The very nature of computers, in which entities must be 100% identical to be recognized by the computer as representing the same concept, creates a need for standardized terminologies. The use of standardized terminologies to describe nursing sensitive tasks and outcomes allows information systems to capture not only the tasks that nurses do but their cognitive processes. It is the cognitive tasks that separate a registered nurse from an unlicensed person. Standardized languages will also enable nursing to have cost-center-based charges added to patient records, with the result that nurses may be reimbursed for their real value instead of being considered part of room and board. When properly implemented, nursing informatics can bridge the gap between the art and science of nursing (Saba, 2001). Informatics offers nursing the chance to look at our practice from an information science perspective. This will allow us to determine which information-processing tasks we do best and which the computer performs better that humans (Ozbolt, 1996).

 ## Summary

Nursing informatics is a specialty in nursing that involves helping clinicians to acquire and integrate patient care data from many sources. Within nursing informatics, there are many different areas of concentration and roles including project manager, systems manager, and independent contractor. Nursing informatics, however, is not solely the province of nursing informatics specialists; all nurses must be involved if successful information systems are to be developed and implemented.

Display 12-3 • SUMMARY OF NURSING INFORMATICS BENEFITS

Relieve clinicians of some of the frustrating tasks related to paper work.
Improve communications.
Improve patient safety.
Provide decision support systems.
Provide up-to-date data for analysis.
Provide nursing data useful in quantifying cognitive nursing care instead of just tasks.
Provide data to differentiate between tasks the computer does well and those that are better performed by a nurse.

Many different types of programs exist for those who wish to specialize in nursing informatics. They range from graduate degree granting programs to continuing education. No accrediting body for education in this specialty as yet, and the wise prospective student should investigate any program before enrolling.

Informatics has many professional organizations, some more locally based that others. Most interdisciplinary associations have nursing working groups. The benefits that informatics brings to nursing include streamlining paperwork and sharpening communications, improving patient safety, and providing data to support the cognitive activities of the nurse; at the same time, informatics provides a way to assign costs for nursing beyond including those charges in the traditional room and board.

connection For definitions of bolded key terms, visit the online glossary available at http://connection.lww.com/go/thede.

CONSIDERATIONS AND EXERCISES

1. What are the four main areas for patient information?
2. Review the role of the ANA in developing nursing informatics as a specialty.
3. Interview an informatics nursing specialist to discover her or his responsibilities. Into which of the roles discussed in this chapter would you place this person?
4. Identify ways your clinical area could participate in research on one of the research priorities for nursing informatics.
5. Investigate the activities of one of the informatics professional organizations. Methods for accomplishing this include researching their home page, attending a meeting, and/or interviewing a member/officer in any of the groups.
6. Evaluate the use of informatics to benefit nursing in your clinical area and list areas where it could be improved.
   a. Does it streamline paper work and communication? If so, how? If not, what plans are there for improvement?
   b. Does it provide decision support tools? If so, how? If not, what plans are there for improvement?
   c. Does it contribute to patient safety? If so, how? If not, what plans are there for improvement?

REFERENCES

About HIMSS. (2002). Retrieved March 6, 2002 from http://www.himss.org/about/aboutus.asp.
About the NSG. (2001). Retrieved March 6, 2002 from http://www.bcsnsg.org.uk/about.htm.
American Nurses Association. (2001). *Scope and Standards of Nursing Informatics Practice.* Washington, DC: American Nurses Association.
AMIA-NW mission. (2001). Retrieved March 6, 2002 from http://www.amia-niwg.org/Mission.htm.
ANIA. (2001) Retrieved March 6, 2002 from http://www.ania.org/.
ANCC certification (2001). Washington, DC: American Nurses Credentialing Center.
Anderson, B. L. (1992). Nursing informatics: Career opportunities inside and out. *Computers in Nursing, 10*(4), 165–170.

Audain, C. (1998). *Florence Nightingale.* Retrieved September 4, 1999 from http://www.agnesscott.edu/lriddle/women/nitegale.htm.

Bakken, S. (2001). An informatics infrastructure is essential for evidence-based practice. *Journal of the American Medical Association, 8*(3), 199–201.

Caring. (2001). Retrieved March 6, 2002 from http://www.caringonline.org/home.html.

Corcoran-Perry, S., & Graves, J. (1990). Supplemental-information-seeking behavior of cardiovascular nurses. *Research in Nursing & Health, 13*(2), 119–127.

Elfrink, V., Bakken, S., Coenen, A., McNeil, B., & Bickford, C. (2001). Standardized nursing vocabularies: A foundation for quality care. *Seminars in Oncology Nursing, 17*(1), 18–23.

Healthcare Information and Management Systems Society. (1996). Educational paths in clinical informatics. In *Guide to effective health care clinical systems* (pp. 67–76). Chicago: Healthcare Information and Management Systems Society.

Heller, B. R., & Romano, C. A. (1988). Nursing informatics: The pathway to knowledge. *Nursing & Health Care, 9*(9), 483–484.

Hersher, B. S. (1985). The job search and information systems opportunities for nurses. In D. Pocklington, & J. Baron, (Eds.). *Nursing Clinics of North America, 20*(3), 585–603.

Hersher, B. S. (1995) Careers for nurses in healthcare information systems. In M. J. Ball, K. J., Hannah, S. K. Newbold, & J. V. Douglas, (Eds.). *Nursing informatics: Where caring and technology meet,* (2nd ed., pp. 77–83). New York: Springer Verlag.

International Medical Informatics Association. (2002). *Welcome to IMIA.* Retrieved March 6, 2002 from http://www.imia.org/.

Kohn, L. T., Corrigan, J. M., & Donaldson, M. S. (Eds.). (2000a). *To err is human* (pp. 49–68). Washington, DC: National Academy Press. Retrieved March 6, 2002 from http://www.nap.edu/catalog/9728.html.

Kohn, L. T., Corrigan, J. M., & Donaldson, M. S. (Eds.). (2000b). Executive Summary. *To err is human.* Washington, DC: National Academy Press. Retrieved March 6, 2002 from http://www.nap.edu/catalog/9728.html.

Lange, L. (2001). *Categories of nursing informatics programs.* Retrieved March 5, 2002 from http://www.amia-niwg.org/NI_Education/categories_of_programs.htm.

Ozbolt, J. (1996). Nursing and technology: A dialectic. *Holistic Nursing Practice, 11*(1), 1–5.

Pillar, B., & Golumbic, N. (Eds.). (1993). *Nursing informatics: Enhancing patient care.* National Center for Nursing Research. Bethesda, MD: U.S. Department of Health and Human Services.

Romano, C. A., & Heller, B. R. (1990). Nursing informatics: A model curriculum for an emerging role. *Nurse Educator, 15*(2), 16–19.

Romano, C. A., Heller, B. R., & Mills, M. E. C. (1996) Research focus areas in informatics. In M. E. C Mills, C. A. Romano, & B. R. Heller (Eds.) *Information Management in Nursing and Health Care* (pp. 295–302). Springhouse, PA: Springhouse.

Saba, V. (2001). Nursing informatics: yesterday, today and tomorrow. *International Nursing Review, 48,* 177–187.

Nursing Classification Systems: Terminology Does Matter

Objectives

After studying this chapter you will be able to:

1. Compare the focus of documentation of patient care in an agency with the ways patient care data are used.

2. List organizations involved in standardization.

3. Describe the role of the ANA in promoting standardized terminologies.

4. Define terms associated with standardized terminologies.

5. Compare and contrast the 12 ANA-recognized standardized systems.

6. List the benefits of using standardized terminologies.

7. Describe the function of the Unified Medical Language System.

In polls, nursing is called one of the most trusted professions, but how does the public define the nursing activities that lead to this conclusion? How is nursing identified in healthcare planning? Occupational therapy, pharmacists, physical therapists, dieticians, and respiratory therapists all can define their tasks. Nurses, conversely, perform many tasks in various roles, which makes it difficult to define what they do. Nationwide efforts to decrease healthcare costs have intensified the need for nursing to identify its contribution to healthcare outcomes (Larrabee, Boldreghini, Elder-Sorrells, Turner, Wender, Hart, et al., 2001).

Activities that are generally performed by nurses may be divided into three types: managerial, dependent or physician directed, and independent or autonomous (Bowles, 1997). Managerial and dependent activities are fairly well captured by most information systems. The third type of activity (e.g., autonomous tasks) is seldom captured. Without these data, the autonomous activities that nurses perform in patient care cannot be retrieved. This translates into a situation in which autonomous nursing activities are not recognized as having any value, because they have not been identified as chargeable activities.

Data Needs and Nursing Documentation

When the government does large studies that look at outcomes and their relationship to the nurse:patient ratio, they use "outcomes potentially sensitive to nursing"

(OPSN). An OPSN is a characteristic that is *thought* to measure the contributions of nurses in providing inpatient care. Some OPSNs are urinary tract infection, skin pressure ulcers, pneumonia, shock, upper gastrointestinal bleeding, and length-of-stay. Using OPSNs, a study done by the Department of Health and Human Services (DHHS) using data from more than 5 million patients discharged from 799 hospitals in 11 states found that having a greater number of registered nurses involved in therapy produced fewer adverse outcomes (Nurse Staffing, 2001). Although this study identified a relationship between nursing care and medically oriented outcomes, it provided no explanation for what it is that nurses do that causes these outcomes. Additionally, the OPSNs describe only a small portion of nursing-sensitive outcomes. Because of a lack of data, health policy makers ignore such outcomes as the ability of a client to perform unaided the activities of daily living, to engage in wellness behaviors and safety measures, or to control symptoms of a chronic condition such as pain and fatigue (Oermann & Huber, 1999). Yet failure to treat these conditions often increases healthcare costs. The lack of nursing data that demonstrate what a registered nurse does that prevents adverse outcomes makes it impossible to determine the true value of nursing. To quote Clark and Lang (1992), "If we cannot name it, we cannot control it, finance it, research it, or put it into public policy" (p. 128).

It is tempting to think that if one were to analyze nursing documentation, it would be easy to obtain these data, but several problems are inherent to such an approach. Retrieving information from paper records, which is where most nursing documentation is stored, is a labor-intensive, hence expensive, task. Worse, there is seldom a set format for documenting, and nurses are not consistent in either their documentation or terminology. Even if the data are in an electronic information system, the terminology used to collect them is generally not sufficiently standardized to be used for comparisons across different settings and in separate geographical areas.

Present-day nursing documentation is also lost to the purposes that Florence Nightingale envisioned. Nightingale saw documentation as a method for evaluating and enhancing patient care and furthering the profession. In its present state, nursing documentation is seldom used in billing. Nursing care is a hidden charge, usually part of room and board, and it seldom bears any relationship to the actual care provided.

Documentation can be classified as having two foci: the individual patient and the local, regional, national, and international healthcare community. Nursing has for too long focused mainly on the data and information needed for individual patient care without realizing the multiple ways that this documentation is used. Many nurses and administrators still believe that nursing notes are simply a means of communication from nurse to nurse and between the nurse and the doctor or of protecting oneself and one's agency from a lawsuit. Before the age of litigation, nursing notes were often discarded when the patient was discharged. This focus on the use of documentation to provide only individual care has resulted in few people, including nurses, seeing the value in the data that are created by nurses. The consequence is that nursing data are not available for planning the use of healthcare resources. Neither the Uniform Hospital Discharge Data Set (UHDDS) nor the Uniform Minimum Health Data Set (UMHDS) contains specific nursing sensitive data.

Healthcare outcomes, which today have assumed great importance, depend on data. To meet this requirement, it is necessary that the data be retrievable, comparable across settings, and measurable. Unfortunately, in nursing, the traditional ways of documenting toward outcomes do not lend themselves to any of these functions (Elfrink, Bakken, Coenen, McNeil, & Bickford, 2001). Documentation is traditionally narrative text, often

TABLE 13-1 ● *Comparison of Traditional With Data-Driven Outcomes Documentation*

Focus of data	Traditional	Data-Driven
Point of view	Lengthy, descriptive data to a specific patient-based objective.	Structured data entry and focus using a computerized information system.
Measurement of progress	Nurse estimates the optimal progress for a specific patient.	Progress is indicated by the use of specified severity indicators.
Terminology	Natural language used, which is often specific for an agency, or even a unit.	Nursing observations are documented with standardized terminologies.
Use of data	Outcomes are measured for only one person.	Outcome data are used for comparison across settings and populations.

Adapted from Elfrink, V., Bakken, S., Coenen, A., McNeil, B., & Bickford, C. (2001). Standardized nursing vocabularies: A foundation for quality care. *Seminars in Oncology Nursing, 17*(1), 18–23.

lengthy, and focused on a specific patient (Table 13-1). The need for the use of documentation to determine the effect of interventions on outcomes that extend beyond an individual patient is not recognized.

With the introduction of computerized information systems, the need for nursing to identify its data and agree on the terminology to use for documentation has become of paramount importance. Given the push by various outside agencies for computerized information systems, only a small window exists to accomplish this if nursing is to be credited as a valuable asset in healthcare. The good news is that this work has been going on for over three decades. What is needed now is for people to realize the importance of this work and for nurses and administrators to implement documentation systems that use standardized terminologies. When nurses do not use standardized terminologies for documentation, their contribution to patient care does not allow for the multiple uses of healthcare data, placing the survival of the profession at risk (Sibbald, 1998).

 ## Standardized Terminologies

A standard is a documented agreement containing precise criteria and definitions that must be used consistently. When railroads began, there were no standards for the distance between the tracks. This made it impossible for trains owned by companies using different track widths to be widely used. As commerce grew, this became a problem of such magnitude that competing parties agreed on a standard distance between the tracks. Likewise, given the international nature of healthcare, it is imperative that standards be used to record healthcare documentation.

ORGANIZATIONS INVOLVED IN STANDARDIZATION

A nonprofit group known as the International Organization for Standards (ISO) oversees all international standardization.[1] Established in 1947, ISO is a worldwide federation of the national standards bodies from some 140 countries (What Is ISO?, n.d.). Their pur-

---

[1] Despite the actual name of the organization, the terminology used to denote it is ISO. This is not an acronym, but a term derived from the Greek "isos" which means equal.

pose is to expedite standardization to facilitate international commerce and to promote cooperation in intellectual, technological, scientific, and economic activities. The work of creating ISO standards is done by various technical working committees. ISO develops standards in all technical fields except electronics, which is the responsibility of the International Electrotechnical Commission (IEC). Their work results in international agreements that are published as international standards with the prefix ISO and a number. Some areas in which standards are being drafted include healthcare records, electronic messaging and communication, health concept representation, and data security. The U.S. organizational representative to ISO is the American National Standards Institute (ANSI).

NURSING'S NEED FOR STANDARDS

Standards have been developed in all fields, including healthcare, because the benefits of having them in place outweigh any disadvantages. Using standards improves communication, facilitates research, and improves the ability to predict resource needs. Although we, as nurses, make sense of our nursing practices, we are very new at making explicit the value that is embedded in our clinical documentation (Clark & Lang, 1992). Despite more than 30 years of work, there is still a low visibility for the standardized nursing terminologies that could uncover this value. Nurses, and even many involved in informatics, have little knowledge of our present standardized terminologies. This situation exists worldwide, resulting in several problems:

1. Nursing care is inadequately funded and billed.
2. Nursing resources are inadequately planned and allocated.
3. The contribution of nursing to healthcare cannot be calculated.
4. It is very difficult to design decision support systems (Goossen, 2000).

HISTORICAL NURSING CLASSIFICATION

Nursing classification systems, like medical systems, depend on the current state of a discipline's knowledge. Historically, we have used the Nightingale model of diseases when thinking, writing, and speaking about nursing (Gordon, 1998). In the past, we believed that the data needed for coding outcomes were strictly based on medical requirement. The need for data from the nursing point of view becomes apparent when one considers the situation in Table 13-2. Interestingly, in a project using nursing data such as that in Table 13-2, the number of falls that 115 patients had was reduced from 30 to just 4 falls. Two were related to alcohol, whereas the others occurred in clients who were away from home when they fell (Bezon, Echevarria, & Smith, 1999). Unfortunately, data like these are not routinely collected; thus, they are not available for outcomes studies or to demonstrate the savings in healthcare costs.

For nursing data to be routinely captured and used in outcomes or other measurements requires the use of standardized terminologies. Three tasks are involved in standardizing nursing terminology: identifying the necessary data elements, developing the terminology, and classifying the terminology. In the United States, the Nursing Minimum Data Set (NMDS) identifies the data elements needed, whereas standardized terminologies provide the classification and vocabulary to use in recording these data elements.

TABLE 13-2 ● *Comparison of Medical and Nursing Data*	
68-Year-Old Woman	
Medical Data	*Nursing Data*
Osteoporosis, mild	Physical Injury, Potential for due to: 1. Loose carpet edges 2. Bathtub without hand grips 3. Inadequate lighting in bedroom
Treatment	*Treatment*
Calcium 500 mg 3× day Calcitonin 200U intranasally in alternate nostrils daily	Fix carpet edges Install hand grips in shower Use higher wattage bulb in ceiling fixture
Outcome	*Outcome*
Fractured hip from fall	Freedom from falls

- Where will the emphasis of planning be with just medical data?
- With only nursing data?
- Will the outcome of planning considering both medical and nursing data yield a better outcome?

 ## Nursing Minimum Data Set

A *minimum data set* is a list of data elements with uniform definitions and categories that specifies the minimum set of items that will meet the essential needs of multiple data users in a specific area. Thus, the minimum data required depend on how these data will be used. Most minimum data sets are designed to meet the needs of those who make policy. The data they contain does not in most cases suffice to meet the needs of those who provide care. Today, there are many minimum data sets, each serving a different purpose. A minimum data set must meet the following criteria:

- ▼ The data must be useful to most potential users, for example, legislators, health-care professionals, administrators, and regulatory bodies.
- ▼ The items in the set must be readily collectable with reasonable accuracy.
- ▼ The items should not duplicate other available data.
- ▼ Confidentiality must not be violated.

The absence of nursing-sensitive data in the minimum data sets mandated for collection and used for healthcare planning was noted in the early 1970s by several leaders in nursing. The concept of an NMDS originated in discussions at the 1977 Nursing Information Systems Conference (Werley, Ryan, & Zorn, 1995). The concept, however, was not quick to catch on—few nurses had much background in research, and of those, few saw the value in everyday nursing data. Nevertheless, in 1985, Werley and Lang, with the sponsorship of the University of Wisconsin School of Nursing, Hospital Corporation of America, and IBM, invited 65 people to a conference to determine which items to include in an NMDS (Ozbolt, 1996). A post-conference group refined the work of this conference and came up with the present set of 16 items (Table 13-3) in three categories: Demographics, Nursing Care, and Service Elements. All but six of the items are already collected as part of the Uniform Minimum Health Data Set (UMHDS), which is not surprising, given that the NMDS was modeled after this data set.

The purposes of the NMDS are to:

▼ Make it possible to compare data from different clinical settings, populations, and geographical areas.
▼ Describe nursing care in a variety of settings, including institutional and non-institutional settings.
▼ Show or project trends regarding nursing care and resources needed for clients with various nursing diagnoses.
▼ Stimulate nursing research by providing links to data.
▼ Provide nursing data to influence clinical, administrative, and healthcare-policy decision making.

When developed, the elements in the NMDS were those identified as necessary for recognizing nursing care in the United States. Some nursing groups have found that more data elements are needed for their purposes. The American Organization of Nurse Executives, along with researchers from the University of Iowa, have built onto the NMDS and established a Nursing Management Minimum Data Set (NMMDS) that focuses on the nursing environment, nurse resources, and finances (Simpson, 1997).

Many other countries have developed NMDSs. The purpose of the U.S. NMDS was to describe and compare nursing care and allow the analysis and comparison of nursing care across settings and geographical areas. Other countries have developed NMDSs for other purposes (Goossen, et al., 1998). At present, efforts are under way by the International Council of Nurses (ICN) and the nursing informatics working group of the International Medical Informatics Association (IMIA) to create an International Nursing Minimum Dataset (INMDS).

One difficulty in nursing in the United States is differentiating the NMDS from the other minimum data sets seen in Table 13-4. In the United States before the NMDS was developed, there were three patient-focused minimum data sets (Werley, et al. 1995). One

---

TABLE 13-3 • *Elements of the Nursing Minimum Data Set*

Nursing Care Elements	Patient or Client Demographic Elements	Service Elements
1. Nursing diagnosis*	5. Personal identification	10. Unique facility or service agency number
2. Nursing interventions*	6. Date of birth	11. Unique health record number of patient or client*
3. Nursing outcomes*	7. Sex	12. Unique number or principal registered nurse provider*
4. Intensity of nursing care*	8. Race and ethnicity	13. Episode admission or encounter date
	9. Residence	14. Discharge or termination date
		15. Disposition of patient or client
		16. Expected payor for most of this bill (anticipated financial guarantee for services)

*All itmes but these are in the Uniform Hospital Data Discharge Set

Adapted from: Leske, J. S. & Werley, H. H. (1992). Use of the nursing minimum dataset. *Computers in Nursing, 10*(6), 259–263.

TABLE 13-4 ● *Some Non-Nursing Minimum Healthcare Data Sets*	
Data Set	**Acronym**
Minimum Data Set — Post-Acute Care	MDS-PAC
Mental Health Minimum Data Set	MHMDS
Minimum Data Set (for Long-Term Care), Version 2	MDS-2
Uniform Hospital Discharge Data Set	UHDDS
Uniform Ambulatory Care Data Set	UACDS

is the Uniform Hospital Discharge Data Set (UHDDS), which was adopted in 1972 and is now mandated to be collected on all hospitalized Medicare patients. The other two are the Long-Term Health Care Data Set and the Ambulatory Medical Care Minimum Data Set. Given the many healthcare-related minimum data sets, it is not surprising that most people, nurses included, are not aware of the differences between the minimum data sets, nor of the fact that only the NMDS and the NMMDS contain nursing data. Because there is no mandatory collection of the NMDS, nor of the NMMDS, nursing is still invisible in data used for healthcare planning and policies.

Standardized Nursing Terminologies

In the United States, the present NMDS set designates those elements that need to be collected but does not specify the terminology that is needed to collect this data. This task can be accomplished by using the standardized nursing terminologies. At present, many terminologies are in use. Many are locally determined and are thus not available for data comparison purposes outside those agencies.

ROLE OF THE AMERICAN NURSES ASSOCIATION

The American Nurses Association (ANA) has been a prime mover in the United States in the recognition of the value of nursing data. In 1989, the ANA created the Steering Committee to Support Clinical Practice. In 1999, its name was changed to the Committee for Nursing Practice Information Infrastructure (CNPII). One of its activities has been to set criteria for the data sets and classification systems that support nursing practice and to recognize those that meet these criteria. The criteria state that the data set, classification, or nomenclature must provide a rationale for its development and support nursing practice by providing clinically useful terminology. The concepts must be clear and unambiguous, and there must be documentation of utility in practice, as well as validity and reliability. Additionally, there must be a group named who will be responsible for maintaining and revising the system.

In 1995, the Nursing Information and Data Set Evaluation Center (NIDSEC) was established by the ANA Board of Directors to evaluate the use of standardized terminologies in nursing information systems by a vendor. Evaluation criteria include the use of the nomenclature, clinical content, clinical data repository (how the data are stored and retrieved), the general system characteristics, and a coding scheme that provides a unique identifier for each concept. The ANA encourages nursing system developers to have their information systems evaluated in comparison with these standards. The need now is for healthcare agencies to realize the value that standardized nursing data will provide for them and to demand from their vendors systems with NIDSEC recognition. When standardized terminologies are used appropriately, nursing data are available for many uses, among them the uncovering of knowledge embedded in clinical practice, developing decision support systems, and using this information in policy setting.

CONCEPTS BEHIND STANDARDIZED TERMINOLOGIES

The science of developing a language or classification that adequately describes nursing is complex. It is part of a field called **nosology**, or the science of the classification of diagnostic terms. Developing a set of standardized terminologies involves much more than identifying and reaching consensus on the terminology. The terms must be part of a classification system that is based on concepts that are clearly stated and understandable to users. Moreover, the classification must be amenable to coding for use in a computerized system. A classification is a logical arrangement of knowledge that specifies different categories and provides a means to relate the categories to each other.

Taxonomies

A classification system is the final product that results from arranging the terms in a **taxonomy**. A taxonomy is a way of organizing, or classifying items, that follows a set of rules and is focused on a given concept or philosophical base. That is, all items in the taxonomy have some features in common and are part of the group that forms the organizing concept. Members are further subdivided according to given features that are decided on by the developing entity. We are all familiar with taxonomies from our high school biology classes. They are pyramid shaped and everything under a category is a type of the item above it (Figure 13-1). The first level in Figure 13-1 contains fish and birds, each a vertebrate, but different kinds. The **axis**, or organizing concept is vertebrates. This type of taxonomy is known as a **monoaxial taxonomy** because it is organized around only one group, vertebrates.

If the taxonomy in Figure 13-1 were coded, fish would receive the number 1, and birds the number 2. The trout and salmon under fish would be coded using the prefix of the top level, 1, plus a unique number for each one. Thus, trout would be 1.1 and salmon 1.2. The next level would follow this same pattern of absorbing the numbers of its "parent" and adding another number. Thus, brook trout would be coded 1.1.1 and the brown trout

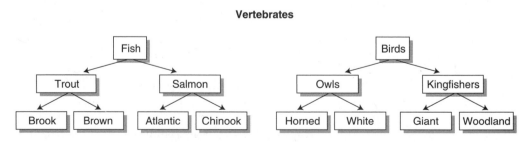

Figure 13-1 • A taxonomy of vertebrates.

1.1.2. This method of coding and classification allows us to look at individual items; at the same time, it is possible to look at characteristics affecting all the items in any category at a given level. For example, it would be possible to study either an individual trout, all trout, or all fish, depending on the need.

In healthcare, a monoaxial taxonomy is not always sufficient to describe the desired element. Some elements require modifiers that would not easily fit into the main axis. In these cases, a **multiaxial taxonomy** is created with users selecting words or phrases from more than one taxonomy to create the terminology to describe the phenomenon. In Figure 13-2, the hypothetical Dot could be described by selecting a criterion from each category; thus, she would be "3A.S.F." In many multiaxial taxonomies terms do not have to be selected from all the taxonomies, but there generally are one or more axes from which a user is required to select a term.

Granularity

When reading about standardized terminologies, one often encounters the term **granularity**. This is a description of the depth of detail that a language system represents. For example, in many cases, using only a nursing diagnosis does not provide a complete picture of a patient; thus, it is not very granular. Adding an etiology would increase its granularity, whereas adding the symptoms that informed that etiology would result in a term that was even more granular. Different purposes require different levels of granularity.

Purpose of Terminology

There are several types of language. We are most familiar with natural language that we use to communicate with one another. Computers, however, require a different approach to language. Clinical data have many uses: the care of an individual patient and functions such as quality assurance, research, policy setting, and locating information. Additionally, many data needs are external to an agency. Comparing data across agencies whose basic data needs differ results in a need to compare data gathered using different standardized languages. In these situations, it is necessary for different data sets to be **mapped** to an overarching data set. To meet these needs, there are two types of stan-

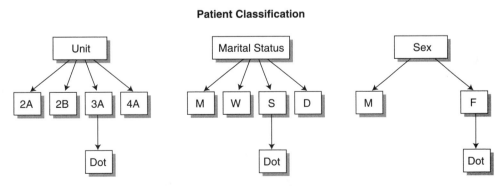

Figure 13-2 • A multi-axial taxonomy.

dardized terminologies: **interface terminologies** and **reference terminologies**. An interface terminology is used by clinicians to enter data and improve care for the patient. It comprises the terms that clinicians use when documenting their care. A reference terminology enables different standardized terminologies to be mapped to each other. In mapping, a relationship is found between the terminology used to describe a condition in one standardized terminology and the terminology used to describe the same condition in another.

ANA-RECOGNIZED STANDARDIZED TERMINOLOGIES

Nursing is a very broad field encompassing many realms: hospital nursing, home-health nursing, community nursing, office nursing, school nursing, and occupational nursing, plus specialties within many of these areas. It is difficult to formulate one standardized terminology that can meet the needs of all these groups; thus, many standard terminologies have been developed. The ANA has recognized 12 of these systems for implementation in the collection of nursing data. These include both the NMDS and the NMMDS and 10 standardized terminology systems, one of which is a reference terminology and another a method of billing-independent nursing practice. They are presented here in roughly the order in which they were recognized by the ANA, with the exception of the North American Nursing Diagnosis Association (NANDA), which is discussed with Nursing Interventions Classification (NIC) and Nursing Outcomes Classification (NOC).

Omaha System

The Omaha System was developed from the efforts of community health nurses in Omaha, Nebraska and agencies in seven other geographical areas to describe and measure community-based practice. Work started in 1970 and was furthered by a federal grant from 1979 to 1983. The present system evolved from many years of effort, the combined work of many healthcare and data processing professionals, and 11 years of federally funded research (Martin & Scheet, 1995). The objective of this system is to provide consistent vocabulary for collecting, sorting, classifying, documenting, and analyzing data pertaining to individual patients, families, or communities. The Omaha System has three components: problems, interventions, and outcomes. These components meet the need to collect three of the four nursing care items in the NMDS.[2]

Home Healthcare Classification System (HHCC)

Another standardized terminology with a community focus is the Home Health Care Classification (HHCC). This grew out of a project conducted at the Georgetown University School of Nursing under the leadership of Dr. Virgina Saba in the late 1980s and early 1990s (Saba, 2002). The objective was to develop a method for assessing and classifying home health Medicare patients in order to predict their needs for nursing and home health services. Like the Omaha system, the HHCC also provides for the collection of three of the four nursing care elements in the NMDS. It has proved useful not only for nursing, but also for other disciplines such as social work, speech therapy, and physical and occupational therapy.

---

[2] Nursing intensity is not at present addressed by most of the ANA-recognized languages.

North American Nursing Diagnosis Association (NANDA)

The organization that in 1982 became NANDA was initiated in the early 1970s by two nurses, Kristine Gebbie and Mary Ann Lavin (Gordon, 1998), who participated in a demonstration project requiring that patient data be computerized (Warren & Hoskins, 1995). They became frustrated when they realized that they were unable to computerize nursing data. This led them to call the first meeting of the National Conference Group for the Classification of Nursing Diagnoses in 1973. The conference objective was to identify terminologies that emphasized the unique role of the nurse. In 1975, the Second National Conference on Classification of Nursing Diagnoses proposed 37 nursing diagnoses to be used in classifying patients' problems. Their first classification system was simply an alphabetical list. As the list grew, a need for classifying the diagnoses became obvious and a taxonomic vocabulary based on Gordon's 11 functional health patterns was created. Later, the classification principles were changed to the nine Human Response Patterns of exchanging, communicating, relating, valuing, choosing, moving, perceiving, knowing, and feeling. The classification in the 2001–2002 NANDA was changed from a monoaxial system to a multi-axial taxonomy. The new system uses the following major concepts within nursing diagnosis: time of duration, population, age, health status, a modifier for the judgment, and the location on the body involved in the diagnosis (NANDA, 2001). To create a diagnosis, users will select terms from the axes necessary to express the term.

Nursing Intervention Classification (NIC)

In 1987, as the work on the NMDS became more widely known, researchers at the University of Iowa started work on the NIC. This was an attempt to standardize the terminology used to describe nursing interventions for use in the NMDS. In 1990, they received a 3-year National Center for Nursing Research grant, and in 1993 they received a 4-year grant for development (Bulechek, McCloskey, & Donahue 1995).

Their work uncovered several interesting facets of nursing. In trying to identify nursing interventions from various sources such as textbooks, care planning guides, and nursing information systems, they discovered that nursing actions are seen as discrete actions rather than as a part of a treatment for a specific condition (McCloskey & Bulechek, 1992). Additionally, the interventions listed for given conditions were not identical from one source to another, so that different terminologies were used for the same interventions. They also found confusion between what is an intervention, an assessment, or an evaluation activity. These difficulties are part of the problem nursing has in deciding which intervention works best with a given phenomenon. More important, they also found that interventions listed were often traditionally versus empirically based. Additionally, there was little record of the history of the decision-making that nurses performed in choosing among interventions. At present, they have identified more than 400 interventions.

Nursing Outcomes Classification (NOC)

A group at the University of Iowa also developed NOC, which is intended to be used with NANDA and the NIC classifications as one large system to collect three of the four nursing care elements in the NMDS. The developers' efforts began in 1991, when a group of 43 nurses representing nursing education and service agencies began to identify and classify nursing-sensitive patient outcomes. For their purposes, they defined outcomes as measurable, variable patient states or behaviors, including patient perceptions, which result from nursing interventions (Johnson & Mass, 1992). Although the outcomes may be stated as goals, they are not intended as such. They used current literature, research instruments, and information systems as the source for identifying the outcomes.

Unified NANDA, NIC, and NOC

Recognizing the need for NANDA, NIC, and NOC to work together, in August of 2001 an invitational conference was held to develop a first draft of a common taxonomic structure for these three classifications. Although the proposed structure is somewhat different from those currently used in the other three standardized terminologies, it does not represent a radical departure from them. Currently, this group is proposing to place this structure in the public domain for use by any interested group.

Although not part of the above group, a current project is under way by a multidisciplinary team at the University of Michigan to develop a methodology for implementing the use of NANDA, NIC, and NOC. Known as the Hands-on Automated Nursing Data System (HANDS), its purpose is to develop a useful system for the gathering, storing, and retrieving of a standardized nursing data set (Keenan, Stocker, Geo-Thomas, Soparkar, Barkauskas. Lee, et al., 2002). The team includes hardware and software experts, a database specialist, a standards specialist in **Health Level-7** (HL7) and the Health Information Portability and Accountability Act (HIPAA), nursing language experts, a statistician, and nurse administrators, researchers, and clinicians.

Phase one of this project revealed the widespread misunderstanding by non-nurse team members about how to integrate standardized languages into documentation systems for the purpose of creating comparable nursing data. (Keenan, Stocker, Geo-Thomas, Soparkar, Barkauskas, & Lee, 2002). One of the lessons learned in this project was that the non-nurse members of the team had many misperceptions about the nature of nursing, believing it to be simple work. This led to difficulties in understanding the complexity of nursing practice. As they worked with the nursing team in this endeavor, these misperceptions were dispelled and they came understand the need to clearly demonstrate what nurses do.

Patient Care Data Set

This system has been under development since 1992 by Ozbolt and colleagues. It was developed primarily for documentation in the acute care area. It consists of nursing diagnosis (many from HHCC and NANDA), nursing interactions termed *patient care actions*, and nursing outcomes. The classification follows that used in HHCC with the addition of two more components to adapt it to the acute care setting. The language consists of clinical terms used in acute care settings by nurses and other non-physician healthcare disciplines to record patient problems, patient care actions, and expected patient outcomes (Ozbolt, 1997). It has been designed to be compliant with HL7.

Perioperative Nursing Data Set (PNDS)

The development of the Peri-Operative Nursing Data Set (PNDS) was started in 1993 by members of the American Operating Room Nurses association. The goal was to make visible to administrators, financial officers, and healthcare policy makers the patient problems that perioperative nurses manage (Beyea, 2000). The system encompasses the entire perioperative experience from preadmission to discharge using standardized elements for nursing diagnoses, interventions, and outcomes. It is intended to provide a framework for documentation for perioperative nurses.

SNOMED CT/RT

Systematized Nomenclature of Medical Clinical Terms (SNOMED CT) is the first terminology recognized by ANA that contained nursing terms but that was not developed exclusively for nursing (Elfrink, et al., 2001). It is a reference terminology, meaning that it will be used to map the different healthcare standardized terminologies for the purpose of comparing data. It grew out of the College of American Pathology's Systematized Nomenclature of Pathology (SNOP), which was first introduced in 1965. In 1977, SNOP was enlarged to include medical terms and became known as the Systematized Nomenclature of Medicine (SNOMED). Development continued with the focus on use in electronic records. In 1999, the ANA recognized SNOMED RT (SNOMED Reference Terminology) as one way to support the integrated electronic medical record for nursing.

In January of 2002, SNOMED CT 1.0 was released. The purpose of this version was to merge SNOMED RT with the Clinical Terms Version 3 (originally known as the Read codes, named for the British general practitioner who devised them in the 1980s to support computer applications). In the 1990s, the U. K. National Health Service obtained the rights and, with participation by 55 British healthcare specialty groups, redeveloped them under the Clinical Terms Project. In 1999, these efforts were combined with SNOMED RT under a joint venture between the U. K. National Health Service and the SNOMED International Group. The new version, now known as SNOMED CT, contains approximately 325,000 concepts linked to clinical knowledge (News, 2002). SNOMED CT allows the user to interpret and link terms from one standardized terminology system to those in another.

SNOMED has been in negotiations with the National Library of Medicine to license SNOMED CT for use without charge by any U.S. healthcare agency that reports to the government. This would include use for Medicare and Medicaid reporting. As this is being written, the diagnoses (nursing problems) from NANDA, HHCC, PNDS, and the Omaha system have been mapped, as have interventions from all these data sets plus NIC. The mapping of outcomes includes not only the above data sets, but also NOC. Standardized terminologies from medicine such as the ninth edition of the International Classification of Diseases (ICD-9) are also mapped in SNOMED CT.

Full dependence on ICD-9 to represent all an agency's data will cause nursing-sensitive data to be omitted from the reports submitted by that agency; this situation leaves nursing in an invisible state. For nursing to be represented in the reports created using SNOMED CT, it will be imperative for one of the ANA recognized terminologies to be used or for an agency to develop its own standardized terminology. The ANA-recognized standardized terminologies will be mapped by SNOMED for use in systems. Those practitioners using their own standardized terminology will need to engage in the complex task of doing their own mapping.

International Classification of Nursing Practice

The International Classification of Nursing Practice (ICNP) is an outgrowth of a failed attempt by the ANA to have the NANDA diagnoses included as part of ICD-10. They were turned down, not for poor content, but because it was considered inappropriate to include work that had been developed within a single country in an international classification

(Clark, 1998). This led the ANA to propose a resolution to the International Council of National Representatives in Seoul in 1989 which led to a project to develop the ICNP.

Begun in 1990, the aims were to develop a standardized vocabulary and classification of nursing phenomena, nursing interventions, and nursing outcomes, which would be useful in both paper and electronic records. Some of the objectives were to establish a common language for nursing practice to enable communication among nurses and others, to describe nursing care in various settings, to stimulate nursing research, and to provide nursing data to influence health policy (ICNP, 1999). The ICNP encompasses nursing diagnoses that they term nursing phenomena, nursing interventions, and outcomes. In this multiaxial taxonomy, nursing phenomena and nursing outcomes use the same eight axes: focus of nursing care, judgment, frequency, duration, topology, body site, likelihood, and bearer. A nursing outcome is simply a new nursing diagnosis. The nursing interventions' taxonomy also has eight axes: activity, target, means, time, topology, location, routes, and beneficiary. Now in the second stage of beta-testing, Version 1 is scheduled for release in 2005.

Alternative Links

This is a vendor system known as the Alternative Billing Codes (ABC Codes) that supports electronic and paper claims processing for providers, healthcare payers, managed care organizations and affiliated organizations. The system is intended for use in coding and support documentation for reimbursement by third parties. It is used for comparing assessment data, nursing outcomes and determining financial outcomes (Elfrink et al., 2001). This system permits accurate reimbursement for Clinical Nurse Specialists, Nurse Midwives, Nurse Practitioners, Licensed Practical Nurses, Registered Midwives, and Registered Nurses and seven other healthcare specialists.

ISSUES IN STANDARDIZED TERMINOLOGIES

None of the previously described standardized terminologies is suitable for every circumstance. Each evolved from a different need, which indicates the breadth of practice in which nurses are involved. The challenge is not to try to develop a one-size-fits-all system, but to select the one that best suits the needs of the institution. The biggest issue in standardized terminologies is to educate nurses and administrators about the use and benefits standardized terminologies can bring to nursing and healthcare. A positive step in this direction is the current HANDS project which seeks to develop methodology implementing the use of NANDA, NIC, and NOC (Keenan, et al., 2002). When standardized terminologies are used, they need to be implemented in such a way that the data are easily retrievable in a usable fashion for comparisons, as well as for state and federal reports.

Additionally, nurses need to be cognizant of the importance of this data. Magistro and Smith (1998) write about nurses who place "anything" in a mandatory field just to be able to move on in the system. This of course renders the data invalid and useless for their intended purposes.

Using a standardized terminology for nursing care involves changes in thinking about documentation. For over a century, nursing documentation has taken a narrative form that follows no set structure, resulting in both over documentation, under-documentation, and documentation that makes following any line of reasoning very difficult, if not impossible. Narrative documentation methods generally preclude the use of data for anything beyond the care of individual patients, and in some cases even preclude this. A great deal of knowledge is currently concealed in nursing data; with the adaptation of standardized terminologies, this information could be uncovered.

BENEFITS OF NURSING STANDARDIZED LANGUAGES

Standardized languages will eliminate inconsistencies in investigating and documenting nursing practice, and they will allow the building of **decision support** systems for nursing. The resulting data will allow the comparison of nursing care among institutions and may demonstrate that institutions with an individualized approach to nursing or that engage in mutual nurse-client decision making have better outcomes with the same interventions than those with a more functional task, oriented approach.

To assume the full role of a professional, it is necessary that nursing services in acute care facilities be billed as a separate entity based on the actual nursing service received. To be paid for services, it is necessary to document in an unambiguous way problems addressed, interventions delivered, and the outcomes achieved (Elfrink, et al., 2001). Proper use of standardized terminologies may facilitate this. Data recorded using standardized terminologies will also facilitate the examination of how nursing care contributes to patient outcomes.

Perhaps, at this point, the most important benefit of using standardized languages is that it will permit nursing data to be included in a computerized patient care record. Because the terminology has exact definitions and is classified, it will be retrievable from clinical systems and able to be used for research as well as for health policy planning. The inclusion of nursing care in health planning will yield a more complete picture of needed resources and can lend support to preventative care. An added benefit is that nursing will cease to be invisible. Although the dependent functions of nursing are important, they do not define nursing. The independent functions of nursing are equally, if not more, important in a healthcare system that is interested in cutting costs. The use of standardized language to document these functions is necessary for the data to be useful for these purposes.

The Unified Medical Language System

Today, in healthcare, many different standardized terminologies are in use (Figure 13-3). Although some express concepts particular to a specific discipline, others are multidisciplinary. It is essential, however, to enable users to find all the information related to a given concept in all machine-readable sources such as clinical records, databases, biomedical literature, and various directories of information sources. To meet this need, in 1986 the National Library of Medicine (NLM) began an ongoing effort to develop the Unified Medical Language System (UMLS). This project involves internal research and input not only by the NLM, but also from the American Medical Association, the ANA, and governmental agencies such as the Agency for Health Care Policy and Research and the Institute of Medicine (Lindberg, 1995). The UMLS is intended as a reference language, not as an interface language or one that is used to enter data. The UMLS consists of three different but related types of information: (1) a metathesaurus of concepts and terms linking terminology from various systems including ICD, SNOMED, and CPT (Blair, 1995); (2) a semantic network that represents a variety of relationships between the concept categories

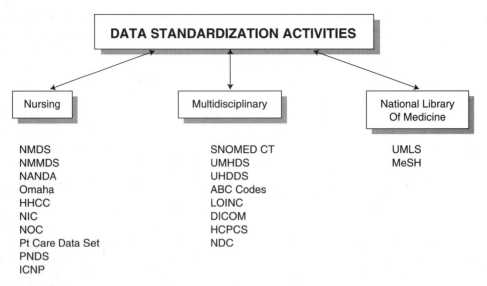

Figure 13-3 • Some Current Date Standardization Activities. Adapted from Simpson, R (1998). *Nursing Informatics: Nursing's Newest Specialty.* Presentation at February 1998 Caring Meeting, Washington, DC. He credits conversations with Kathy Milholland-Hunter as the basis for the figure.

to which the terms in the metathesaurus have been assigned; and (3) an information sources map that contains information about the entire system. The objective is to develop a thesaurus that will allow clinicians from any discipline to search using any of the codes, vocabularies, terms, or concepts familiar to the individual user. The UMLS includes the standardized languages that have been recognized by the ANA.

 Summary

Nursing data are elusive. To determine the benefits of nursing from healthcare data that are currently submitted to reporting agencies, it is necessary to use what are called outcomes *potentially* sensitive to nursing. Most nursing documentation makes it difficult to find the nursing actions that produce these or other outcomes. Additionally, outcomes definitively sensitive to nursing are not easy to locate. None of these finds its way into the mandated data collection that is used to plan healthcare. Changing this requires that nursing identify the interventions, the nursing phenomenon to which they are directed, and the related outcomes. To make these available for research and policy planning, they must be expressed using standardized nursing terminologies so that they can be entered into and retrieved from a computerized information system.

The science of developing and maintaining standardized healthcare languages is known as *nosology*. Standardized terminologies are classified into a taxonomy which may be monoaxial or multiaxial. The classifying principle will depend on the purpose of the taxonomy. The granularity of a language determines the level of detail that a language will capture.

In the 1980s, the ANA recognized the need for nursing to standardize the data it uses in documentation. They have devised criteria for standardized technologies to be useful.

Using these criteria, 12 different standardized systems have been recognized. Two of these recognized systems are minimum data sets that designate the data elements that need to be collected, whereas eight are actual interface terminologies that can be used by clinicians to enter data into a computerized system.[3] One is a reference language, and one is a set of codes intended for billing. Benefits to be gained from using standardized terminologies in nursing include the ability to develop nursing decision support systems, to discover the best interventions for phenomena that are part of the independent functions of nursing, and to have nursing data present in a computerized information system.

Many different standardized terminologies exist in healthcare in addition to nursing terminologies. The UMLS is being developed by the NLM to allow users familiar with any standardized terminology to find all the information on a given topic while still using the language familiar to their discipline. For nursing to gain the benefits of this and other uses of data, it must adjust its point of view about documentation so that it includes both providing individual care and providing data for many other uses. If nursing is to move from its invisible status, a condition identified in a 1990 article in the *Journal of the American Medical Association*, individual nurses will need to unite behind the efforts to develop and use standardized terminologies.

connection—— **For definitions of bolded key terms, visit the online glossary available at http://connection.lww.com/go/thede.**

CONSIDERATIONS AND EXERCISES

1. List the uses of patient documentation for health planning. Compare these purposes with the documentation format used in a clinical area with which you are familiar. What conclusions can be drawn?

2. Match the data that you collect from a patient with potential uses beyond the care of an individual patient. Which of these data could be used to document:
   a. A nursing phenomenon that is part of the independent practice of nursing
   b. A nursing intervention directed to that phenomenon
   c. An outcome of this intervention

3. Investigate the many functions of the ISO at http://www.iso.ch/iso/en/ISOOnline.frontpage.

4. List organizations involved in standardization.

5. Describe the role of the ANA in the development of standardized terminologies.

6. Define the following terms:
   a. Minimum data set
   b. Taxonomy
   c. Axis
   d. Monoaxial
   e. Multiaxial
   f. Granular
   g. Interface terminology

[3] Those responsible for the NMMDS are currently developing standardized terminologies to be used in collecting this data.

h. Reference terminology
  i. Mapping of a term
7. Compare and contrast the 12 ANA recognized language systems.
8. List the benefits of using standardized terminologies.
9. Describe the function of the Unified Medical Language System.

REFERENCES

About HCPCS. (2001). Retrieved March 19, 2002 from http://www.ahacentraloffice.org/coding/hcpcs_about.asp.

American Medical Association. (1990). Trouble past of "invisible" profession. *Journal of American Medical Association, 264*(22), 2851–2857.

Beyea, S. (2000). Standardized nursing vocabularies and the peri-operative nursing data set. *CIN Plus, 3*(2), 1;5–6.

Bezon, B. J., Echevarria, K. H., & Smith, G. B. (1999). Nursing outcome indicator: preventing galls for elderly people. *Outcomes Management for Nursing Practice, 3*(3), 132–127.

Blair, J. (1995). An overview of healthcare information standards. Retrieved April 2, 2002 from http://www.hipaanet.com/cpri.htm.

Bowles, K. (1997). The barriers and benefits of nursing information systems. *Computers in Nursing, 15*(4), 191–196.

Bulechek, G. M., McCloskey, J. C., & Donahue, W. J. (1995). Nursing interventions classification (NIC): A language to describe nursing treatments. In American Nurses Association. *An emerging framework: Data system advances for clinical nursing practice* (pp. 115–131). Washington, DC: Author.

Clark, J., & Lang, N. (1992). Nursing's next advance: An international classification for nursing practice. *International Nursing Review, 39*, 109–112, 128.

Clark, J. (1998). The International Classification For Nursing Practice Project, Online Journal of Issues in Nursing, Retrieved March 9, 2002 from http://www.nursingworld.org/ojin/tpc7/tpc7_3.htm.

Elfrink, V., Bakken, S., Coenen, A., McNeil, B., & Bickford, C. (2001). Standardized nursing vocabularies: A foundation for quality care. *Seminars in Oncology Nursing, 17*(1), 18–23.

Goossen, W. T. F. (2000). *Towards strategic use of nursing information in the Netherlands.* Amsterdam, Netherlands: Gegevens Køninlijke Bibliltheek Den Haag.

Goossen, W. T. F., Epping, P. J. M., Feuth, T., Dassen T. W. N., Hasman, A. R., & van den Heuvel, W. J. A. (1998). A comparison of nursing minimal data sets. *Journal of the American Medical Informatics Association, 5*(2), 152–163.

Gordon, M. (Sept. 30, 1998). Nursing nomenclature and classification system development. *Online Journal of Issues in Nursing.* Retrieved June 21, 2002 from http://www.nursingworld.org/ojin/tpc7/tpc7_1.htm.

International Classification for Nursing Practice (ICNP). *Project: Information sheet* (1999). Retrieved March 21, 2002 from http://icn.ch/icnp.htm.

Johnson, M., & Mass, M. (Eds.). (1992). *Nursing outcomes classification (NOC).* St. Louis: Mosby Year Book.

Keenan, G. M., Stocker, J. R., Geo-Thomas, A. T., Soparkar, N. R., Barkauskas, B. H., & Lee, L. L. (2002). The HANDS project: Studying and refining the automated collection of a cross-setting clinical data set. *CIN: Computers Informatics Nursing, 20*(3), 89–100.

Larrabee, J. H., Boldreghini, S., Elder-Sorrells, K., Turner, Z. M., Wender, R. G., Hart, J. M., & Lenz, P. S. (2001). Evaluation of documentation before and after implementation of a nursing information system in an acute care hospital. *Computers in Nursing, 19*(2), 56–65.

Lindberg, D. A. B. (1995). The UMLS Knowledge Sources: Tools for building better user interfaces. In Lang, N. (Ed.) *Nursing data systems: The emerging framework* (pp. 151–159). Washington, DC: American Nurses Publishing.

Magistro, D., & Smith, K. (1998). Defining nursing informatics. *Caring, 13*(4), 2, 5.

Martin, K. S., & Scheet, N. J., (1995). The Omaha System: Nursing diagnoses, interventions, and client outcomes. In N. M. Lang (Ed.). *Nursing data systems: The emerging framework* (pp. 105–113). Washington, DC: American Nurses Association.

McCloskey, J. C., & Bulechek, G. (1992). *Nursing interventions classifications (NIC)*. St. Louis: Mosby Year Book.

NANDA. (2001). *Nursing diagnoses: Definitions and classification 2001–2002,* (4th ed.). Philadelphia: Author.

NEWS: SNOMED International Introduces the Comprehensive Healthcare Terminology. (2002). *CIN: Computers Informatics Nursing, 20*(3), 84–85.

Oermann M., & Huber, D. (1999). Patient outcomes: A measure of nursing's value. *American Journal of Nursing, 99*(9), 40–47.

Ozbolt, J. (1997, October). Multiple attributes for patient care data: Toward a multiaxial combination vocabulary. In CD-ROM version of *Proceedings of the AMIA fall symposium*, Nashville, TN, October 25–28, 1997.

Ozbolt, J. (1996). From minimum data to maximum impact: Using clinical data to strengthen patient care. *Advanced Practice Nursing Quarterly, 1*(4), 62–69.

Saba, V. K. (1988). Classification schemes for nursing information systems. In N. Daly, & K. J. Hannah, (Eds.). *Proceedings of nursing and computers: Third international symposium on nursing use of computers and information science.* (pp. 184–193). St. Louis: C.V. Mosby.

Saba, V. (2002). Nursing classifications: Home Health Care Classification System (HHCC): An overview. *Online Journal of Issues in Nursing.* Retrieved September 9, 2002 from http://nursingworld..org/ojin/tpc7/tpc7_7.htm.

Sibbald, B. J. (1998). Canadian pioneer of nursing informatics. *Canadian Nurse, 94*(4), 60; 59.

Simpson, R. L. (1997). Technology: Nursing the system, the nursing management minimum data set. *Nursing Management, 26*(6), 20–21.

Simpson, R. (1998). *Nursing informatics: Nursing's newest specialty.* Presentation at February 1998 Caring Meeting, Washington, DC.

U. S. Department of Health and Human Services Health Resources and Services Administration. (2001). *Nurse staffing and patient outcomes in hospitals. Executive summary, final report.* Washington, D. C.: Author.

Warren, J. J., & Hoskins, L. M. (1995). NANDA's nursing diagnosis taxonomy: A nursing database. In N. M. Lang, (Ed.) *American Nurses Association framework: Data system advances for clinical nursing practice* (pp. 49–59). Washington, DC: American Nurses Association.

Werley, H. H., Ryan, P., & Zorn, C. R. (1995). In N. M. Lang,(Ed.) *American Nurses Association framework: Data system advances for clinical nursing practice* (pp. 19–30). Washington, DC: American Nurses Association.

What is ISO? (n.d.). Retrieved March 19, 2002 from http://www.iso.ch/iso/en/ISOOnline.frontpage.

Informatics in Practice: Clinical Information Systems

Margaret Hassett, MS, RN, BC[1] and Linda Q. Thede, PhD, RN, BC

Objectives

After studying this chapter you will be able to:

1. Describe the need for an integrated electronic patient record.

2. Interpret the responsibilities of end users during each phase of the systems life cycle that facilitate the development and implementation of a successful system.

3. Describe the Patient-Centered Information Model.

4. List benefits from electronic information systems.

Information management has been a prime requisite of healthcare and decision making since healthcare became the province of professionals. In the 19th century and first half of the 20th century, healthcare in the United States was a charitable, community-based effort to care for the sick and needy (Staggers, Thompson, & Snyder-Halpern, 2001). Its focus was episodic; acute care was provided in stand-alone healthcare facilities (Staggers, et al., 2001). People often were born, raised, and died in the same community; their health records were in one physician's office and the one hospital where that physician practiced. Although information was important, there was little need to share this information because the physician easily had access to both sources of his or her patient's healthcare information. Additionally, few specialties were practiced, so patients generally had only one physician.

The last part of the 20th century changed this. Hospitals and other care facilities proliferated while specialties grew. The Hill-Burton Act of 1948 provided the money for the building of hospitals. In the 1960s, Medicare and Medicaid provided reimbursement for services to many individual patients, and the health insurance industry grew. This provision of funding allowed many new innovations to develop: new drugs, advanced surgical procedures, new technologies and equipment, and sophisticated diagnostic procedures. All of which led to the development of medical specialties, each treating a different part of a patient and creating its own record for that

[1] Manager, Clinical Applications, PatientKeeper, Inc, Brighton, Massachusetts

patient. It is not unusual to find a patient being treated by several physicians at the same time. These physicians share little information; they may duplicate tests or prescribe medications that are not compatible with those prescribed by another physician. Despite these and other problems, the current healthcare system relies primarily on paper records that are oriented to episode and provider.

The need for healthcare providers to manage information in an integrated manner and to provide high-quality care in a cost-effective manner has never been greater. Yet the healthcare industry continues to struggle to determine how best to adapt and integrate information technology to manage its data. To provide high-quality care it is necessary to have an up-to-date clinical record with accurate and detailed clinical information. The sheer size and complexity of the healthcare system today demand computerized information systems to provide this information.

Healthcare Information Systems

Like all modern businesses, healthcare depends on information. For more than a century, the main healthcare information system for clinical information management has been the paper record. This record is theoretically the repository of all information and data concerning a patient's health history.

STRENGTHS OF PAPER RECORDS

Paper records have many attributes that have led to their longevity. They are familiar, relatively easy to use, and very easy to customize. A paper record also can accommodate all necessary data and offers relatively good security against unauthorized access (McHugh, 1992). Additionally, these records are portable, allow flexibility in recording data, and accommodate subjective data easily; in addition, if not too large, they can glanced through quickly (Dick & Steen, 1991).

WEAKNESSES OF PAPER RECORDS

Many sources document the weakness of the paper record in today's information-intensive healthcare system. One problem is the difficulty in reliably summarizing information for discharge because the organization of the record is by department instead of by problem (Dick & Steen, 1991). Additionally, records are often illegible or incomplete and have inaccurate data and information. Lack of standardization of terms in the clinical documentation process contributes to the expense of coding the paper records to generate required reports to support both clinical practice and healthcare business needs.

Paper records also take a great deal of nursing time (McHugh, 1992). Estimates in the literature note that they consume between 25% and 50% of a nurse's time (Dick & Steen, 1991). Additionally, paper records often require the same data to be entered in more than one place. Clinicians may scribble notes on whatever paper is available, including paper towels and worse, then transcribe the data later, a process that may lead to data being entered incorrectly either for the wrong patient or being lost entirely. Unavailability of the record may also lead to errors or omissions in data entry or to clinician time lost waiting to use the record.

Perhaps the biggest weakness of paper records is the difficulty of retrieving information. Not only is a requested record often not available, but finding information in a record can be frustrating. For research purposes, access to information in paper records is very labor intensive. Before any analysis can be conducted, one must identify the records that contain the needed data, search the record to find the data, and manually enter it into a computer. All these steps offer the potential for error, as well as increase the cost. They also prohibit timely reporting of needed data for making clinical and business decisions.

NEED FOR AN ELECTRONIC PATIENT RECORD

The need for healthcare data, both from within and without an organization, is increasing. These demands are difficult to meet with paper patient records. Externally, government and other third-party payers are requiring data from patient records. The Joint Commission on Accreditation of Health Care Organizations (JCAHO) requires information from patient records to show compliance with their quality assurance program. Internally, healthcare administrators require timely data from patient records to allocate resources and develop effective strategic plans.

Meeting the needs of various healthcare professionals with paper charts is becoming increasingly difficult. Charts often become so large that busy professionals do not have the time to hunt for needed pieces of data. Various healthcare professionals need patient care data to be formatted to meet the needs of their particular discipline. For example, the primary physician needs a view that will facilitate the management of the medical aspects of care, the pharmacist needs to see data about medications the patient is receiving, and nurses need a view of information that facilitates nursing care (Dick & Steen, 1991). To meet these informational and practice needs effectively requires electronic multi-application systems that are interfaced to share data and networked to support communication of the information not only between practitioners but also between different institutions in one healthcare organization.

TYPES OF INFORMATION SYSTEMS

Patient care facilities need many different types of information systems to support and communicate the variety of information necessary to maintain proper care of patients. In a well-designed system, there is an interface, or an exchange of information, between systems to support the sharing of data so that the data does not have to be reentered. An order entry system, for instance, would combine the order with patient demographic information from the admission, discharge, and transfer system; send the information to the department responsible for discharging the order; and send the information to the fiscal system, where a cost would be attached and a bill generated.

Admission, Discharge, and Transfer

The admission, discharge, and transfer (ADT) application is the backbone of the clinical and business portion of most hospital systems. This application provides and tracks patient details, such as demographic and insurance information, medical record number, care provider, next of kin, and so on. All patient interactions are tracked or linked to this basic information. Laboratory results find their way to the appropriate provider or care area based on the information contained in this portion of the **hospital information system** (HIS). It is important, therefore, that the data in this system should e updated and verified on a regular basis.

Financial Systems

Financial systems are another distinct application in the HIS. They are considered by some as the second backbone of the HIS because they track financial interactions and provide the fiscal reporting necessary to manage an institution.

Order Entry

Order entry applications, which are in use in many healthcare institutions, are usually the second application with which clinicians must regularly interact, the first being the ADT system. An order entry system allows a clinician to place an order by simply selecting a patient and the needed service from a computer screen. When the selection is made, the order is immediately sent to the appropriate department. This saves time because the order is immediately transmitted to the appropriate department, and transcription errors are prevented. Additionally, order entry systems allow financial information to be captured easily.

Some opinion suggests that order entry systems ought to function in something of a **decision-support** mode. That is, if a medication order is entered and the dosage exceeds normal limits for that medication, the provider will be given this information. The system should also provide information about any potential drug incompatibilities and patients' allergies.

Ancillary Systems

Ancillary applications, such as those for physical therapy, laboratory, or radiology that integrate or share information with other systems, provide for some specific informational needs of these ancillary services. Ancillary applications may provide quality control, testing in a laboratory, assessment write up, equipment billing in a physical therapy department, or film tracking in a radiology system. Use of these systems can also improve reporting and documentation efforts.

Clinical Documentation

Clinical documentation applications are available in various formats. A good documentation system, whether for nursing or another discipline, is part of the clinical workflow and provides communication of real-time information. These systems remove the need to go find the chart and allow all who must use the chart to access it whenever and wherever it is needed.

Screens can be designed to support assessment documentation by listing systems, or practitioners can be cued by the system with a pop-up box to complete or verify vital information, such as allergies. In a well-planned documentation system, there is little need for entry of free text, although the ability to do so should be there if necessary for the occasional time when there is no place to input needed information. When these systems work well, it is because the healthcare professionals who will use the system were involved in the system's planning, design, implementation, and evaluation.

Nursing information systems sometimes use the nursing process approach with nursing diagnoses as the organizing framework. When properly designed, data collection supports clinical workflow instead of distracting from it. It should provide flexibility in both data entry and in viewing data necessary for patient care. Additionally, it should provide easy access to additional information, such as policies and procedures, as well as to literature available online. Clinical documentation systems should also provide for retrieval of data for use in long-range planning and research. Use of clinical data by practicing nurses can be facilitated by easy availability of **aggregated data**, which can prove useful in determining best practices as well as forming the basis for **decision support** systems.

Scheduling

Scheduling applications are another type of application often found in a healthcare information network. They can schedule patients, staff, or services with a department of the facility. Staff scheduling systems can share information with hospital personnel and the fiscal system. Patient scheduling systems are enhanced when they share information with materials management for supplies related to the scheduled procedure, the ADT system for patient demographics, and the financial system for cost accounting purposes.

Acuity

Acuity applications, which have been in use in some form for two decades, provide for the classification of patients or services in an attempt to predict and provide the appropriate resources. Given the unpredictable nature of healthcare, they are not always satisfactory. In a cost-conscious healthcare system, however, they are necessary. An acuity system may be integrated with other systems such as ADT, staffing, and documentation, in an effort to create more accurate predictions and to provide adequate staffing.

Specialty Systems

Many patient care units have special needs that cannot be met by a generalized system, such as the integration of a fetal monitor from a labor and delivery area. Additionally, intensive care units (ICUs) engage in many automatic physiological monitoring activities. These monitors are capable of continuously collecting patient data, setting off alarms for abnormal results, generating decisions, trending results, and interfacing with an electronic information system to provide coordination with other patient data. Additionally, when interfaced with a computerized system, they provide electronic storage for the record that is generated.

One of the biggest challenges associated with most specialty systems is integration of information between systems. Ideally, patient information should be provided automatically from the ADT system. Data should be provided to the practitioners through the results reporting system, and bills should be generated by the financial system. Many specialty systems are unable to provide for this exchange of information. The specialty system, therefore, must generate reports and billing information in an alternate form, such as a hard copy of a report. This information is then distributed to the appropriate places and, in many cases, reentered into a system—a method that is prone to errors.

Communication Systems

Communication systems, such as e-mail and Internet connections, facilitate exchange of information needed by the various healthcare disciplines. Although these systems are not usually integrated with the already mentioned systems, they enhance information flow in an organization and are already having an impact on clinical practice.

Critical Pathways

Information systems also allow for the construction of critical pathways. Critical pathways provide a foundation for multidisciplinary documentation that focuses on the attainment of a specific outcome within a given length of time. The pathway identifies the patient and desired outcomes. The outcomes and time required for their achievement are predetermined by representatives of the multidisciplinary groups involved in the care of patients with that diagnosis. The structure of the path allows for documentation of assessment elements, interventions, patient response to interventions, and coordination of documentation by all disciplines. The development of a critical path should be based on a review of the literature and a synthesis of the findings.

For critical pathways, all disciplines document on the same tool, which is focused on the desired outcome. In the case of a total knee replacement, the desired patient outcome is discharge to home in 3 days. Specific criteria include pain control, range of motion, ambulation, and medication knowledge met by a stated time. The respective practitioners note the element of care that is their personal responsibility. For example, physical therapy would document progress in range of motion and ambulation, nursing would record the results of pain control and the client's medication knowledge, and the physician would document related medication changes.

This form of documentation permits more cost-efficient care through better communication. Representatives of each discipline participating in the patient's treatment plan can see the whole picture and know the patient's current status. Care provider documentation is used to compare the patient's progress by noting results or patient responses in a progressive and interrelated format. This type of record keeping also allows for comparison of clinical data regarding interventions, outcomes, and multidisciplinary approaches.

Systems Life Cycle

To provide effective information systems, all healthcare agencies need a strategic information plan that details the function of information technology in the mission of the institution. This plan should be based on the mission of the organization as well as on the strategic business plan. It includes the results of both enterprise-wide needs assessment and problem/solution methods to meet these needs (Craig, 2001). The plan is driven not only by organizational needs, but also by technology and factors outside an organization that affect healthcare. Under this master plan, individual information management needs can be identified and met. The ideal strategic plan will be geared towards producing a totally integrated electronic patient record.

Each identified need is met as part of this overall plan. The system is developed using a process known as the **systems life cycle**. The steps in this process are very similar to those of the nursing process. The number of steps and the name used for each stage varies with the authors, but they all involve basically the same steps: needs assessment, planning, implementation, and evaluation/maintenance. In this cycle, progress is often backwards as well as forward, that is, as a new phase is being performed, there may be a need to revisit decisions made during an earlier phase.

NEEDS ASSESSMENT/ANALYSIS

The first step in the systems life cycle, needs assessment, is a broad category. The obvious information management problems for the specific system should be identified. An attempt should also be made to identify information needs that are not being met but which, if met, would be beneficial to the agency. This process will be more effective if a high-level executive is involved during this phase. The level of administrative backing often determines what can be accomplished with the information system, both in terms of finances and support for needed changes.

Identifying information needs is integrated with analyzing the present information systems, which may or may not be computerized. What is the current flow of information? Where are the bottlenecks? Who beyond those in one area needs access to specific information? When new systems are being planned, clinicians may express a desire to follow the present system. In the case of paper records, this is usually a recipe for failure. In paper records, the data recorded, information created, and its use follow the form of the record, but in a computerized system, data entry, uses, and flow can and should follow many pathways.

At this stage, it is an excellent idea to create a first draft of an evaluation plan. Overall evaluation requires asking whether the stated needs were met. There are other items that it may help to evaluate that can provide evidence of improvements in patient care and demonstrate return on investment (ROI). For this to happen, it is necessary to establish current standards for such things as the amount of time documentation takes, the number of errors and the patient safety issues generated through illegible or incorrect drug orders, and the length of delays in treatment because of an inability to get a medical record. The evaluation plan should also include items to evaluate at each step of the cycle. When the evaluation plan is used at each step of the systems life cycle, it can reveal the weaknesses in earlier steps that need revisiting.

Beyond identifying information needs, questions such as the following need to be answered by the planning team:

▼ What is to be accomplished or provided by the information system?
▼ What impact will the new system have on current workflow?
▼ What are the costs and benefits of the system?
▼ Can the system be supported and maintained with current organizational structures and personnel?

During this step, one will also want to determine the level of training that will be needed by the staff—not only the users, but the information technology (IT) support and maintenance staff. Initiating a computerized system for the first time will be smoother if employees can concentrate on learning the system and its issues rather than gaining IT or computer skills. Moving from a text-based system to a graphical interface that uses a mouse may also require additional training of some personnel.

Clinical users should be consulted about their information needs. They need to voice their expectations of the system, explain their workflow (including how, when, and where they use given pieces of data), and listen to what is being proposed. Often this step is difficult because clinicians have a difficult time expressing their needs in IT matters. An informatics nurse specialist can be very helpful in this process by helping end users voice their needs and by facilitating a communication bridge between IT and clinicians.

Clinicians with a basic understanding of the possibilities for IT management are very valuable in this process. A request for patient teaching materials, policies and procedures, as well as access to literature available in a system, although it may not be part of the current plan, can alert those responsible about information needs beyond immediate patient documentation. Being aware of standardized terminologies and asking that they be included in a new system may also be something that needs to come from the clinicians. Needs no one knows about can never be met.

After the initial expectations, needs, and current workflow impact have been determined, efforts in the analysis phase challenge the analyst to be creative and open to new ways of doing the work. This phase requires an effective melding between an appreciation for the users' needs, the required workflow, and the limits of the technology or organization's capabilities. During this phase, open communication between clinicians and those responsible for the assessment will assist IT specialists in completing an accurate assessment and provide clinicians with a realistic picture of what to expect.

PLANNING

This phase comprises several tasks, such as selecting a system and designing the parts (e.g., screen) that can be individualized. It is also necessary to plan for testing the system and training. Some of these tasks will be done concurrently; others will need to precede another task (e.g., it is necessary to select a system before training can be done). The planning phase is vitally important. The relative cost of fixing an error in the project increases exponentially as the development and implementation progress to later stages. The cost of fixing an error that is not found until the system is operational can be as much as 40 to 1000 times what it would cost to fix it in the analysis or planning phase (Douglas, 1995).

Selecting a System

In this part of the planning phase, data and information from the first phase are put together and translated to the needs for the system. The team identifies what features are essential to the new system and which would just be nice features to have. At this point, a team member may go back to the clinicians and ask them to differentiate their needs from their wants. Some teams will use a rating scale to determine the necessity of a feature. These criteria may then be incorporated into a request for information (RFI) or even into a request for a proposal (RFP). The usual procedure is to send an RFI to many different vendors then narrow the selection to two or three from whom to request an RFP. Note that preparing an RFP on the part of a vendor can be very costly, so one should not be requested unless the agency is seriously considering buying from the vendor.

At some point during this phase, site visits may be made to agencies that use the system being considered. Before selecting sites to visit, it is important to talk with several agencies and listen to both bad and good features. No system is perfect, and the success of a system may have as much to do with the agency as with the vendor. Site visits are best made without the prospective vendor present. During a site visit, talking with clinical users as well as with the information services people and administrative people will provide the most knowledge.

The site visitation team should include several potential users, not just IT services or administrative personnel. Creating, for each team member, a list of questions that will be used for all visits will allow comparisons between the different sites. Visitors should also be sure to see the system in operation. The staff nurse may find herself or himself functioning either as a member of the visitation team or as the nurse at the site being visited. In either position, it is important to be open-minded and listen carefully, not only to what is being said, but to what is *not* being said. Ask the prepared questions, and follow up on those questions when necessary. As a nurse at a visited site, be honest but fair in talking about the system.

System Feature Design

In the planning stage, partly in conjunction with system selection, concerns such as security, data sharing, and screen design will start to be worked out. The end user, or clinician, should work in conjunction with the development team on these properties. A large part of security depends on the end user, and the ways that he or she can contribute to this can be discussed. The physical layout of the agency will affect security needs as well as the functions of the unit. A unit in which emergencies cases are common will need one method of **logging in** and **logging out**, whereas a long-term care facility may be able to implement a different system. Home health agencies will have other security considerations.

Screen design is a feature that affects greatly how a system is received by users. In this endeavor, clinicians need to work closely with the designer. The clinician should think not only in terms of how data are entered now, but in terms of how the data are used both during data entry and for patient care. That is, when vital signs are entered, what other information would it be helpful to be able to see? And when vital signs are viewed, what other information is also examined? Trying out a prototype of a proposed screen will identify its pluses and minuses when it is still relatively inexpensive to change.

Adherence to standards in the system design and data collection enhances data sharing and aggregation among other systems, practices, and organizations and greatly expands the ability to create reports. Standardizing collection and reporting of data allow for increased benchmarking across institutional structures. Standards may be technical, such as **Health Level 7 (HL-7)** (the communication standard for exchanging healthcare data), or practice languages, such as the Nursing Intervention Classifications (NICs) (Zielstorff, Hudgings, & Grobe, 1994).

IMPLEMENTATION

Tasks from the planning stage overlap with implementation as system testing takes place simultaneously with other activities. Actual testing can be better organized after at least part of the system has been installed and is functioning. Some planning for training also occurs in an earlier stage, but it cannot be finalized until the system is somewhat operational. Training must, however, take place before the "**go live**" day or the day when the system becomes available to users. Another important feature is system documentation. This should be started in development and continued with each change made in the system. The need for up-to-date and complete system documentation cannot be overstressed.

Testing

Before the "go live date" or date when the system is put into use, much testing is done. This testing needs to include features and expected functionality of the IT system, hardware, backups, downtime, restarts, data capture and storage, network communication, among other factors. A set of situations is devised to depict normal and abnormal events that could occur. Clinicians may be involved in devising the features and functionality scenarios and in the actual testing. During this period, many "bugs" are discovered and worked out. The participation of end users in initial testing provides the design team with valuable developmental information. Users can verify that the system is functioning appropriately for inclusion in a workflow. Observing users during testing can also highlight training needs. Many times, something that is considered intuitive by the design team may prove confusing for the user.

Training

The need for basic computer training that is uncovered in the needs assessment phase should be met before training for the actual system occurs. Well-prepared users are vital to the system's success. Training is best done with a "play" hospital, sometimes called a training environment, in which trainees can work with the system but are not working with actual data. This enables them to enter data, make changes, and do all the things that they will be required to do in practice. The same scenarios used in testing can be used for training. The ideal time for training generally is within 3 weeks of the "go live" date. If training must be done earlier, it is likely that clinicians will need to review what they were taught. This can be accomplished by having a computer terminal that can access the training environment on the unit, or by release time to visit the training laboratory.

For the system to best serve users' needs, during training end users should take responsibility for learning to use a system by asking questions and providing feedback on functionality and features. Training activities should be viewed as multipurpose activities. The trainer not only teaches intended users how to use a system but also determines specific system support required by the users, as well as system design or function issues missed in earlier steps. During the training sessions, security and data accuracy must be addressed. By discussing the issues in the context of system use, the user responsibilities related to security are more meaningful.

Training should also include instructions on how to obtain help for the system. An ideal system will contain context-sensitive help, or help that is modified based on where in the system help is accessed. Providing easy-to-use flip charts securely fastened to the terminals can also assist clinicians in using the system. Many agencies also make use of "super users." These are clinicians who have indicated an interest in and aptitude for the system and have received a longer training period. Their job is to assist other users when there are problems. They may also be involved in training other clinicians.

Go Live

There are several different methods of going live. The one chosen depends on the needs of the agency and personal preferences.

The Big-Bang Approach. In this approach, or direct or crash conversion, the entire institution implements a new system at the same time. This method can be the most disruptive to an environment. It is used most frequently when there is no initial system, the system in use is old, or there is a requirement for implementation on a specific date, such as the beginning of a new fiscal year.

Pilot Conversion. This approach enables the testing of a system on a smaller scale. For instance, a new documentation system or point-of-care device may be implemented on one care unit for a period of time for the purpose of evaluation. If overall implementation is to be successful, it requires that specific evaluation criteria be established and that the pilot testing be completed within a defined time period. Usually a pilot implementation is used to determine operational or training needs for future implementation of the system.

Phased Conversion.   This approach requires the operation and support of the new and the old system for designated period. The implementation plan will normally address the specific operational needs and define the timing of the implementation. Specific departments or care units may be targeted with specific dates for a switch over to the new system. This method allows an organization to allocate resources in a more efficient manner.

Support for Go Live.   Regardless of the method of implementation, adequate system and user support are crucial for successful implementation of the system. It may be necessary to schedule additional staff for the first few days or weeks, depending on the number of users affected and the workflow impact. Initially, 24-hour on-site support may be required, with later support provided from a help desk. Vendor support is important in the initial stages of implementation to troubleshoot unforeseen issues that need to be resolved quickly, especially if the method used is the big-bang approach.

MAINTENANCE/EVALUATION

Although evaluation should be a part of every phase of the cycle, there should be a planned evaluation 6 months after implementation. Before that, improvements may be difficult to identify due to issues related to adjusting to new methods of working. If a pre-evaluation was done before implementation, comparisons can be made. In many tasks in this phase, evaluation and maintenance are often one and the same. Clinicians may find that there are some changes that would make the system easier to use. In such cases, clinicians should provide a thorough explanation of the needed change and the rationale behind it. In addition to these recommendations, information from the help desk concerning common problems will lead to the need for more changes. Established teams and analysts must continually evaluate any system and deal with identified issues.

OVERVIEW OF LIFE SYSTEMS CYCLE

Figure 14-1 provides a review of the systems life cycle. Notice that all during the cycle, evaluation and revisions occur that require changes in earlier phases. The systems life cycle is never completed. Systems will need upgrading, new features will be requested and implemented, and problems or requests will arise, be resolved, and probably spawn other problems or requests. Eventually, identified needs will lead to a new round of the cycle as these needs become too great for the present system or new technology becomes available. An information system is an open, living arrangement of applications, and it embodies all the characteristics of a product as outlined by the systems theory.

 Patient Centered Informatics Model (PCIM)

Today many agencies are involved in moving away from the departmentalized systems that have arisen in the past. Many unacknowledged factors contributed to the departmentalized approach to information systems. Healthcare is a composite of separate disciplines, each with its own level of power and influence in the system and a point of view usually reflected in the organization of a paper record and in the power structure of the institution. Lack of familiarity with computers by decision makers was another factor that worked against integrated information systems; many decision makers simply did not un-

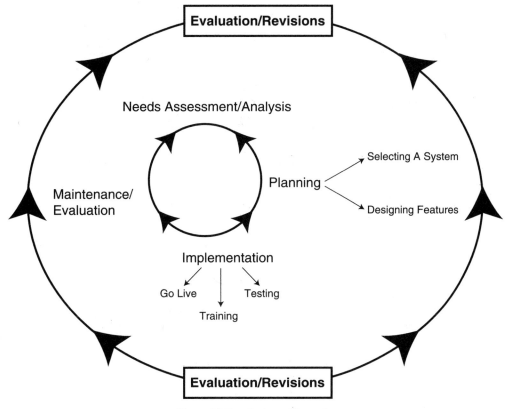

Figure 14-1 • Systems life cycle.

derstand the capabilities of a system, in fact, some saw the computer as just an expensive substitute for paper and pen.

This departmentalized view is changing to meet the current focus on outcomes and other needs for healthcare data beyond the care provided to an individual patient. Healthcare is an interdisciplinary endeavor in which different professional groups share the task of treating the same patient. Different disciplines all need some of the same data, but the data with which they need to be combined, as well as the presentation format, usually varies by discipline (Schoop & Wastell, 2001). Capturing this data more than once is not cost effective and leads to errors.

The need to help executives approach information systems with this broad focus as well as to make the patient the center of information management became very clear to Staggers, Thomas, and Happ (1999) after working with many large enterprises as they selected and implemented new systems. Based on their observations and concepts from previous models, they developed a framework to meet this need: the Patient-Centered Informatics Model (PCIM). Using systems theory as a basis, and taking into account maintaining the data, information, and knowledge foundation, this model considers information systems not as just another departmental or institutional need, but instead as an entity that must consider the world in which the enterprise itself exists.

The model (Figure 14-2) is intended to show the relationships of all elements involved in clinical information systems. Inputs are the influencing factors, the patient represents processing, and outputs are the results. As can be seen in the model, many factors outside an agency influence the design of an information system. These include regulations issued by JCAHO and other regulatory authorities, laws, standards of practice for all the disciplines, agency policies, and the healthcare model of the agency itself. For example, if the agency supports patient self-care methods such as health promotion and disease prevention, the design will need to include a large educational component (Staggers, Thomas, & Happ, 1999). These factors are often underemphasized in analyzing the needs a system must meet.

The processing involves taking data and converting them into information and potential knowledge; in addition, it involves communicating needed data and information to people in various locations. In this stage, the patient stands on technology because it forms the base on which the entire model rests. The various healthcare processes (e.g., managed care) represent one factor to be considered in processing, as does identifying information about the provider and the location where the care is delivered. Processing requirements also include providing real-time access to a knowledge base such as to care guidelines and current research, an area that remains one of the most underdeveloped areas in information systems. The processing system must, of course, keep the patient at the heart of the system and support a consistent identification using something such as a master patient index.

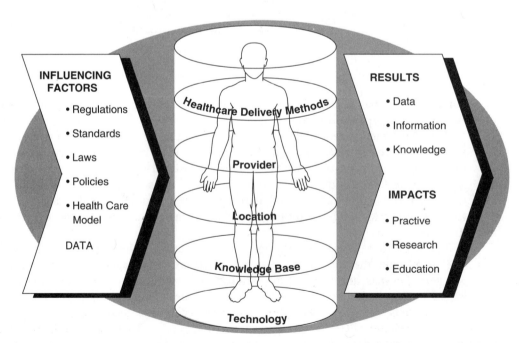

Figure 14-2 • Patient-Centered Information Model. Used with permission from Staggers, N., Thomas, C. R., & Happ, B. (1999). An operational model for patient-centered informatics. *Computers in Nursing, 17*(6), 278–285.

The outputs are the provision of data and information in real time as and when required by the end user. Outputs include measurable outputs, discrete data, synthesized information, and knowledge that is arrayed for maximum ease of comprehension. These outputs will not only be useful in practice, but they can also provide data for research and education. The aim of the PCIM is to facilitate a change in the point of view of executives, clinicians, and informaticists. Instead of a focus on individual departmental systems, this model promotes seeing an information system as an integrating, synthesizing force that is affected by and affects the entire healthcare community. This community includes the patient, individual practitioners, and the outside factors in the community, region, nation, and world that affect healthcare. This approach does not change the key ingredient in implementing a successful information system, which is that the system meet user needs and match the way information flows in an organization.

Benefits of an Electronic Patient Care Record

Electronic information systems permit healthcare providers to collect and communicate patient data in a more effective and efficient manner. One of the most frequently realized benefits is that more complete, legible information is easily available. Another benefit seen in a well-designed integrated information system is that the organizational time and money spent on tracking physicians' orders, telephone calls, and change of shift reports decrease (Bowles, 1997). Shortening the time wasted waiting for information and eliminating unnecessary services are advantages seen regularly. Problems that arise when a patient is in one location and the chart is in another will also be eliminated. Information can be easily shared between involved disciplines to facilitate high-quality patient care.

Information systems can also provide access to the patients' charts regardless of the physical location of the patient. For instance, when a patient is scheduled for an x-ray, the radiology department personnel can view patient demographics, the patient's health history and insurance information without ever leaving the department. Meanwhile, the physician can be notified that an order directing nothing be given to the patient orally (NPO) and orders for preparation for the procedure are needed. Once given, they can be automatically communicated to the dietary, pharmacy, and nursing staff.

REAL-TIME INFORMATION

Another benefit of an integrated electronic information system is the ability to get information in real time. An example is the patient who is referred to a facility for an outpatient test, such as magnetic resonance imaging (MRI). The referring office, if it is connected to the same information system, will be able to view available appointments and schedule the patient for the MRI before the patient leaves the office. When tests are completed, results can then be communicated directly back to the referring doctor in a timely fashion. In addition to providing a copy to the physician, the results can be placed in the patient's record; this will ensure that they will not become lost or misfiled. Treatment plans are enhanced with this type of rapid information exchange; it supports efficient and informed practitioner decision-making. Quality management and risk management needs can also be meet with real time data and on-line reports.

IMPROVED QUALITY

In non-computerized systems, the Institute of Medicine (IOM) reported that 11% of test results are lost, thus requiring repeating the test; 30% of ordered treatments are never documented; and in 40% of cases, a diagnosis is never recorded (Song, Ho, & Ho, 1997). An electronic information system can improve quality of care by preventing these all too common difficulties. Computerized systems also have the potential to prevent errors. When physicians enter orders directly into the system, transcription errors are eliminated. Additionally, the order can be compared with recommended dosages stored in the database, and the physician can be provided with information about the drug prescribed. When this order is integrated with patient information about the drugs the patient is concurrently receiving, as well as the patient's allergies, drug mismatches can be better avoided. Other clinical reminders can be used to ensure that a patient is receiving the correct drug. The Health Evaluation Logical Processing (HELP) system at Latter Day Saints hospital in Salt Lake City, Utah, combines the results of microbiology cultures for antibiotic susceptibility with a physician's order (Goldszmidt, 1996). If the patient is not receiving an antibiotic effective against that particular pathogen, the system issues an antibiotic alert to the clinical pharmacist. In 1 year, 49% of the physicians contacted about these alerts were unaware that the prescribed drug was ineffective against the pathogen for which it was prescribed. The system also monitors for adverse drug reactions by looking at all drug orders, results of certain laboratory tests, and drug levels. If a problem is found, an alert is printed which is verified by either the pharmacist or a nurse. In the first year that this part of the system was operational, it facilitated the identification of 401 problems.

The collection of information relative to the effectiveness of patient care is another advantage to automated patient and treatment documentation. Documentation systems can be structured behind the screens to aggregate data input for specific reports. One is able to easily extract information that previously could be obtained only through exhaustive chart reviews. This will enable clinicians to use clinical data to enlarge their focus of patient care from individual patients to recommendations for overall improvements in patient care. When standardized nursing terminologies are used in the system, nurses and others will be able to locate and use information identifying the autonomous activities that nursing adds to healthcare.

FINANCIAL SAVINGS

Installing information systems is expensive, but few methods have been developed to measure ROI. Part of this may be due to the low value placed on information and informatics by the health industry (Stead & Lorenzi, 1999). This view does not lend itself to easily identifying the measurements that demonstrate cost savings. A well-designed, successful system, however, can show benefits in many areas, which adds to the difficulty in calculating ROI (Display 14-1). Which costs and benefits have been calculated greatly affect reported ROI. Some costs, such as time saved, can be calculated only if the tasks have been timed before the computerized patient record was installed. Others, like paper costs, can be measured and have been. A study at the Princeton Medical Center found the paper costs for charts was $41,795 in the last year that was measured before they went completely paperless (Raygor, 1994). Many institutions report savings from using computerized records instead of paper (Adderley, Hyde, & Mauseth 1997).

Display 14-1 • CONSIDERATIONS IN CALCULATING THE BENEFITS OF AN ELECTRONIC HEALTH RECORD (EHR)

Some things to be considered in calculating return on investment (ROI) on an EHR (dependent on the features installed):

- Is there an improvement in patient care?
  Are antibiotics that are not effective against a specific microbe no longer being administered?
  Are drug incompatibilities uncovered?
  Is length of stay (LOS) decreased and outcomes improved by the availability of patient information and access to a knowledge base/decision support system?
  Is there a reduction in lost data?
  Are there fewer costly errors in care?

- Is time saved by:
  Recording information by all disciplines?
  Retrieving information (including decrease in number of telephone calls, or gaining access to a chart)?
  Preparing data required for various internal and external reports?

  Follow up time for incomplete records because records are more complete?
  Monitoring quality and outcomes?
  Newly ordered drugs being sent to the unit?
  Receiving reports from other departments?
  Not having to look for a chart?
  Being able to easily read the chart?

- Do the time savings increase patient satisfaction?

- Is there a reduction in staff frustration due to inability to retrieve needed information? Does this reduce employee sick time or turnover?

- Are charges reported more accurately?

- Is there a reduction in incidents, such as medication errors or patient falls, because of better monitoring?

- How much money is saved buying less paper?

Other savings are illustrated by the experience of the Maimonides Medical Center in New York where a system was implemented with the goal of empowering healthcare professionals by providing the information they needed when and where they needed it (Sullivan, 2002). This agency found that this system, by improving physicians' diagnostic interpretations and leading to more accurate and efficient treatment, reduced the average length of stay by 2.21 days. Additionally, they found a decrease in the period of time from when a drug was ordered until it was delivered to the unit (from 275 to 88 minutes), a 58% decrease in problem medication orders, and a 20% reduction in ancillary test orders.

Results at the Maimonides Medical Center also demonstrated that time savings in communication needs to be considered in calculating an ROI. One early study demonstrated that electronic communications systems can save up to 1 hour per nurse per shift (Barrett, Barnum, Gordon & Pesut cited in Hendrickson & Kovner, 1990). Other published studies demonstrate that nursing information systems save nursing time (K.H. Bowles, 1997). Some published studies, however, refute these findings (Hendrickson & Kovner, 1990). Some of the differences may be due to the features that the information system supports. For example, those that support communication seem to have a labor saving factor, whereas those emphasizing charting or physiological monitoring do not. This may be because the measurements of time involved in this task do not take into account the time saved in locating information. Evaluation of time saved must take into account the affects that a given task has on other tasks; time cannot be evaluated as a stand-alone factor.

Summary

The original healthcare computerized systems met financial and billing needs. As computerized systems moved into the clinical area, individual systems that focused on a department or a process became the norm. Healthcare information, however, needs to serve not only individual clinicians or departments. It needs to be a tool for auditing the quality of care and uncovering practice knowledge. Additionally, it needs to serve healthcare planners, researchers, lawyers, and third-party payers.

To meet this need, healthcare agencies need a strategic information plan to be used as a guide to selecting and implementing necessary information systems. Carrying out this plan involves the individual systems that are implemented in a process known as the systems life cycle that parallels the steps in the nursing process. The involvement of end users, such as practicing nurses, in all stages of this cycle is imperative to a successful implementation and system. A well-planned and implemented system can provide many benefits, including improved efficiency in both communication and documentation. Information systems can also provide aggregated data for use in improving clinical practices. When standardized nursing languages are included in a documentation system, nursing data will be available for unit, institutional, and regional uses, and it will demonstrate the value that nurses add to healthcare.

One factor that has slowed down implementation of information systems has been concern about ROI. Healthcare agencies that adopt systems that improve communication seem to have more success in creating savings than those in which systems are concerned more with documentation. Still, there are few agreed upon output measures on which to base this, but some agencies have found savings when a broad outlook is taken.

connection For definitions of bolded key terms, visit the online glossary available at http://connection.lww.com/go/thede.

CONSIDERATIONS AND EXERCISES

1. In two to three pages, describe the need for an integrated electronic patient record. Include examples from your experience as a patient and/or healthcare provider.

2. Give examples of behaviors that end users should demonstrate during each phase of the systems life cycle and that will affect the success of a system.

3. List factors that you see necessary for inclusion in the Patient-Centered Information Model.

4. Which benefits from an information system do you see, and which do you not see, in an agency with which you are familiar? Give some possible reasons for any discrepancies.

REFERENCES

Adderley, D., Hyde, C., & Mauseth, P. (1997). The computer age impacts nurses. *Computers in Nursing, 15*(1), 43–46.

Barrett, J. P., Barnum R. A., Gordon, B. B., & Pesut, R. N. (1975). *Evaluation of the implementation of a medical information system in a general community hospital.* Columbus, OH: Battelle Columbus Laboratories (NTIS #PB 248 340).

Bowles, K. H. (1997). The barriers and benefits of nursing information systems. *Computers in Nursing, 15*(4), 191–196.

Craig, J. B. The life cycle of a health information system. In S. Engelbardt & R. Nelson (Eds.) *Health Care Informatics: An interdisciplinary approach* (pp. 181–208). St. Louis: Mosby.

Dick, R., & Steen, E. V. (Eds.). (1991). *The computer-based patient record.* Washington, D.C.: National Academy Press.

Douglas, M. (1995). Butterflies, bonsai, and buonarroti: Images for the nurse analyst. In M. J. Ball, K. J. Hannah, S. Newbold, & J. V. Douglas (Eds.). *Nursing and informatics: Where caring and technology meet* (2nd ed.; pp. 84–94) New York: Springer-Verlag.

Goldszmidt, E. (1996). Applicatio*ns of medical informatics in antibiotic therapy.* Available online at http://mystic.biomed.mcgill.ca/~goldszmi/camel-2.html. Retrieved March 5, 1998.

Hendrickson, G. & Koner, C. T. (1990). Effects of computers on nursing resources. *Computers in Nursing, 8*(1), 16–32.

McHugh, M. (1992). Nurses' needs for computer-based patient records. In M. J. Ball & M. F. Cohen (Eds.). *Aspects of the computer-based patient record* (pp. 16–29). New York: Springer-Verlag.

Raygor, A. J. (1994). A study of the paper chart and its potential for computerization. *Computers in Nursing, 12*(1), 23–28.

Schoop, M. & Wastell, D. G. (2001). Effective multidisciplinary communications in health care: Cooperative documentation systems. In R. Haxu & C. Kulikowski (Eds.) *Yearbook of medical informatics 01* (pp. 379–387). New York: Schattauer.

Song, L., Ho, J., & Ho, S. (1997). The integrated patient information system. *Computers in Nursing, 15*(2 Supplement), S14–S22.

Staggers, N., Thomas, C. R., & Happ, B. (1999). An operational model for patient-centered informatics. *Computers in Nursing, 17*(6), 278–285.

Stead, W. & Lorenzi, N. M. (1999). Health informatics. *Journal of the American Medical Informatics Association, 6*(5), 341–348.

Sullivan, A. (2002) Connected EMRs Yield Measurable ROI. *Health Care Informatics, 19*(5), 65–66.

Thomas & Happ (1999)

Zielstorff, R. D., Hudgings, C. I., & Grobe, S. J. (1994). *Next-generation nursing information systems.* Washington, DC: American Nurses Publishing.

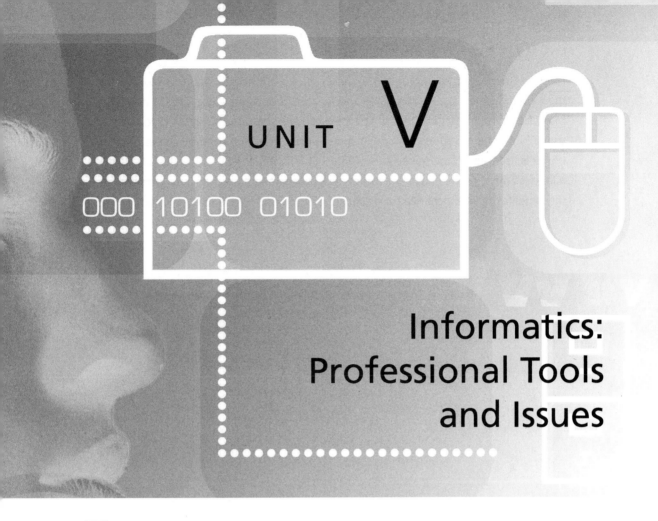

UNIT V

000 10100 01010

Informatics: Professional Tools and Issues

THE end product of informatics is knowledge. The process of transforming data into knowledge is the crux of informatics, but it does not end there. Using the products made possible by informatics is one of the themes of this unit. This, of course, is the main opportunity in informatics, but like all opportunities, there are many challenges associated with achieving these ends.

The first three chapters in this unit are interdependent. They are structured to focus on different aspects of using and finding information, but to gain a full persective they must be viewed as a whole. Chapter 15 provides background information that will facilitate the knowledge work that nurses, and all healthcare professionals, must do. Knowledge work requires information literacy and the use of technology, which are examined along with a brief discription of the critical thinking necessary in this process. Also included in this chapter is information about the use of informatics in research and administration. Chapter 16 examines another tool for knowledge work: databases, which can enable the uncovering of knowledge hidden in the current black hole of patient care documentation. Bibliographic databases are the subject of Chapter 17. Written by the well-known healthcare librarian Peg Allen, this chapter provides insights about the many bibliographic databases and tips for successful searching. Chapter 18 looks at the use of informatics in education and includes a discussion of the various types of CAI, how it is used, and some pointers for using it. The final chapter in this unit and this book addresses many of the issues that informatics professionals are confronting, including the benefits of a universal healthcare record, privacy concerns, and ergonomics.

Other Facets of Informatics: A Wide Impact

Linda Q. Thede, PhD, RN, BC; Susan Pierce, EdD, RN;
and Margaret (Peg) Allen, MLS-AHIP

Objectives

After studying this chapter you will be able to:

1. Interpret the nurse's knowledge worker role.

2. Interpret the relationship between information technology and information literacy.

3. Discuss the steps in information literacy.

4. Interpret the place of critical thinking in nursing.

5. Discuss the different types of knowledge-based information systems.

Informatics is valuable to healthcare in many ways. Too often it is only considered in terms of computers and information systems; the end product, data, is ignored. These data, provided by and transformed into information through informatics, support improved patient care practices. Transforming this information into knowledge, however, is not the sole province of informatics; it requires the involvement of all healthcare professionals. This participation depends on skills in **information literacy**, the appreciation, development, and use of evidence-based practice (EBP), the use of knowledge-based systems, and the use of special purpose software. Not all healthcare workers need specialized skills in each area, but all need to have an appreciation of how each area contributes to the goal of improved patient care.

Nurses and Healthcare Workers as Knowledge Workers

Today, the changes in the healthcare environment are demanding more information management tasks from nurses and other healthcare professionals than ever before. These changes are rooted in changes in society and healthcare. In developed countries, people over 65 are the fastest growing group; the U.S. population is more diverse than ever before; world population is increasing; and incidences of chronic illness and infectious disease are increasing (American Association of Colleges of Nursing, 1998). Additionally, today's ease of travel increases the likelihood of patients presenting with unfamiliar diseases, and the threat of bioterrorism creates an environment in which one must constantly be alert to a sudden onrush of patients presenting with similar infectious symptoms. Furthermore, the characteristics of the healthcare consumer have changed. No longer content to be passive patients, consumers now have easy Internet access to medical knowledge. This has changed consumer expectations about healthcare.

Healthcare workers must provide care to diverse clients in various settings, demonstrate accountability for quality of care and cost containment, and become life-long learners in response to the information explosion. All of these changes require nurses and other healthcare workers to acquire and use previously unknown healthcare knowledge—information that must be located, evaluated, synthesized, and applied. Information needs can be related to a model developed by Graves and Corcoran (1988), where sources of information for a clinical decision are shown as coming from both patient-specific data found in the patient record, from domain knowledge, expert personal (or colleague) knowledge, and knowledge found in published information (Figure 15-1).

The frequency and use of information serve as evidence to administrative officials and other healthcare disciplines of the essential nature of the information needed to support nursing practice. Identifying the types of information used contributes to recognition of the specific information resources needed at the point of care and the types of client problems encountered in specific care settings. Nurses must become aware of their information needs and be active in meeting them. This involves seeking out research information to make clinical practice decisions and developing a value for the use of this information. This value is essential for engagement in evidence-based-practice (Pierce, 2000).

Information systems that facilitate access to knowledge resources at the point of care are a first step in meeting practice information needs. These may consist of:

▾ **Decision-support systems**
▾ Bibliographic databases that provide access to published literature including original research and reviews of individual research, as well as standard care plans, critical paths, practice guidelines, protocols or other tools designed to enhance patient care

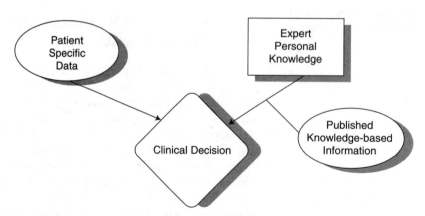

Figure 15-1 • Data use in clinical decisions. Adapted from Graves, J., & Corcoran, S. (1988). Design of nursing information systems: conceptual and practice elements. *Journal of Professional Nursing, 4* (3), 168–177.

▼ Factual databases that provide information about drugs, diagnostic tests, and treatments, as well as resource directories

Access in the care setting is vital; without convenient access to information, nurses and other health professionals usually rely on either personal or colleague "expert" knowledge, which may or not be current or valid.

 ## Information Literacy

Having additional sources of information easily availabe is helpful, but these sources cannot provide all the knowledge that a nurse needs. To meet these knowledge-based information needs, healthcare workers need information literacy, which can be described as the ability to define a need for information and the possession of the skills to locate, evaluate, and synthesize information to meet this need. It was recognized by the American Association of Colleges of Nursing (1999) as one of the fourteen essential content strands for nursing education programs. Being information literate is an expected competency for the beginning or experienced nurse (American Nurses Association, 2001) because it is through application of the information literacy process that research-based information is acquired and used (Display 15-1). In addition, information literacy skills are necessary to continue life-long learning.

INFORMATION TECHNOLOGY

Information technology skills are necessary to support the application of information literacy. Information literacy is concerned with information seeking, access, content, communication, analysis, and evaluation, whereas information technology is concerned with an understanding of the technology and skills necessary for using it productively. Information technology skills require three kinds of knowledge: current skills, foundational concepts, and intellectual abilities (Committee on Information Technology Literacy, 1999). Current skills imply the ability to use up-to-date computer applications such as desktop applications and search engines, as well as the ability to understand the underlying principles of computers, networks, and information. These two skill areas provide insight into the abilities as well as the limitations of this technology in information man-

---

**Display 15-1 • INFORMATION LITERACY
BEHAVIORS**

People who are information literate:
• Access information efficiently and effectively.
• Evaluate information critically and competently.
• Use information accurately and creatively.

Adapted from American Library Association (1998). Information literacy standards for student learning. In *Information Power: Building Partnerships for Learning*. Retrieved May 28, 2002 from http://www.ala.org/aasl/ip_nine.html.

TABLE 15-1 ● *Information Literacy Process*	
Step	**Activity**
1	Become aware of the need for information
2	Develop a searchable question or statement, then plan and implement the search
3	Retrieve the needed information
4	Organize, synthesize, and evaluate the information
5	Apply knowledge gained to patient care and evaluate results

Adapted from Elfrink, V., Bakken, S., Coenen, A., McNeil, B., & Bickford, C. (2001). Standardized nursing vocabularies: A foundation for quality care. *Seminars in Oncology Nursing, 17*(1), 18–23.

agement. Additionally, they provide the raw material for adapting to new information technology. The ability to apply information technology to problem solving requires intellectual capabilities that encompass abstract thinking about information and the ability to manipulate it to produce new understanding. Along with information literacy, these skills enable people to cope with unintended and unexpected problems when they occur.

STEPS IN INFORMATION LITERACY

Information literacy is a five-step process. It is based on the principles of information (library) science and is adaptable to all disciplines (American Library Association, 1989). These steps range from discovering a need for information to applying knowledge in practice (Table 15-1).

Discovering a need for information—the first step in this process—involves the nurse's developing recognition of when and how information can be used to improve the quality and cost-effectiveness of patient care. From this awareness comes identification of specific needs for more information to solve a problem. The next step involves planning how to obtain this information. This step involves two procedures. First, the problem that needs to be resolved must be formally identified and clearly stated; then, a search plan for finding this information must be devised. For a search to be successful, it is important to frame the searchable clinical question adequately so that it defines and describes the problem to be resolved.

To illustrate, a 16-year-old girl has been admitted to the pediatric unit because of complaints of headaches that have increased in frequency for 4 months. Organic causes have been ruled out and medications she has taken either have unpleasant side effects or offer little relief. To find information to meet the specialized needs of this client, the nurse must determine three variables or elements. The use of a template such as the one in Figure 15-2 is helpful at this stage. The first variable identified is that of outcome—what change in the patient's status is desired? In this example, this nurse has identified that the desired outcome is a reduction in the frequencies of tension headaches. She or he has decided to investigate the effects of structured relaxation on tension headaches. The desired population is identified as girls 13 to 19 years old.

With this template completed, the nurse is ready to plan the search strategies using these three variables as key words for the search. The nurse must now think about how to use and combine the terms to yield the most effective results and then which literature databases would be most useful for the search. The greater the nurse's proficiency

What is the effect of	**Structure relaxation**
	X Intervention (Predictor Variable)

On	**Reducing the frequency of tension headaches**
	Given Characteristic (Outcome)

For	**Females ages 13 to 19**
	Specific group of patients (Patient Characteristics)

Figure 15-2 • Example of use of a template to develop a searchable question.

in developing search strategies, the greater the value will be of the information re-trieved. Search competency in combining question variables into search terms is criti-cal in identifying the best available current information that can be used to guide clin-ical decision-making. A health sciences librarian can be very helpful with this and the next step (Pike, 2001; Pond, 1999).

With the question developed and the search strategy planned, the nurse is prepared for step three, which is locating and retrieving the needed information. This step combines the skills of information technology with those of information literacy. Selecting appro-priate databases among the many available for searching is the first part in locating needed information. (Chapter 17 addresses selecting and searching bibliographic databases.) Us-ing several bibliographic databases is helpful to ensure that the resources are varied and derived from different viewpoints.

After a search has been completed and the necessary resources have been identified, they must be retrieved. The nurse may find some of the resources in online journals, some of which are free, but others require a paid subscription. Additionally, a few print journals make some or all of their articles from back issues freely available on the Internet. Others may be available online to subscribers or as part of the full-text databases that are licensed by library systems and healthcare providers for access by their authorized users. Many re-sources, however, are still found in a library. If the library does not have the resource, it may be available through interlibrary loan.

When the identification and retrieval of information are complete, appraise the infor-mation resources for their relevance to practice. During this step, the literature is read to find and organize relevant information and to establish the accuracy and comprehensive-ness of the information. For help with evaluation, see articles such as "How to Assess a Research Study" (Rankin & Esteves, 1996) and research-based texts such as *Knowledge for Healthcare Practice: A Guide for Using Research Evidence* (Brown, 1999). When the eval-uation of the information is complete, the information must be synthesized and translated into an action plan.

The final step of the information literacy process is the actual application of this plan. Administrative support may be needed at this point, especially when it is necessary to de-velop new procedures before implementation. The results of the intervention must also be documented. If it is to be used with multiple patients, the best plan is to document with an electronic database, either an established information system or a database from one of the office suites. This will allow easy retrieval of the data for further decision-making and provide evidence to increase the body of nursing knowledge.

PLUSES FOR INFORMATION LITERACY

Synthesizing the results of a literature search is an important consideration for improving the quality of patient care and must be the first step in any research study. Research has shown that the information provided by literature searches changes clinical decisions (King, 1987). Other researchers have found that when searches were done early during a patient's hospitalization, the results shortened the length of stay (Klein, Ross, Adams, & Gilbert, 1994). A study conducted in the United Kingdom determined that information from searches was usefully applied not only to immediate clinical decisions, but also to the evaluation of practice outcomes and the design of practice guidelines and educational offerings (Urquhart & Davies, 1997). Studies such as these support Joint Commission on the Accreditation of Healthcare Organizations (JCAHO) and other healthcare accreditation requirements for access to knowledge-based information resources. Information literacy is essential for EBP.

CRITICAL THINKING

Information literacy is supported by critical thinking. Critical thinking is, however, a difficult concept to define. It is a little like good nursing care; we know it when we see it, but defining it in objective terms is complex. Consequently, it has been defined using several different perspectives. Some say it is thinking *about* thinking *while* you are thinking to facilitate more precise, fair, and accurate thinking (Paul, 1988 quoted in Wilkinson, 2000). Others believe that it is thinking that is purposeful, that is goal directed, and that requires the use of cognitive strategies to increase the probability of a desired outcome. Most would agree that it is rational thinking that recognizes a need for more information, is without bias, and with a goal to reach the most accurate conclusion possible. It is supported by information literacy. Breivik (1991, p. 226) related information literacy to critical thinking stating, "In this information age, it does not matter how well people can analyze or synthesize if they do not start with an adequate, accurate, and up-to-date body of information, they will not come up with a good answer."

Critical thinking is not the acquisition and retention of information, but a plan to acquire, analyze, evaluate, synthesize, and apply such information (Scriven & Paul, n.d.). It has two components: the skill set necessary to process and generate information and the intellectual commitment to use those skills to guide behavior. Critical thinkers approach a problem from multiple angles, but always in a logical manner. A vital part of critical thinking includes knowing when one needs more information, developing, and applying a plan for acquiring this information, and using this plan to generate knowledge. This plan can encompass searching for information in established databases, creating a database for the purpose of creating information and knowledge, or both. Either way, the result is directed toward improved outcomes based on information and knowledge.

KNOWLEDGE GENERATION

Integrating the published literature with **aggregated data** from computerized clinical information systems creates new knowledge. Knowledge generation has two parts. In terms of clinical informatics, knowledge generation refers to knowledge developed from turning nursing data into information and interpreting that to reach a new conclusion. From the research perspective, knowledge generation starts with the application of the steps of information literacy—identifying, retrieving, appraising, and synthesizing nursing literature to solve nursing problems in new and more useful ways. Recognition of the nurse's role as a knowledge worker evolves from understanding both parts and their relationships to nursing practice. Information literacy and informatics are keys to knowledge work and generation.

KNOWLEDGE DISSEMINATION ACTIVITIES

When data are changed into information and information is transformed into knowledge by nurses, such conclusions only maintain value if they are shared among the members of the profession to have an impact across practice settings. Knowledge sharing allows nurses to influence not only nursing but also to drive health policy and influence interdisciplinary health practices. The computer is a tool that facilitates knowledge dissemination in many ways. In a broad sense, raw data can be transferred between settings to facilitate use in different ways by different nurse groups. For example, spreadsheets and databases are software applications used to "crunch" new data or cluster it for interpretation; e-mail can be used to share these files between users.

After data have been transformed into information and interpreted, the findings can be published for dissemination across the profession. This can be accomplished by using desktop software such as:

- ▼ Word processing to create a manuscript
- ▼ Presentation and graphics programs to develop drawings or create a presentation or poster presentation
- ▼ Spreadsheets to create graphs
- ▼ Web development software to create Web documents and databases

Whether information is shared between two nurses or more widely across other members of the profession, information technology is helpful.

 ## Informatics and Clinical Practice

Knowledge generation and knowledge dissemination activities are an integral part of all nursing roles. Few nurses will become informatics nursing specialists, but all nurses need an awareness and general understanding of the potential of informatics. The nurse as a knowledge worker should embrace those activities and processes that are role appropriate.

EVIDENCE-BASED PRACTICE

The emphasis on outcomes and efficiency in the healthcare environment has changed the focus of clinical information systems from data gathering to the use of data (i.e., evidence) both from the literature and clinical documentation. The outcome emphasis has also contributed to the desire for best practices derived from EBP to increase the likelihood of efficacy of care.

"Evidence based medicine is the conscientious, explicit, and judicious use of current best evidence in making decisions about the care of individual patients. The

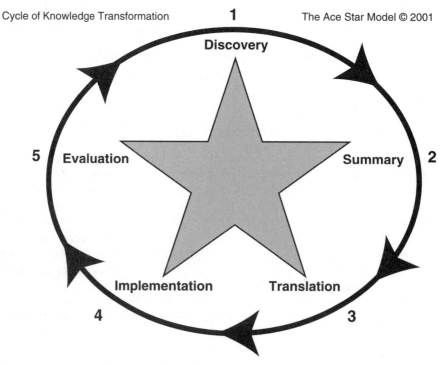

Figure 15-3 • ACE star model of evidence-based practice—the cycle of knowledge transformation. Used with permission from Stevens, K. R. (2001). ACE star model of EBP: The cycle of knowledge transformation. Academic Center for Evidence-based Practice. Retrieved June 4, 2002 from http://www.acestar.uthscsa.edu.

practice of evidence based medicine means integrating individual clinical expertise with the best available external clinical evidence from systematic research. By individual clinical expertise we mean the proficiency and judgment that individual clinicians acquire through clinical experience and clinical practice... By best available external clinical evidence we mean clinically relevant research, often from the basic sciences of medicine, but especially from patient centered clinical research into the accuracy and precision of diagnostic tests (including the clinical examination), the power of prognostic markers, and the efficacy and safety of therapeutic, rehabilitative, and preventive regimens." (Sackett, Gray, Haynes, & Richardson, 1996, p. 71)

The Star Model of EBP seen in Figure 15-3 (Stevens, 2001) depicts EBP as a cyclical process of moving knowledge from original research into patient care. In the first step of this process, original research studies are synthesized to produce an evidence summary. The goal of an evidence summary is to provide the best evidence of effectiveness by summarizing an entire body of studies. The process involves identifying pertinent research evidence through a critical appraisal of original studies using defined questions. The evidence is then translated into practice guidelines for use in the clinical setting, and it is often combined with clinical expertise to produce a set of recommendations of best practice. These best practices are then implemented into practice and evaluated in terms of patient outcomes, health status, efficiency, satisfaction, and economic factors. Conclusions from the evaluation stage may lead to more research.

EBP is about *using* rather than *doing* research. It is a tool for clinical decision making aimed at improving healthcare delivery. Its goal is to bridge the gap between research and clinical practice. In EBP, clinical observations must be systematically recorded without bias and synthesized with original research that has been subjected to a systematic review.

KNOWLEDGE-BASED DECISION SUPPORT SYSTEMS

A nurse, like all other healthcare professionals, is primarily a knowledge worker. To practice effectively, nursing must be supported in this role. Snyder-Halpern, Corcoran-Perry, and Narayan (2001) described nurses as data gatherers, information users, knowledge builders, and knowledge users. The nurse collects clinical data, structures these data, and transforms them into information that is interpreted with the nurse's specialty information and used in clinical decision making. When clinical data are collected and used to create knowledge, the nurse functions as a knowledge builder. In the knowledge user role, the nurse combines her specialty knowledge with the clinical data as part of both information use and knowledge building. These functions are supported within the clinical area by informatics.

When clinical data are made available and combined with synthesized research, knowledge-based systems can be created. A knowledge-based decision system is one that assists users in making clinical decisions. These systems range from those that assist a user to formulate a problem and consider the alternative courses to those that combine user inputs with a knowledge base from experts to make suggestions for courses of action. Little agreement exists about the appropriate terminology for this type of system; terms such as **decision support**, **expert system**, and **artificial intelligence** are often used interchangeably (Turley, 1993). If a distinction is to be made, it is generally based on the part played by the computer, with decision support systems having the greatest user input and the smallest role for the computer, and artificial intelligence having the greatest computer role and smallest user input. Theoretically, a decision support system will make suggestions based mostly on user input, whereas the suggestions of an expert system will have the recommendation and authority of an expert. Artificial intelligence software may or may not be programmed to act on input without user guidance. In reality, these distinctions often become blurred, and for the purpose of aiding the clinician, are probably not important. How these systems can help the practitioner is what is really important. In this chapter, we consider a decision support system as one that allows a user to consider alternatives; an expert system is one that uses a knowledge base to make suggestions.

Decision Support System

The purpose of a decision support system is to extend decision-making abilities, not replace them. There are different approaches to decision-support, each with a different application. One approach is to assist the user in formatting the problem. This type of software facilitates the identification, reduction, and summarization of information. Spreadsheets are excellent tools for this task. They allow the essentials in a decision to be formatted in such a way that the user can play "what if" by changing data in cells and viewing the result. Spreadsheets also include built in functions, such as basic statistical tools and financial formulas, and a sophisticated tool to allow users to rotate rows and columns to see different summaries of the source data. They also facilitate the production of graphs to allow the user to visualize the elements of a problem. Databases are also useful in formatting data and can produce reports for different groups about the same characteristic.

Making a decision involves analyzing and synthesizing known information while guessing at unknown conditions. An analysis approach to decision-support is useful in these situations. When using this type of software, a user is asked to identify all the variables involved and to assign a specific weight to each one (Meehan, 1996). These weights are then used to determine priorities.

Another type of decision-support software is an optimization program. Users input all the facts about a situation into the software, which will then generate a number of possible solutions (McHugh, 2001). The program then simulates the implementation of the various solutions, allowing the user to see the results and select the best solution based on calculated outcome. Scheduling software is often based on this model. The usefulness of this type of software depends on the user's being able to identify all the impinging variables.

EXPERT SYSTEMS

The purpose of an expert system is to evaluate data and make a recommendation that an expert would make, given the same information and situation. The expert system accomplishes this by combining inputs from clinicians with its knowledge base in a way that mimics the reasoning of a human expert. Expert systems have three overall parts: a database or knowledge base that contains the information needed for the domain of the system; a model base, or inference engine, which includes statistical and analytical methods for processing the data; and a user interface, or procedures for use in interacting with the system (Brennan, 1985). Several expert systems have been developed in medicine that focus on the diagnosis of disease (Pillar & Golumbic, 1993).

There have been several expert systems developed in nursing such as the Creighton Online Multiple Modular Expert system (COMMES) developed at Creighton University and the Computer-Aided Nursing Diagnosis and Intervention (CANDI) system developed at the University of Michigan. None of these has been widely used in clinical settings. Several problems remain inherent in developing an expert system for a domain as large as nursing. One difficulty is the existence of a multitude of conceptual and philosophical models that are different and potentially incompatible (Ozbolt, 1995). Another difficulty is the development of a knowledge base in nursing; this involves identifying and defining the phenomena that comprise nursing and then determining how they are related.

Nevertheless, some systems that work only within limited areas have been developed and successfully tested. One, in Thailand, assists nurses in making nursing diagnoses in the care of mechanically ventilated neonates (Jirapaet, 2001). Another system that supports family physicians and nurse practitioners in the management of patients with outer eye complaints has been found to perform nearly as well as an experienced ophthalmologist (Martin, 2001). This system is being distributed to primary care for use in managing this specific type of complaint.

As can be seen with these two examples, expert systems perform best in a situation in which the "depth of knowledge is greater than the breadth of knowledge, and where the content is specific and knowledge well understood. In these areas rules can be applied to restricted knowledge domains" (Turley, 1993). As standardized nursing terminologies become more common in information systems, it will become possible to use not only expert knowledge, but to combine it with data from actual clinical practice.

 ## Informatics and Research

Research is integrated and aided by informatics. Most information management needs in research are met by adapting word processing, spreadsheet, statistical package, database, or presentation software. There are, however, some special purpose software packages that can facilitate research, such as the reference management tools discussed in Chapter 17. Additionally, electronic literature searches are part of a researcher's tool box. All these tools are discussed in other chapters.

PREPARING AND ANALYZING DATA

Software for analyzing quantitative data is discussed in Chapter 11. Qualitative research, however, requires many different tasks and approaches, necessitating several different types of software. Deciding which software package to use involves investigating different types of software and obtaining a detailed description of what each software application does (or does not do). There are software tools that assist in recording, analyzing, and transcribing audio and video data; there are others that specialize in the collection, analysis, and management of observational data (QDA Resources, 2002). Text analysis is supported by three different types of software: text retrievers, code-and-retrieve packages, and theory-building software (Fielding, 1994). Text retrievers use keywords from the data to recover data that is determined pertinent to each category. A code-and-retrieve package facilitates dividing text into chunks, attaching code to the chunks, and displaying all the chunks with a given code. Theory building software usually includes the features of code-and-retrieve, but then it assists in making connections between codes for the purpose of formulating propositions.

RESEARCH USING THE WORLD WIDE WEB

The use of the Internet and the World Wide Web (WWW) has vastly increased in the last few years. The Internet and the WWW are natural additions to a researcher's tools. The WWW lends itself well to survey research, although it has also been successfully used in qualitative research through electronic mailing lists, forums, or a Web page inviting participants to respond in narrative format to questions. There are numerous advantages to using the WWW. The most obvious is the savings involved in not having to print and mail questionnaires. One study found a 38% savings over mail-based methods (Schleyer & Forrest, 2000). The pool of possible study subjects is also large. This worldwide pool could increase the generalizability of the research (Thomas, Stamler, Lafreniere, & Dumala, 2000), even though one study found differences in disease activity between a WWW-based population and patients surveyed in a clinical practice. In the study, the patients selected from the WWW were sicker than those in the clinic population (Soetikno, Mrad, Pao, & Lenert, 1997). Another advantage is the elimination of the laborious step of entering data. Data entered into WWW forms can be saved and moved to an application package, such as a database or spreadsheet, and then exported to a data analysis package.

One of the disadvantages of using the WWW is the possibility of multiple submissions of the survey by one person, although this is also possible with mailed surveys that do not have an identifying number. Additionally, the pool of study subjects is of necessity limited to those subjects who have Internet access. The demographics of this group tend to show a higher level of education and income. Other difficulties can be technical, but as the WWW and browsers for use in it have been upgraded, these difficulties have decreased. They can be kept to a minimum by designing Web pages that are accessible by older versions of browsers, particularly if study subjects are sought in less developed countries.

Creating a successful WWW survey often depends on the design of both the site and the survey. Using expertise in website design and letting respondents know the expected time required to complete the survey are good practices (Thomas, et al., 2000). The use of a security expert to protect respondent anonymity as well as to inform users of the privacy policies is also helpful. Marketing is often done using mailing lists to publicize the study. Before selecting a list, it should be monitored to ascertain that it is active. Asking organizations with web pages who have an interest in the topic of the research for publicity on their web page is another excellent marketing tool.

 ## Informatics and Administration

One of the primary roles of nursing administration is the management of both business and clinical information. This involves many tasks such as staffing, budgeting, reporting, and supporting the clinical practitioner. Fluency in the use of desktop application programs can assist in many administrative tasks. Other more specialized software packages can assist nurse managers.

PERSONNEL MANAGEMENT

Personnel management is one of the most important jobs a nurse manager has. Nursing personnel, staffing, and employment data can be managed with personnel management systems, which generally include four categories: personnel profiles including demographic data; daily work schedule and time-off requests; payroll data; and educational and skill qualifications as well as licensure information. They can also produce qualitative data useful in assessing the skills and qualifications of nursing personnel.

Staffing is one of the most difficult decision-making roles a nurse manager fulfills. To try to arrange staff scheduling needs accurately, patient acuity systems have been developed. Most patient acuity systems generate data to calculate the number of full-time equivalents needed for a nursing unit (Saba, Johnson, & Simpson, 1994). Some look at self-care deficits such as those related to activities of daily living, treatments, medications, and patient teaching. Another approach, known as time-based activities, is to assign each task a time based on hospital-specific, predetermined measures. Another method is the use of specified nursing diagnoses based on patient dependency. This approach uses decisions made by the primary nursing care provider. All depend on accurate data input.

PATIENT CARE MANAGEMENT

Most patient care systems are subsystems of larger information systems (Saba, Johnson, & Simpson, 1994). Some examples of these systems are nursing care planning, quality assurance, inventory systems, and discharge planning systems. They all add to the ability of a nurse manager to improve patient care.

Nursing care planning systems have been available for the last 25 years. Several approaches are used in such systems (Saba, Johnson, & Simpson, 1994). The older traditional approach generates a plan based on medical diagnoses. Newer systems of this type may even generate the nursing diagnoses commonly seen with a given medical diagnosis. A third approach is to base care planning on the nursing process. Advantages of the latter type of system include improved quality of information, reduced errors, and increased interdepartmental communication. A major disadvantage for a nursing process-based approach is development time. Schemes must be developed for each phase of the process.

Quality assurance systems can evaluate the quantity and quality of nursing services (Saba, Johnson, & Simpson, 1994). They use data from sources such as patient records, nursing care plans, and patient observations and can compare nursing performance against predetermined goals to facilitate making quality improvements. Inventory systems assist in the task of ordering, dispensing, and billing for supplies. Discharge planning systems include items such as a summary of the patient's learning needs at discharge, requirements for exercise and physical therapy, and a medication and problem list. They provide an excellent report for admission of a patient to home care or to a long-term care facility.

PROJECT MANAGEMENT

Project management is a task faced by both researchers and administrators. Many software programs exist that can assist in this task. They generally fall into one of three categories: bar charts (Gantt), critical path method (CPM), and program evaluation review technique (PERT). A Gantt chart uses a bar representing the amount of time each task will take placed on a time line for the dates when this task is scheduled. CPM and PERT are very similar (Project Management Tools, n.d.). They use a graphic representation called a project network or CPM diagram to visualize the interrelationships of project elements and the time element determined in advance for each activity. They both lead to a critical path. The differences rest in how they treat the time for each activity and their focus. PERT's main focus is the time variable, whereas the focus of CPM includes an analysis of the time/cost trade-off.

INFORMATICS AND EDUCATION

In the education environment, faculty and student can use informatics in different ways to enhance the teaching-learning process. These applications include the development of both information literacy and technology literacy. For a thorough understanding of the integration of informatics into nursing education, refer to Chapter 18.

 ## Summary

The pervasiveness of technology and the importance of information management in nursing cannot be overemphasized. Information literacy facilitates the access and use of research in guiding practice. Using evidence to validate practice provides nurses with a means for accountability and for clinical decision making. Generation and dissemination of new understanding increase the knowledge base of the profession and define the value of nursing care in developing positive client outcomes. The nurse's ability to manipulate information assures the place of the profession in direct care delivery and healthcare policy making.

Many needs in both research and administration can be met by desktop applications, but other tools are available to meet more specialized needs, such as qualitative research. Many of theses systems are often part of a total information system that assists the nurse manager in personnel management and in improving patient care.

connection—— **For definitions of bolded key terms, visit the online glossary available at http://connection.lww.com/go/thede.**

CONSIDERATIONS AND EXERCISES

1. Identify and discuss areas in clinical practice that demand knowledge work.

2. Describe the relationship between information technology and information literacy.

3. Employ the steps in information literacy used to solve a clinical problem.

4. Describe your use of critical thinking in a clinical situation.

5. Identify the differences between the various types of knowledge-based systems.

6. Write two or three paragraphs illustrating the use of informatics in administration and research.

7. One of the items in the list of Considerations and Exercises at the end of Chapter 1 asked you to "Think of the act of giving a medication. What data would you tell a systems developer was needed for this act? How should it be processed?" You were asked to save this answer and compare it to an answer you write after studying Chapter 15. Now that you've read information about an expert system, what would you now like to have included in this system?

REFERENCES

American Association of Colleges of Nursing. (1999). *Nursing education's agenda for the 21st century.* Retrieved June 3, 2002 from http://www.aacn.nche.edu/Publications/positions/nrsgedag.htm.

American Library Association. (1989). *American Library Association presidential committee on information literacy final report.* Chicago: Author.

American Library Association. (1998). Information literacy standards for student learning. In *Information power: Building partnerships for learning.* Retrieved May 28, 2002 from http://www.ala.org/aasl/ip_nine.html.

American Nurses Association. (2001). *Scope and standards of nursing informatics practice.* Washington, DC: Author.

American Association of Colleges of Nursing. (1998). *Essentials of baccalaureate education for professional nursing practice.* Washington, DC: Author.

Breivik, P. (1991). Information literacy. *Bulletin of the Medical Library Association, 79*(2), 226–229

Brennan, P. F. (1985). Decision support for nursing practice: The challenge and the promise. In K. E. Hannah, E. Guillemin, & D. Conklin, (Eds.), *Nursing uses of computers and information science* (pp. 315–319). Amsterdam: Elsevier Science Publishers.

Brown, S. J. (1999). *Knowledge for healthcare practice: A guide for using research evidence.* Philadelphia: W. B. Saunders.

Committee on Information Technology Literacy, National Research Council. (1999). *Being fluent with information technology.* Retrieved May 28, 2002 from http://www.nap.edu/catalog/6482.html.

Fielding, N. (1994). *Getting into computer-aided qualitative data analysis.* Retrieved May 29, 2002 from http://caqdas.soc.surrey.ac.uk/getting.htm.

Graves, J., & Corcoran, S. (1988). Design of nursing information systems: conceptual and practice elements. *Journal of Professional Nursing, 4*(3), 168–177.

Jirapaet, V. (2001). A computer expert system prototype for mechanically ventilated neonates: Development and impact on clinical judgment and information access capability of nurses. *Computers in Nursing, 19*(5). 194–203.

King, D. N. (1987). The contribution of hospital library information services to clinical care: a study in eight hospitals. *Bulletin of the Medical Library Association, 75*(4), 291–301.

Klein, M. S., Ross, F. V., Adams, D. L., & Gilbert, C. M. (1994). Effect of online literature searching on length of stay and patient care costs. *Academic Medicine, 69*(6), 489–495.

Martin, L. (2001). Knowledge acquisition and evaluation of an expert system for managing disorders of the outer eye. *Computers in Nursing, 19*(3), 114–117.

McHugh, M. (2001). Computer systems. In V. K. Saba & K. A. McCormick (Eds.) *Essentials of Computers for Nurses: Informatics for the New Millennium* (3rd ed., pp. 101–121). New York: McGraw-Hill.

Meehan, N. K. (1996). Decision-support systems for nurse managers. In M. E. C. Mills, C. A. Romano, & B. R. Heller, (Eds.). *Information management in nursing and healthcare* (pp. 45-53). Springhouse, PA: Springhouse.

Ozbolt, J. (1995). Knowledge-based systems for supporting clinical nursing decisions. In M. J. Ball, & M. F. Cohen (Eds.), *Aspects of the computer-based patient record* (pp. 274–285). New York: Springer-Verlag.

Paul, R. (1988). What, then, is critical thinking? *The Eighth Annual and Sixth International Conference on Critical Thinking and Educational Reform.* Rohnert Park, CA: The Center for Critical Thinking and Moral Critique, Sonoma State University.

Pierce, S. T. (2000). *Readiness for evidence-based practice: Information literacy needs of nurse faculty and students in a southern U. S. state.* Dissertation Abstracts International, UMI #3035514, 62-12B, p. 5645.

Pike, E. (2001). Librarian as resource. *Canadian Nurse, 97*(8), 6.

Pillar, B., & Golumbic, N. (Eds.) (1993). Acquiring and delivering knowledge from and for patient care. In B. Pillar & N. Golumbic, (Eds.) *Nursing informatics: Enhancing patient care.* Betheseda. MD: National Center for Nursing Research, U.S. Department of Health and Human Services. Also available at http://www.nih.gov/ninr/research/vol4/Chapter3.html.

Pond, F. (1999). Searching for studies. In S. J. Brown (Ed.), *Knowledge for Healthcare Practice: A guide for using research evidence.* Philadelphia: W. B. Saunders.

Project management tools. (n.d.) Retrieved May 30, 2002 from http://www.snc.edu/socsci/chair/333/numbers.html.

QDA Resources (2002). Retrieved May 29, 2002 from http://www.ualberta.ca/~jrnorris/qda.html.

Rankin, M. & Esteves, M. D. (1996, December). How to assess a research study. *American Journal of Nursing, 96*, 32–37.

Saba, V., Johnson, J. E., & Simpson, R. L. (1994). *Computers in nursing management.* Washington, DC: American Nurses Publishing.

Sackett, D. L., Rosenberg, W. M. C., Gray, J .A. M, Haynes, R. B., & Richardson, W. S. (1996). Evidence based medicine: what it is and what it isn't. [electronic version] *British Medical Journal 312*, 71–72.

Schleyer, T. I. L., & Forrest, J. L. (2000). Methods for the design and administration of web-based surveys, *Journal of the American Medical Association, 7*, 416–425.

Scriven, M., & Paul, R. (n.d.) *A working definition of critical thinking.* Retrieved May 28, 2002 from http://lonestar.texas.net/~mseifert/crit2.html.

Snyder-Halpern, R. Corcoran-Perry, S., & Narayan, S.(2001). Developing clinical practice environments supporting the knowledge work of nurses. *Computers in Nursing, 19*(1), 17–23.

Soetikno, R. M., Mrad, R., Pao V., & Lenert, L. A. (1997). Quality-of-life research on the internet: Feasibility and potential biases in patients with ulcerative colitis. *Journal of the American Medical Association, 4,* 426–435.

Stevens, K. R. (2001). ACE star model of EBP: The cycle of knowledge transformation. Academic Center for Evidence-based Practice. Retrieved June 4, 2002 from http://www.acestar.uthscsa.edu.

Thomas, B., Stamler, L. L, Lafreniere, K., & Dumala, R. (2000). The Internet: An effective tool for nursing research with women. *Computers in Nursing, 18*(3), 13–17.

Turley, J. (1993). *The use of artificial intelligence in nursing information systems.* Retrieved April 7, 2002 from http://www.hisavic.aus.net/hisa/mag/may93/the.htm.

Urquhart, C., & Davies, R. (1997). EVINCE: The value of information in developing nursing knowledge and competence. *Health Libraries Review, 14*(2), 61–72.

Wilkinson, J. M. (2001). *Nursing process and critical thinking* (3rd ed.). Upper Saddle River, NJ: Prentice-Hall.

Databases: Creating Information From Data

Objectives

After studying this chapter you will be able to:

1. Explain the role of databases in improving patient care.

2. Define parts of a database.

3. Normalize a database table.

4. Use query operators appropriately.

5. Plan a small database.

6. Discuss the limitations of databases.

Does hospitalization of patients whose diabetes is newly diagnosed prevent future hospitalizations for diabetic complications? Do certain approaches to pain management shorten hospital stays? Is the incidence of preventable illnesses higher in children whose mothers received postpartum visits from a nurse? The literature can provide some answers to these questions, but true evidence-based practice requires clinical data.[1] The clinical data that could be used in conjunction with the literature to answer these questions are recorded but are very infrequently used to answer these questions.

We record patient care information in the proper place in the patient's record, and there it stays. Any thought of using data **aggregated** from many medical records to answer clinical questions and gain a broader understanding of a condition is generally discarded because the format of most of the data makes this type of data retrieval difficult. Medical records provide a wonderful individualized record for one patient, but because the data lack structure and are too often on paper, comparisons with similar patients are exceedingly difficult. Given the long history of the use of paper records, it is not surprising that even when data are in an electronic format and could be used to answer clinical questions, we are unaware of the possibilities for using these data. This picture will change only when we gain an understanding of how a database works. This knowledge can come from learning about the databases that are part of all major office suites.

Nursing and Databases

We are all familiar with databases. The telephone book, an address book, and the *Physician's Desk Reference* are all databases. A database is simply a collection of **data** that are organized or structured in such a way that selections from it are easily retrievable, either singly or as a group. Paper databases, however, are organized, or indexed, by only one bit of data (e.g., a name in the phone book). Owing to this type of indexing, finding a name connected with a number is not an easy process. If a phone book were in an electronic database, one could easily either re-sort the **records** by number or request that the database produce the record that contained the number in question. Electronic databases, however, have many more capabilities than reordering records or finding an isolated piece of information. Databases are a tool than can assist nurses and other healthcare personnel in uncovering knowledge in any subset of data from an information system and in managing this information.

Nurses use data from many sources every day. In planning care for a patient, a nurse processes information about the patient's condition, data about the patient from assessments and the patient's chart, as well as data about the policies of the agency. During this processing, a nurse may also add data from other resources (e.g., a colleague, drug reference, or an article). When making a decision about how to care for the patient, the nurse transforms data to information, information to knowledge, and acts using a synthesis of all this data, information, and knowledge. After taking care of the patient, as the nurse reflects on what was learned, this experience may be combined with other experiences to increase a personal knowledge bank. The nurse puts together similar data from different experiences and comes to conclusions that are used to update his or her personal knowledge database. The next time the nurse takes care of a similar patient, this personal database will be called on, along with anything learned since. All of this information is synthesized and used in patient care.

Everyone has these personal databases; without them, we would be unable to function. When we find ourselves in a strange situation in which we are uncomfortable, the feeling of discomfort often springs from the insufficiency of our present personal database to cope with the situation. When we gain the needed data and transform the information into knowledge, we once again feel comfortable. We know what to do because our personal database now provides us with the information to allow us to act in the appropriate manner.

Although parts of a personal knowledge database may be shared with colleagues and new nurses, it is not in a format that can be used by others to promote quality nursing care, nor is it in a format that can be used objectively to determine whether one's experiences are similar to those of other nurses in other institutions and geographical areas. Additionally, the human mind is limited in the amount of data it can hold or work with at one time; thus, there are limits to a personal database. The data that we in healthcare need to recall and synthesize are both prodigious and complex. Living in the information age as we do, it is impossible to manage all this information manually and effectively. Electronic databases serve several needs for nurses and healthcare professionals. They can help us to locate and use data needed to increase a personal database as well as allow us to collect and analyze data to improve patient care.

DATABASE DEFINITION

A **database** is a collection of related information about a subject that is structured in such a way to permit procedures such as retrieving information, drawing conclusions ,and making decisions. *Database management* refers to those tasks necessary to create, maintain, and retrieve information from a database. A **database management system** (DBMS) is an application program that provides the tools for creating a database, entering data, retrieving, manipulating, and reporting information contained within the data. The tools available within a DBMS vary. A simple address book requires very few tools, whereas a clinical information system requires a DBMS with many tools. A middle of the road tool is contained in the professional version of all the office software suites: Access in Microsoft, Approach in Lotus, and Paradox in Corel. These tools are quite powerful and can be used by non-informatics healthcare professionals as well as by informatics personnel.

BIBLIOGRAPHIC DATABASES

One database format with which all healthcare personnel are familiar is the bibliographic database. These databases have been helping people find information for as long as libraries have existed, and they have grown to include specialized databases for various disciplines. Starting with paper card catalogs, bibliographical databases have now progressed to computerized databases, yet the same principles of data structure and organization exist. The difference is that with an electronic database the search capabilities are vastly enlarged. Structuring data in an electronic format increases exponentially the ability to find information from those data.

DATABASE CAPABILITIES

A database can perform many tasks. Often, data are available in an agency information system, but a lack of knowledge about how to use them keeps hidden information that could improve practice. Databases permit a user to massage data in many different ways. **Reports** can be designed once and printed monthly using the new data, and raw data (e.g., birth date) can be transformed into an age.

Database capabilities can be helpful in many places in nursing. One area in which a database could be very effective is infection control. All too often, the reports are done manually by leafing through paper records and counting occurrences. A nurse who knows how to use a database can easily produce reports and discover information that might not otherwise be visible. For example, the nurse could discover how many times a given physician's patients had the same nosocomial infection, or how many patients who had surgery in Operating Room Number 3 developed an infection from the same pathogen. Patterns can be looked at for a day, a week, a month, a year, or for any length of time for which the data are available. Falls could also be studied, as could the type of mattress used by patients who develop pressure ulcers as well as other variables that affect pressure ulcers.

Database Basics

The essence of any database is the data. Data are elements that have not been interpreted. The word *nurse* and the number 37 are data. They are out of context; although one may have a general idea of what they are, one does not know how they are being used or interpreted. The basic data in a database are based on this kind of raw data and are referred to as **atomic level data.** For example, a temperature reading of 37 is atomic level data, but a blood pressure reading of 120/70 contains two pieces of atomic-level data: the systolic (120) and the diastolic (70). Only at the atomic level are data flexible enough for manipulation.

The basic structure for data in most databases is a table. In a database table, each row is called a **record,** and each column is referred to as a **field.** Table 16-1 is a fictitious database for clients who have had some type of hip surgery. The labels across the top of each column or field are called **field names.** The first record, which has record number 1122, is for the patient Forest Green. In that record, Forest is the **field entry** for the field First Name. In that record, the field entry for the field Age is 23. All field entries in the first record are data elements that are information about Forest Green. They are part of Forest Green's record. The fields, or columns, however, contain data representing the same element for many patients. For example, ORIF—Rt hip, Rt hip arthroplasty, and Lt hip arthroplasty are entries in the surgery field (ORIF is open reduction—internal fixation, Rt is right, Lt is left). The entire set of records is a table. In some databases a table is referred to as a file. All of the tables involved in a project are called a database. The software used to manage databases is referred to as a DBMS.

Data seen in a table format are in the aggregate; you are seeing the entries in the same fields from many different records. In this format, it is possible to learn things about patient experiences as a whole. Database users can learn the minimum, maximum, and average length of stay (LOS) for patients who have had a left hip arthroplasty; they can count the numbers of patients for each type of surgery; or they can average the LOS for all clients

TABLE 16-1 ● *A Client Table in a Database*

Rec #	First Name	Last Name	Age (y)	Gender	Surgery	LOS (d)	← Field Names
1122	Forest	Green	23	M	ORIF-Rt hip	4	← Record
1212	Summer	Day	78	F	Rt hip arthroplasty	4	← Record
1234	Sea	Shore	65	F	Lt hip arthroplasty	3	← Record
1331	Will	Coyote	82	M	Lt hip arthroplasty	7	← Record
1357	Jersey	Farmer	55	M	ORIF-Rt hip	3	← Record
1441	Storm	Wave	68	M	Rt hip arthroplasty	4	← Record
2121	Star	Bright	33	F	ORIF-Rt hip	6	← Record
2211	Glen	Springs	70	M	Lt hip arthroplasty	3	← Record
2323	Tuesday	Night	77	F	ORIF-Lt hip	4	← Record
3113	Spring	Flower	73	F	ORIF-Lt hip	3	← Record
3232	Pearl	White	81	F	Rt hip arthroplasty	4	← Record
4114	Tiffany	Light	69	F	Lt hip arthroplasty	3	← Record
4321	Misty	Mountain	72	F	Rt hip arthroplasty	6	← Record
4567	Caspar	White	59	M	Rt hip arthroplasty	3	← Record
7654	Mark	Time	70	M	Lt hip arthroplasty	4	← Record
↑	↑	↑	↑	↑	↑	↑	
Field	Field	Field	Field	Field	Field	Field	

← ← ← ← ← ← ← ← ← ← ← Table→ → → → → → → → → → → → →

LOS = length of stay.

for all surgeries. With a small number of patients and only a few fields, this could be done manually. In real patient care situations, however, the number of patients and amount of data make this impractical.

For the data in a database to be used in this type of report, it is necessary that the entries in each field that denote a condition or other entity be identical. For example, in Table 16-1 the entries for the surgery "hip arthroplasty" are not all identical. One group starts with "Lt" and another starts with "Rt." Computers have difficulties dealing with differences; thus, to the computer the entries "Lt hip arthroplasty" and "Rt hip arthroplasty" are just as different as "tonsillectomy" and "cholecystectomy." This is one reason that the standardized terminologies discussed in Chapter 13 are necessary.

Database Models

The term *database model* refers to the way in which the tables in a database are organized. Several models exist: hierarchical, network, flat, relational, and object oriented. Each has advantages and disadvantages. The choice of which model to use is based on the tasks that the database must perform. Today, many operational databases, instead of belonging to one class, have characteristics developed from more than one model.

HIERARCHICAL

The hierarchical database was an early database models. This type of database (Figure 16-1) is a database with tables that are organized in the shape of an inverted tree like a taxonomy or the file structure of a disk as described in Chapter 5. In this organizational plan, often called a *tree structure*, records are linked to a base, or root, but through successive layers. In Figure 16-1, the Record Number table would be the root table. The Demographics table would be a child of the root as would the LOS table. Nursing Diagnosis and Surgery would be the children of the parent LOS table. Each child in a hierarchical database can have only one parent, whereas a parent may have no, one, or many children. The difficulty with the hierarchical structure is that it is hard to link data from one branch of the tree with another (e.g., Nursing Diagnoses with Demographics). When the hierarchical structure is used, it is important to consider the challenge of multiple relationships.

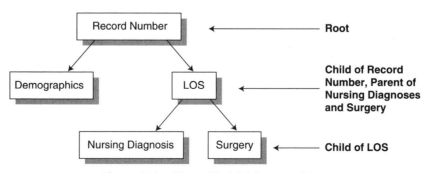

Figure 16-1 • Hierarchical database model.

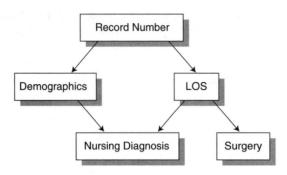

Figure 16-2 • Network database model.

NETWORK DATABASE

The network model of database organization was developed in part to address some problems with the hierarchical model (Hernandez, 1997). The basic structure is similar to that of the hierarchical model, but the trees can share branches. In Figure 16-2, the child Nursing Diagnosis has two parents, Demographics, and LOS.

OBJECT-ORIENTED DATABASE

The object-oriented database model uses "objects" that encompass both data and the data's behaviors. The behaviors consist of information about the use and processing of a piece of data. Each object relates to a parent or child, making it resemble the network model (Which Client/Server Database Technology Fits?, 2001). An object-oriented paradigm exists in most of today's desktop applications; right clicking on an object presents a menu of the behaviors (i.e., features) that one can apply to the selected object. The database programs in the desktop applications have the functionality of both object-oriented and relational models and are sometimes referred to as *object/relational databases*.

FLAT DATABASE

A **flat database** is a database in which the data are all in one table. Table16-1 shows a flat database. The address book in a word processor is another example of a flat database. Flat databases are very simple to construct and use, but they have limitations when it comes to tracking items that belong to the subject of a table when there are more than one. For example, if one wanted to track the children of people in an address table, to keep data at the atomic level it would be necessary to repeat all the information in all the fields for each child named in the address table (Table 16-2). This duplicates data, which not only wastes memory but more important is prone to error when the person doing data input does not enter the same information for each field. In Table 16-2, the name in the second record and the zip in the address field do not match the original, which often happens when duplicate entries of the same data are made.

Other attempts to preserve the flat database model may involve the creation of more than one field for a child. The problem with this approach is that the number of children a person has is an unknown variable; thus, the question becomes how many extra fields to create. When the same data are in more than one field, it becomes difficult to look at

TABLE 16-2 ● *Flat Database Problems*				
Rec #	**Name**	**Address**	**City, State and Zip**	**Child**
1234	Sea Shore	25 East Deer Run	Placido, AZ 88887	Laura
1234	Sea Q. Shore	25 East Deer Run	Placido, AZ 88878	Brian
1234	Sea Shore	25 East Deer Run	Placido, AZ 88887	Douglas
1212	Summer Day	210 Lake View	Asuza, NM 72172	Adam
1212	Summer Day	210 Lake View	Asuza, NM 72172	Brent
2211	Glen Springs	34 Mountain Side	Springs, CO 71717	

The fields in these tables do not represent atomic-level data but are used here to save space in the illustrations. In a real database, the name field would be two fields, and the city field would be three fields.

them in the aggregate. Another work-around involves entering more than one entry into the field (e.g., entering Laura, Brian, and Douglas all in the Child field). These data are not at the atomic level and will interfere with full functioning of the database.

RELATIONAL DATABASE

The relational database model uses fields known as **key fields** to relate two or more tables. This allows data from more than one table to be used to produce information. All of the databases in the desktop office software suites are relational, although they also incorporate many features of the object-oriented database model. One advantage of relational databases is that the tables can be related in many different ways; they do not depend on the tree structure (Figure 16-3). When presented with a problem such as that shown in Table 16-2, the table should be broken into two tables, as shown in Table 16-3 on page 267.

Breaking Table 16-2 into the two tables as shown in Table 16-3 is called **normalizing** data. Normalization means avoiding duplication in fields. It often involves creating another table to hold details that cannot be accommodated in a flat database and still maintain atomic level data or that would make it necessary to enter the same data more than once. Although technically there are five levels of normalization, being certain that there is no duplication of data, or fields containing the same item, usually fully normalizes small databases.

A relationship like that in Table 16-3 is called a one-to-many relationship; that is, one record in the parent table in Table 16-3 relates to many records in the child table. In relational database vocabulary, the main table in Table 16-3 is sometimes referred to as the *parent table*; it may also be called the **master table**. The table supplying the names of the children of the people in the master table can be referred to as a child table or a **detail table**; it contains details for a record in the master table. The relationship is through the key field, or the Rec # field, which is a field in both tables. To summarize, the relational database model consists of two or more tables that are related through a key field; the entries in both tables in the key fields are identical for matching records.

Using a Database

As stated, databases have many uses. Although a spreadsheet can perform some rudimentary database functions, using a spreadsheet to track nonnumerical data helps the

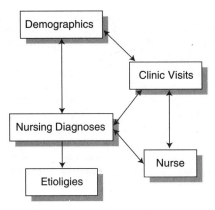

Tables can be related in any order as long as there are key fields that can be used to retrieve the needed records.

Figure 16-3 • Relational database model depicting the many possible relationships.

user to find only a small percentage of the information that could be discovered. Both databases and spreadsheets can sort data and create graphs and reports. Although a spreadsheet allows users to ask simple questions of the data, it is a database that permits users to create the more complex queries that uncover information hidden in the data.

OBTAINING DATA

Entering data in a database is one of the most onerous chores involved with databases. Another possible source of data is data that have already been collected, such as those from a large information system. Raw data from an information system will be American Standard Code for Information Interchange (ASCII) data. They will be in one of two formats: fixed format field or delimited file format (Display 16-1).

When users have to enter data, the database designer can facilitate data accuracy in several ways. One method involves providing a format for how the data should be entered. For example, a phone number might be entered as (335) 672-9875 or 335/672-9875. The field can be designed so that all the user need do is enter the numbers; they are then automatically formatted by the computer. Another method involves providing a **look-up table** of possible terminologies, which can be made to pop up when a user enters a field, allowing the user to click on the appropriate entry. Alternatively, the entry can automatically fill in when the first letters are typed. When numbers will be entered, the field can be set to accept only numbers within a given range; an error message will appear for incorrect entries that advises the user of the range of data needed. These types of fields should be used whenever possible.

Although data can be entered in a table, it is also possible to enter it in a form. Forms are used for data entry in a clinical information system. A **form** is a view of data that, instead of always showing data as a table, shows just the fields for a record that needs data entry. Figure 16-4 illustrates a form for entering the LOS for a patient. This form shows one record for the data represented in Table 16-4. Notice that on the form the field name "Rec #" has been changed to read "Record Number." In addition, instructions for finding

TABLE 16-3 ● *Relational Model*

Parent or Master Table

Rec #	Name	Address	City, State, Zip
1234	Sea Shore	25 East Deer Run	Placido, AZ 88887
1234	Sea Q. Shore	25 East Deer Run	Placido, AZ 88887
1234	Sea Shore	25 East Deer Run	Placido, AZ 88887
1212	Summer Day	210 Lake View	Asuza, NM 72172
1212	Summer Day	210 Lake View	Asuza, NM 72172
2211	Glen Springs	34 Mountain Side	Springs, CO 71717

Child or Detail Table

Rec #	Child
1234	Laura
1234	Brian
1234	Douglas
1212	Adam
1212	Brent

Table 16-2 would be divided into two tables in a relational model, related by the record number, which would be called a *key field*. Looking at both of these tables it is easy to see who is the parent of Douglas by matching the Rec # field. Using the key field, the relational database can place any of the fields in either table together to produce a table, such as Table 16-2. The difference is that all the entries in the name, address, and city, state, and zip fields will come from the one record in the parent table, meaning they will be identical, and only have to be entered once. Creating two tables normalizes the data.

the appropriate record are seen on the form, as well as a button for accessing the previous or next record in the database. A well-designed form provides information that makes it easier for the person entering data. The easier a designer makes the job of entering data, the better the chance will be of obtaining complete and accurate data.

The form view of data illustrates one of the advantages of electronic databases: they provide different views of the data. Not only can fields for entry of data be structured in different ways, but once captured, data may be presented in many different ways. The data can be used as part of a form letter in the same way that data are used for mail merge in word processing. Selected pieces from one record can be arranged in any form that aids the reader's understanding. The data can also be processed; that is, used as a basis for calculations that provide information. One principle of good database design is that no piece of data is ever entered twice. In a large information system, this would mean that after the patient's history is entered, needed pieces can be used to populate any screen for which it is needed. If vital signs are entered as atomic level data, they can be used to produce a graphic view of the data.

TRANSFORMING DATA INTO INFORMATION: SORTING AND QUERYING

When data are aggregated and processed, they yield the information they contain. There are several ways of processing, as well as presenting, data. The two main methods, sorting and querying, are often used together. Both can be used as a basis for a report.

Display 16-1 • ILLUSTRATION OF ASCII FILE FORMATS

In the fixed format, the fields will all begin at a given column and be a given number of characters in length. If imported into a word processor, they will look like columns. For example, in the fixed format data below the first name field starts at column 1 and is 5 columns long. The age field starts at column 16 and is 2 columns long.

1	2	3	4	5	6	7	8	9	10	11	12	13	14	15	16	17
W	i	l	l			C	o	y	o	t	e				2	3
M	i	s	t	y		M	o	u	n	t	a	i	n		7	2

In a delimited ASCII file, each piece of data is separated by a given symbol. Generally, non-numeric data are enclosed in quotation marks, whereas numeric data are not. In the example below, data are separated by commas. This would be called a comma-delimited format. Other characters may also be used, but the comma is the most common delimiter.

"Will","Coyote",23
"Misty","Mountain",72

When one knows the defining characteristics of an ASCII data file format, the data are easily imported into any of the databases in commercially available office suites.

Sorting

The simplest of the two techniques is resorting, which is reordering the records in the database. A simple or primary sort can reorder the records on a given field. For example, data from Table 16-1 could be resorted by any of the other fields in that table: first name, last name, age, gender, surgery, or LOS. It is also possible to perform what are called secondary sorts, or a resorting of data in a group that results from a primary sort. The records in Table 16-4 have been resorted using a primary sort of surgery that groups all the records with the same entry in the surgery field together. A secondary sort has then been performed on the LOS field. The records are now ordered from the longest to the shortest LOS within each group. These groupings can be used as a basis for a calculation; for example, one could calculate the average LOS for each type of surgery.

In the records in Table 16-4, the calculation for LOS for hip arthroplasty would be faulty because there are two different entries for hip arthroplasty. To prevent this, the users and designer of the database must agree on a method for categorizing these data. One method would be to eliminate the "Lt" and "Rt" entirely. Another would be to have a field for body location, or perhaps a field for right or left. The final decision needs to be based on the use to which the data will be put, and it must also be workable for the user. These are some of the decisions that must be made when an information system is designed.

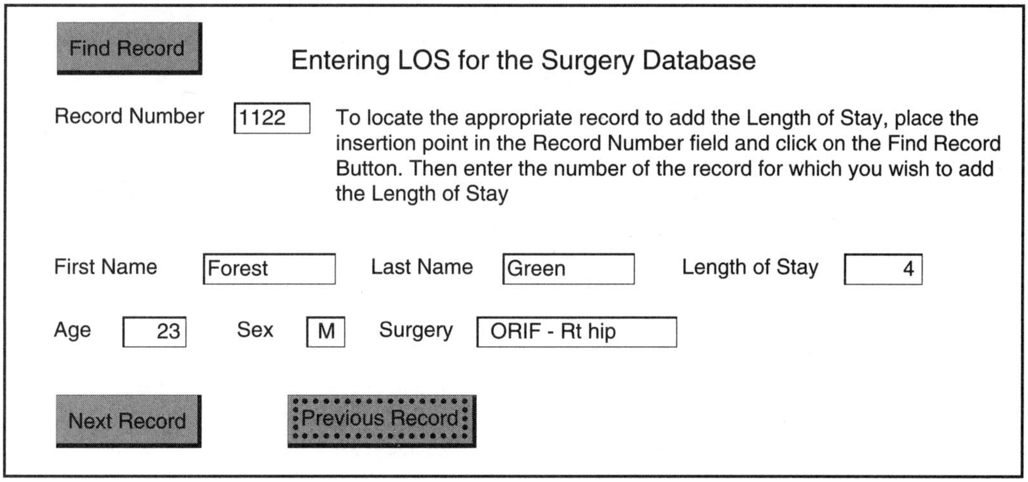

Figure 16-4 • Form view of data in the surgery table.

Querying

A table is the heart of a relational database, but the *query* is the feature that shapes the data into meaningful patterns. Queries can produce a subset of records based on fields that meet given criteria, or they can report on the entire database. Additionally, queries can be performed on the results of another query. The only limiting factors are the data available and the user's imagination and ability to use the criteria selectors, known as *operators*.

Queries are based on Boolean logic, which is named after the nineteenth-century mathematician George Boole. It is a form of algebra in which returns are either true or false. There are three Boolean operators: AND, OR, and NOT. They are used extensively in searching bibliographic databases. Using AND with criteria will narrow the results be-

Rec #	First Name	Last Name	Age	Gender	Surgery	LOS
1331	Will	Coyote	82	M	Lt hip arthroplasty	7
7654	Mark	Time	70	M	Lt hip arthroplasty	4
1234	Sea	Shore	65	F	Lt hip arthroplasty	3
2211	Glen	Springs	70	M	Lt hip arthroplasty	3
4114	Tiffany	Light	69	F	Lt hip arthroplasty	3
2121	Star	Bright	33	F	ORIF-Rt hip	6
2323	Tuesday	Night	77	F	ORIF-Lt hip	4
1122	Forest	Green	23	M	ORIF-Rt hip	4
1357	Jersey	Farmer	55	M	ORIF-Rt hip	3
3113	Spring	Flower	73	F	ORIF-Lt hip	3
4321	Misty	Mountain	72	F	Rt hip arthroplasty	6
1212	Summer	Day	78	F	Rt hip arthroplasty	4
1441	Storm	Wave	68	M	Rt hip arthroplasty	4
3232	Pearl	White	81	F	Rt hip arthroplasty	4
4567	Caspar	White	59	M	Rt hip arthroplasty	3

TABLE 16-4 • *Primary Sort (Surgery) and Secondary Sort (LOS) of Records From Table 16-1*

TABLE 16–5 ● *Mathematical Operators for Querying*

Operator	Query Criteria in Age Field	Returns
> (greater than)	>50	Records in which the entry in the age field is greater than 50
< (less than)	<50	Records in which the entry in the age field is less than 50
<> (not equal to)	<>50	Records in which the entry in the age field is any number but 50
>= (greater than or equal to)	>=50	Records in which the entry in the age field is greater than or equal to 50
<= (less than or equal to)	<=50	Records in which the entry in the age field is less than or equal to 50
Between	Between 30 and 40	Records in which the entry in the age field is between 30 and 40 (inclusive)
Null or blank (field is empty)	Null (or Blank)	Records in which the entry in the age field is empty.

cause the record must meet both conditions to be returned. When OR is used, a search is broadened, because a search can meet either condition. NOT returns records that do not meet the stated condition. These conditions may be used alone or in combination.

Although not strictly part of Boolean logic, other mathematical operators are also used in querying (Table 16-5). Like Boolean logic, these operators may be used in combination with each other or with Boolean logic. For example, a user may wish to see the names of the patients who were male, 55 years of age or older, AND had ORIF-Rt hip surgery (Table 16-6). In a relational database, queries may be constructed that ask questions of the data in all tables that have a relationship. For example, with a table of nursing diagnoses for the patients in Table 16-4, questions could be asked that show the nursing diagnoses for those patients whose LOS was the longest or the shortest.[2]

One other querying feature is available: wildcards. Databases use two types of wildcards. One can be used to find entries with only one character difference; the other represents the search for many character differences. The exact symbols used vary with the database. For example, suppose we wanted to find all the clients in Table 16-4 who had an arthroplasty. If the wildcard symbol for many characters was an asterisk (*), we would enter "*arthroplasty" to find all the records that contain arthroplasty in the surgery field. To find all those who had an open reduction internal fixation (ORIF) we would enter "ORIF*."[3]

Although it may seem self-evident, it is not unusual for beginners to want to answer questions for which data are not present. For example, the data in Table 16-4 could not provide an answer to who the physician was for each patient nor tell what the primary medical di-

---

[2] The tables from Table 16-1 and a related table of nursing diagnoses will be available on the text web page for downloading and using for practicing queries or doing reports in a relational database. See http://connection.lww.com/go/thede

[3] In application programs, wildcards have one symbol to designate one character and another to designate one or more characters. In bibliographical databases, the only wildcard is a symbol that represents one or many characters and a wildcard is used only at the end of a word.

TABLE 16-6 ● *Query Result of Table 16-4*				

The query below shows the records for those patients who were male, 55 years of age or older, and had open-reduction internal fixation, right (ORIF-Rt) hip surgery.

First Name	Last Name	Gender	Age	Surgery
Jersey	Farmer	M	55	ORIF-Rt hip

agnosis was for each patient. When planning a database, or asking for data to be downloaded from an information system, one must anticipate the questions that one will want to answer and be certain that the needed data are available. Queries can quickly become complex. For this reason, it is necessary to test a query with a subset of data for which you can easily determine the answers before trusting the results on a large set of data.

REPORTING

Reports can be viewed on the screen or printed out on paper. In an information system, when a user asks to see a graph of vital signs, a prewritten report is used to create the graph from the vital sign data. In databases from one of the office software suites, a form is used for data entry and to post data to the screen. A report is usually a printed format of the data, although it can also be seen on the screen. Reports, like forms, can represent many different views of the data; they are not just the data in the aggregate format of the table. In a relational database, reports can be built from the data in more than one table as well as from a query. The objective is to print the data in a format that will be the easiest for the user to understand. If a person is used to a given format for reports, the data from a database can be presented in a report styled to match that format. Data from either a table or a query can also be used as the data for a mail-merge document in a word processor.

Reports may include graphs as well as permit calculations on data. Additionally, it is not necessary to include all the fields in a table or query in the report. Display 16-2 is a report that uses data in Table 16-4. The report uses the grouping principles (based on primary and secondary sorts) and calculates an average LOS for each type of surgery, as well as the average LOS for all the records. Because the terminology for the surgeries is not the same, however, groupings and averages are seen for each terminology used in the field, not for the type of surgery. Notice that the report contains only the fields for surgery, LOS, and first and last names. In addition, the field names have been edited to represent the actual contents of a field.

After a report has been designed, it can be used many times. Each time the report is printed, it retrieves current data in a table to produce a report that reflects current content. Thus, the same report will differ whenever the data in the table change. For example, if every month we use the same report that produced the output seen in Display 16-2, the results will report the current data, not the data that were in the database when the report was designed. If date is one of the fields in the base table, the same report design could be used to print this report each month using only those data for that month simply by changing the query criteria. At the end of the year, a report for the entire year could be printed.

Display 16-2 • REPORT OF AVERAGE LENGTH OF STAY FOR SURGERIES

SURGERY	LT HIP ARTHROPLASTY
LENGTH OF STAY (DAYS)	PATIENT NAME
3	Light, Tiffany
3	Shore, Sea
3	Springs, Glen
4	Time, Mark
7	Coyote, Will
Average length of stay for Lt hip arthroplasty: 4 days	

SURGERY	ORIF-LT HIP
LENGTH OF STAY (DAYS)	PATIENT NAME
3	Flower, Spring
4	Night, Tuesday
Average length of stay for ORIF-Lt hip: 3.5 days	

SURGERY	ORIF-RT HIP
LENGTH OF STAY (DAYS)	PATIENT NAME
3	Farmer, Jersey
4	Green, Forest
6	Bright, Star
Average length of stay for ORIF-Rt hip: 4.33 days	

SURGERY	RT HIP ARTHROPLASTY
LENGTH OF STAY (DAYS)	PATIENT NAME
3	White, Caspar
4	Day, Summer
4	Wave, Storm
4	White, Pearl
6	Mountain, Misty
Average length of stay for Rt hip arthroplasty: 4.2 days	

AVERAGE LENGTH OF STAY FOR ALL PATIENTS: 4.07 DAYS

 ## Planning a Database

When one learns to use one of the databases in an office software suite, one wants to start creating a database by deciding what to capture. Comments are made, such as "I want to track X," but no preliminary thought is given to why and how to track X. Unfortunately, these efforts often result in a database that does not provide the needed information.

Some of the steps necessary to design a database[4]:

- ▼ Stating the questions the database needs to answer or describing the reports that will be based on the data
- ▼ Identifying the data needed to accomplish these goals and the methods for obtaining the data
- ▼ Identifying the tables into which data will be organized in a manner that will normalize data
- ▼ Planning data manipulation necessary to produce the output
- ▼ Planning how data will be entered
- ▼ Creating the database

If the database will contain any data that might be construed as protected (i.e., confidential) health information, contact information services and ask their help in securing the data before starting on a database project.

In the next section, we will follow a nurse manager in implementing these steps and in planning a database that will assist in managing information for the unit. Part of the nurse

---

[4] The steps listed here are at a very elementary level, but they will suffice for a simple database.

manager's job is to maintain a list of phone numbers for the personnel on the unit, keep a record of the mandatory educational programs that each employee attends, and notify each employee when the program is due again. The nurse manager decides that using a relational database would make this job easier.

STATING NEEDS THE DATABASE SHOULD MEET

The nurse manager decides that the database should meet the following needs:

1. Provide a printed list of phone numbers
2. Provide a list of which mandatory programs need to be completed by an employee each month grouped by program (e.g., those needing Fire Safety would be listed together)
3. Print an individual note to each employee who is due to complete a mandatory educational program or programs in the coming month

IDENTIFYING THE DATA NEEDED TO ACCOMPLISH THESE GOALS AND METHODS FOR OBTAINING THE DATA

This nurse manager identifies the needed data as those seen in the first column in Table 16-7. She also identifies field names for each piece of data and the field type. For the computer to know what to do with the data in a field, each field must be designated a specific type of field. The specific field types vary for the various databases in the office suites, but some general types of fields are common to all databases (Table 16-8). Most fields are text fields. Because numeric fields will allow only numbers as entries and will delete any leading zeros, fields such as phone numbers and zip codes should be text fields. There are many different kinds of numeric fields, such as those that will accept only whole numbers (integers) and those that will add a "$" to each entry. The nurse manager planning this database identifies the Mandatory Program Name field as a look-up field. To meet this need, a table that contains the names of the mandatory programs will be created from which the user will select an entry for the Mandatory Program Name field. This will ensure that all the entries in that field for a given program are identical.

The nurse manager plans to ask the human resources department to give her a list of current employees in the unit along with their phone numbers in an ASCII fixed file or comma delimited format. The nurse realizes that some of the phone numbers are proba-

TABLE 16-7 • *Data Needed for Database*

Data Needed	Field Name	Field Type and Length	Table Assigned
First name	Fname	Text – 15	Employees
Last name	Lname	Text – 20	Employees
Phone number	Phone	Text – 14	Employees
Mandatory program name	ProgName	Look-up	MandatoryPrograms
Date program completed	DateComplete	Date	MandatoryPrograms
Date for repeating program	DateRepeat	Date	MandatoryPrograms

TABLE 16-8 ● *General Field Database Types*	
General Field Type	**Description**
Text	Can contain any character entered from the keyboard, up to 255 characters including spaces. Length must be declared.
Numeric	Will accept as data only numbers, deletes leading zeroes.
Date	Accepts only date entries in an appropriate format. Permits calculations based on dates.
Memo	A text field that permits very long entries.
Look-up	A variation of a text field that allows a user to select an entry from a predetermined list.
Auto-number	Automatically generates a number for each record. Very useful for key fields when no other obvious choice, such as medical record number exists.

bly not up-to-date and makes a note to have the unit clerk check the phone numbers and forward any corrections back to human resources. Any updates will be made on the unit and forwarded to human resources.[5]

IDENTIFYING THE TABLES

Next, the nurse manager looks at her data and decides that two tables are needed. They are identified as Employees and Mandatory Programs as seen in the fourth column of Table 16-7. At this point, she must decide how the tables will be related and add any necessary key fields. Looking at the tables, the nurse realizes that the Mandatory Programs table provides details for the Demographic table; hence it will be the detail table in a one-to-many relationship. A key field is now needed for each table. A key field in the master table must be a unique identifier; no other record in the table may have the same datum in that field. The nurse realizes that employee number is a unique identifier for each person in the database. Thus, this field is added to both the Demographic and Mandatory Programs tables. Realizing that human resources had not been asked to provide the employee number, she adds this to the request.

PLANNING DATA MANIPULATION NECESSARY TO PRODUCE THE OUTPUT

In planning output, it is necessary to consider how data will be manipulated and queried as well as how they will be presented. Using a pattern such as that in Display 16-3 can help to organize one's thoughts. This nurse probably also made some sketches of how the reports should look to be sure that all necessary data and processing were included in the planning.

PLANNING HOW DATA WILL BE ENTERED

The nurse manager has already planned how to obtain some of the data. For the rest, the nurse sketches a design for the data-entry forms. In doing this, the nurse finds that it is possible to have one form that will display all the data for an employee from both

---

[5] In an ideal situation, only one database would be used. When there is more than one database with the same data, at least one of the databases generally contains inaccurate entries.

Display 16-3 • **PLANNING DATABASE OUTPUT**

Report 1: Provide printed list of phone numbers

Tables needed:	Employees (Fields needed: first name, last name, telephone number)
Query needed:	None
Manipulation:	Sort by last name

Report 2: Provide list of mandatory programs for each month

Tables needed:	Employees (Fields needed: first name, last name) Mandatory Programs (Fields needed: name of program, repeat date)
Query needed:	Query to select the fields from both tables, select only those records in which the repeat date is the month for which the report will be needed.
Manipulation:	In the report, group by name of program with a secondary grouping by the last name. Title the report for the month and year. Do not include repeat date on the report.

Report 3: Note to each employee needing to complete a mandatory offering

Tables needed:	Employees (Fields needed: first name, last name) Mandatory Programs (Fields needed: name of program, repeat date)
Query needed:	Query to select the fields from both tables, select only those records in which the repeat date is the following month.
Manipulation:	In the report grouped by name of employee with a secondary grouping by the program need. Create a page break between each primary group so notes for each individual are all printed on a separate page. Include the date by which the program needs to be repeated and the name of the program.

---

tables. To create this form, the nurse manager first creates a form for the detail table (Mandatory Programs) to serve as a **subform**. Then, a form for the master table (Employees) is created and the detail table subform is placed on it. When completed, it looks like Figure 16-5.

DATA FLOW DIAGRAM

Some database designers do a **data flow diagram** (DFD), which is especially helpful for complex databases. A DFD is a tool that allows one to visualize how data will flow through a system and where processing or analyzing of the data needs to occur. DFDs can be at a very abstract level, such as for an entire system, or at a basic level, detailing which data are required for a specific function and how they should be manipulated. There are many variations on constructing a DFD, but they must represent four entities: data flow, where the data are stored, how they are processed, and their eventual destination (Kozar, 1997). The symbols used to represent these entities may vary from DFD to DFD. The nurse manager decides to create a DFD (Figure 16-6) and uses the following symbols:

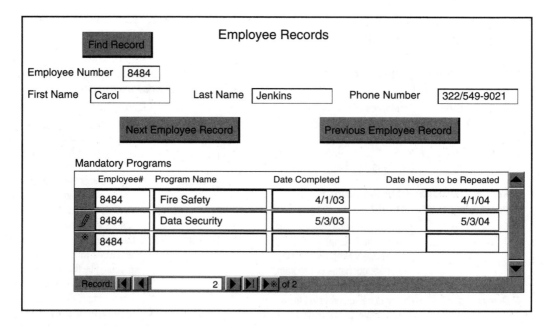

Figure 16-5 • Form for entering data.

- ▼ Input—rounded rectangle
- ▼ Data flows—movement of data in the system—arrows (→)
- ▼ Data stores—data repositories for data (a table in our situation)—rectangle open on top
- ▼ Processes—transformation of data, a circle (○)
- ▼ External entities—sources or destinations outside the specified system boundary — a rectangle (□)

CREATING THE DATABASE

When all the planning has been done on paper, it is time to create the database. Professional database designers each have their own system and series of steps, but they all use paper to plan. In a more complex database, it is common to create a few tables, enter some dummy data, and try some queries to see whether the data structure is correct. Just as in the systems life cycle, each of the steps above is iterative; that is, as one progresses one finds errors or omissions in the preceding steps and returns to that step to make corrections. Not only will overall time be saved when a database is thoroughly planned, but the frustration involved in having to redo the database when errors or omissions are discovered will be avoided.

 Data Mining

Creating information and knowledge in a small database such as the ones discussed in this chapter is often a matter of asking the right questions and being able to create the query. Although the thinking process involved in developing questions to ask of data will always be helpful, in clinical information systems, it is often impossible to consider all possible relationships. Consider a situation in which one is interested in the factors that affect outcomes

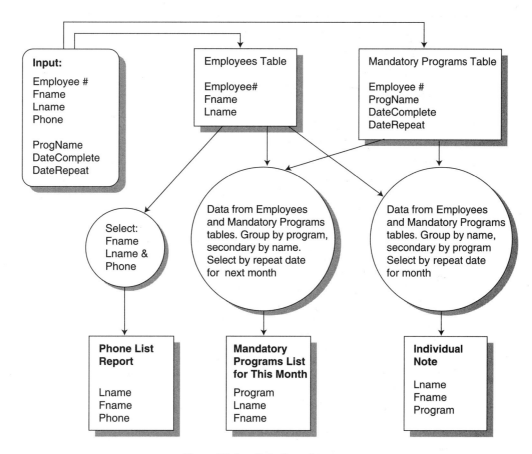

Figure 16-6 • Data flow diagram.

in hip replacement surgery. There may be 40 or more variables that affect this. **Data mining** is the process that allows users to get at the information that is hidden in this data. In short, data mining can be defined as the automated processes that permit the conversion of data to information and knowledge by finding hidden relationships within data. These processes use complex statistical techniques to uncover hidden relationships that are predictive of some behavior. They are supported by three factors: massive data collection, powerful multiprocessor computers, and data mining algorithms (An introduction to data mining, 2002).

There are many different approaches to data mining. Although a form of research, this is research in a retrospective manner; existing data is used to see what, if any, predictive relationships are present. Although data mining tools can operate outside a data warehouse, when they do, they require extra steps for extracting, importing, and analyzing the data (Bourgoin, Smith, Stone, Thearling, &Yarmus, 1996). A data warehouse is a collection of data that presents a coherent picture of the entire enterprise. Developing a data warehouse involves processes that extract the data, then clean and date it. Barriers that impede the use of data mining in healthcare are a lack of standardized clinical vocabularies and differing work processes among healthcare facilities that make it difficult to maintain clean and useful data (Gillespie, 2000).

Conclusions Reached Using Databases

In this chapter, the idea of gaining information and knowledge from data has been discussed. The final step in this process, wisdom, needs to be addressed when drawing conclusions from data. For example, if an infection database showed that a given surgeon's patients had a large number of nosocomial infections from *Staphylococcus*, it would be easy to draw the conclusion that this surgeon was to blame. Wisdom, however, dictates that one be sure one has all the necessary data. Certainly, one would investigate the physician, but there could be other factors. What other things do the patients of this surgeon have in common? The same operating room, the same postoperative unit, the same nurse? The data have provided the information that a problem exists and suggests one investigative avenue, but wisdom dictates that one consider all variables.

Databases do not necessarily mirror reality completely. Data that are collected and the structure of the data are based on assumptions that represent the world view of those responsible for the database. Thus, those who design databases must make decisions. The view of healthcare held by the people deciding on what a healthcare information system will produce determines what information is captured and what is ignored. Assumptions in themselves are not bad, but they should be acknowledged. The information from a database is only as objective as the data that it contains. To rely on output from a database without any understanding of the data that were used to create the information is to make decisions with inadequate knowledge. For this reason, nursing needs to be a part of deciding which data are included in an information system. When a database captures only procedures, without any indication of the outcome or the critical thinking needed to perform them safely, the value of nursing care to healthcare is hidden and patient safety is jeopardized. Nurses need to be proactive in seeing that nursing-sensitive data are part of an information system. To fulfill this need, they must familiarize themselves with the American Nurses Association's recognized standardized terminologies and select one of them to use to capture nursing data.

Summary

Databases are the underpinning of all healthcare information systems. Data at the atomic level are the basis for the tables that are the structure on which a database is built. There are several different database models: hierarchical, network, object-oriented, flat, and relational. The databases that come in the professional version of the office software suites are a hybrid combination of the object-oriented and relational models. In a relational database, the tables are related by a key field that is present in both tables. Getting data into a database is one of the most difficult tasks in the process. Importing data from a larger information system into a desktop database can provide data for analysis at the unit level.

Information is produced from a database by querying. Boolean and mathematical operators can be used with criteria either singly or in combination. Before trusting outcomes, query results should always be tested with a subset of data for which the answers have be obtained manually. When conclusions are drawn from data, it is advisable to consider whether all the data needed for that conclusion are present in the database.

Effective databases are planned on paper before being created on the computer. The first step is to identify what outcomes the database should provide. Using that information, the data necessary to meet these needs are determined, along with the methods for manipulating and reporting those data. These steps are iterative; it is often necessary to make corrections or additions to a prior step as planning progresses.

connection——⌣ For definitions of bolded key terms, visit the online glossary available at http://connection.lww.com/go/thede.

CONSIDERATIONS AND EXERCISES

1. List some clinical conditions that it would be possible to investigate by importing data from a healthcare information system.

2. In the database below, identify a field, field name, and record.

Patient	Unit	Pathogen
Sylvia Forest	2A	Steptococcus

3. What is a function of a key field?

4. What fields would be needed in a database to record the five (include pain) vital signs?

5. You have a table with the fields in the table below. Reduce this table to atomic level and normalize the database (BP, blood pressure).

Name	Date	8a BP	12p BP	4p BP	8p BP

6. What questions could you ask of a database with the following fields? Which Boolean or mathematical operators would you use for the query?

First Name	Last Name	Primary Medical Diagnosis	Nursing Diagnosis

7. Download a database from the Chapter 16 page on the text Web page (http://connection.lww.com/go/thede) and query it using a desktop database (Corel Paradox or Microsoft Access).

8. Plan a database to provide information for a topic of your choosing. Keep it simple!

9. Discuss the limitations of a database.

10. Evaluate the data re collected by an information system for nursing-sensitive data.

REFERENCES

An introduction to data mining. (2002). Retrieved May 5, 2002 from
http://www3.shore.net/~kht/text/dmwhite/dmwhite.shtml.

Bourgoin, M., Smith, S., Stone, E., Thearling, K., &Yarmus, J.(1996). *An introduction to data mining.*
Retrieved May 5, 2002 from http://www3.shore.net/~kht/text/dmwhite/dmwhite.shtml.

Gillespie, G. (2000). There's gold in them thar' databases. *Health Data Management, 8*(11), 40–42, 44,
46, 48–50, 52.

Hernadez, M. J. (1997). *Database design for mere mortals.* Reading, MA: Addison-Wesley Developers Press.

Kozar, K. F. (1997). *Systems with data flow diagrams.* Retrieved May 8, 2002 from
http://spot.colorado.edu/~kozar/DFD.html.

Which client/server database technology fits? Experts and practitioners describe alternatives. (2001).
Retrieved May 5, 2002 from http://www.pds-site.com/WhitePapers/wp_wdbfits.htm.

Nursing Knowledge: Access Via Bibliographic and Factual Databases

Margaret (Peg) Allen, MLS-AHIP[1]

Objectives

After studying this chapter you will be able to:

1. Access nursing knowledge using bibliographic and factual databases.

2. Identify bibliographic and factual databases useful to nurses.

3. Understand the structure of a bibliographic database record.

4. Select databases appropriate for various informational needs.

5. Search bibliographical databases using thesaurus terms and limit functions.

6. Plan literature search strategies to support evidence-based practice.

7. Describe the use of bibliographic management software.

Given the vast amount of information published, it is impossible to know everything applicable to nursing practice. According to one author, "[to read] everything of possible importance to medicine, one would need to read 6,000 articles each day" (Arndt, 1992). To help find the information resources patrons need, librarians have created indexes that serve as guides to the literature. Originally developed in print formats, such as the card catalog and annual indexes of the periodical literature, these systems are now produced as bibliographic databases that can be searched electronically. Electronic databases are more flexible than print indexes and often contain more information, including the abstracts for journal articles. Print databases, which required one card or entry for each item, were limited by space and generally did not offer as many different "terms" to use in searching for a topic. Many types of information resources are indexed in online databases. Besides being able to search these databases for information, the user can develop personal bibliographic databases using bibliographic management software.

Electronic Bibliographic Databases

An electronic knowledge-based bibliographic database is a collection of bibliographic records describing published information such as journal articles, books and chapters in books, audiovisual materials, web resources, and other miscellaneous publications. Many include the complete text of some of these publications or links to the full-text

[1] Library Consultant; Cinahl Information Systems, Inc. and Wisconsin Area Health Education Centers.

article. The bibliographic records in these databases include information that allows one to find the actual information resources; whereas full-text means that the database includes both the citation and the complete text of the indexed document. The distinction between bibliographic databases and full-text databases, however, is starting to blur. Factual databases are those that replace books, such as telephone directories and drug references, with easily updated online information. Although they may contain some citations to the literature, their primary purpose is to provide easy access to the facts needed. Access to these databases may be provided via a local area network, an intranet, or networked access to Internet resources. For example, a collection of reference books on CD-ROM may be networked on your hospital or college information network. This makes them accessible from any computer connected to the network or even using a personal digital assistant.

NURSING KNOWLEDGE ONLINE LIBRARY CATALOGS

Online library catalogs can be searched by author, title, or subject headings, just as in the old card catalog. Some systems allow searching in additional fields, such as by call number. In addition, you can usually search by words anywhere in the record, so you do not need to know the first word in a title you want to find. Many online catalogs are accessible using the Internet. For example, using a Web browser one can search LOCATOR*plus* (http://locatorplus.gov), the online catalog for books, audiovisuals, and journal titles available at the National Library of Medicine (NLM). The information in LOCATOR*plus* can also be searched through the NLM Gateway (http://gateway.nlm.nih.gov/gw/Cmd), which includes *all* NLM databases and Web resources.

KEY DATABASES FOR NURSING KNOWLEDGE

NLM has the mission of making the knowledge derived from biomedical research accessible to all health professionals. With funding from the U.S. government, NLM developed the online MEDical Literature Analysis and Retrieval System (MEDLARS), and produced MEDLINE (MEDlars onLINE), the first online database indexing journal articles (MEDLINE, 2001). MEDLINE records begin with 1966 journals; experimental records from 1964 and 1965 are now available as OLDMEDLINE.

MEDLINE was initially planned to include all journals indexed for *Index Medicus*, which in the early 1960s included just six nursing journals (Henderson, 1968). When MEDLINE was in the planning stages, both the American Nurses Association and the American Dental Association were invited to participate in its development, significantly increasing the journal coverage for these professions. In 1997 MEDLINE evolved from a fee-for-service database searched only by librarians to its current worldwide availability as PubMed (http://pubmed.gov) and the NLM Gateway. Search interfaces for journal article databases such as MEDLINE are constantly evolving and changing, but the basic record structure remains essentially the same. One can also search MEDLINE using search interfaces from commercial vendors, such as EBSCO, Ovid, and SilverPlatter.

MEDLINE now includes NLM's entire journal article indexing from 1966 to the present, covering titles originally selected for *Index Medicus* and several other journal article indexes. For example, the American Hospital Association published the *Hospital Administration and Planning Index* (HealthSTAR database) in cooperation with NLM from 1977 to 2000 ("Hospital and Health Administration Index: Now Quickly Accessed by its Subscribers at No

Cost," 2000). The titles selected for that index now comprise the Health Care Administration subset of MEDLINE. The author's Web site (http://www.pegallen.net) includes a diagram on the *Search Help* page illustrating some of the relevant subsets in MEDLINE.

International Nursing Index (INI), most recently published by Lippincott Williams & Wilkins, is no longer in production ("Nurses, librarians, and publishers making a difference" 2002). INI was based on the nursing journal subset of MEDLINE and a nursing articles search strategy. A comprehensive international index, the print version of INI included additional material not in MEDLINE, such as a list of doctoral dissertations in nursing. The print volumes (1966–2000) should be consulted for these non-journal citations. For access to the journal literature, INI included the MEDLINE indexing for approximately 300 nursing journals, including the 51 nursing journals now included in *Index Medicus*. INI also included indexing of nursing content from any of the more than 4,600 periodical titles indexed for MEDLINE and the former HealthSTAR database. MEDLINE searches include only the journal indexing from INI.

The CINAHL database is a comprehensive guide for nursing, as well as allied health, alternative and complementary therapies, and consumer health. As an integrated nursing subject database, it includes information in all formats—not just journal articles or library holdings. Its print counterpart is the Cumulative Index of Nursing and Allied Health Literature, which does not include all the publication formats indexed in the CINAHL database. CINAHL includes some unique fields in its database records, such as the *Instrumentation* field, which lists research tools used in a study. CINAHL also includes a *References* field for most of the regularly indexed journals, which includes the full-text of the cited references. The full text of the references is included only if the publisher gives permission. Like the NLM databases, CINAHL is available from multiple online vendors, but for a fee. Many libraries and organizations subscribe to CINAHL via one of these vendors.

FULL-TEXT DATABASES

In addition to bibliographic citation databases that help find information resources, some databases, known as full-text databases, also include the content of these resources. Because of copyright laws, database producers must either obtain permission to include these copyrighted information resources or create their own original copyrighted content for inclusion in the database. CINAHL includes a limited amount of full-text information, such as:

▼ Articles from a few nursing journals, particularly state nursing journals
▼ Critical paths
▼ Government publications in the public domain
▼ Research instrument records, which may include the full-text of the instrument
▼ Original documents written for Cinahl Information Systems, such as drug records, clinical innovations, and continuing education modules

Other databases may either include full-text articles as part of the indexed content, or link to a collection of full-text journals.

FACTUAL DATABASES

Factual databases are another type of knowledge database available through the Internet or other networked systems. Examples of factual databases include the directory of researchers in the Sigma Theta Tau Registry of Nursing Research and other online directories, encyclopedias, and reference works, such as drug information databases. Many of these databases limit access to subscribers or members of the sponsoring organization, and thus require a password or access through an intranet. Factual databases are expensive to produce and require income from subscribers or sponsors to support their maintenance and development. This is also true for bibliographic full-text journal databases. Many libraries and several states subscribe to factual and full-text databases that can be used by authorized individuals.

Bibliographic Database Structure

The record structure of a bibliographic database includes fields for both descriptive and subjective data. It is helpful to review the record format used in library catalogs. In the book record format, the author, title, edition, publisher, date, and description fields are used to describe the information resource. Recording this information is considered descriptive cataloging. Subjective data fields include those for subjects and the call number. A cataloger assigns subject headings and a call number by examining the book and determining the main subject or subjects covered in the book, using a standard list of subject headings. The call number is then determined by the classification scheme used by the library, such as the Dewey Decimal system which is used by most public and high school libraries; the Library of Congress scheme, used by most academic and special purpose libraries; or the NLM classification, used by most hospital and health science libraries.

SUBJECT HEADINGS

Subject headings are also standardized, so that the indexer or cataloger will always use the same words to describe a subject, not one of many synonyms for the same concept. Each library chooses a standard subject authority or thesaurus for all its cataloging. Libraries using the NLM classification use the subject headings found in NLM's Medical Subject Headings (MeSH), which is the controlled vocabulary NLM uses for cataloging books and other holdings and for indexing journal articles in MEDLINE (http://www.nlm.nih.gov/mesh/meshhome.html). MeSH differs from many other subject heading lists because it is based on a hierarchical structure. Because of this factor, searches on a broad subject can be constructed to include the narrower subjects in the MeSH tree structure for the broader term. This is known as "exploding" the broader term to include all the terms under it in the hierarchy.

ORGANIZATION OF THE SUBJECT HEADINGS

Both MeSH and the CINAHL subject heading lists use this hierarchical tree structure. See Figure 17-1 for an example. Each indent indicates a lower level of specificity. Using terms at lower levels will generally find fewer items, but these items should be closer to the more specific topic. MeSH subject headings can be found online in the MeSH Browser (on the left side of the PubMed search screen). This Find MeSH feature in the PubMed MEDLINE search interface uses the UMLS (United Medical Language System) Metathesaurus, which includes terms from nursing and other medical classification systems. Other search systems for MEDLINE and CINAHL have varying means of leading from the users' search terms to the for-

```
        Anatomy (MeSH Category)
          Body Regions (Non-MeSH)
            Extremities
              Amputation Stumps
              Arm (+ more specific terms)
              Leg
                Ankle
                Foot
                  Forefoot, Human
                    Metatarsus
                      Toes
                        Hallux
                  Heel
                    Tarsus
              Hip
              Knee
              Thigh
```

Figure 17-1 • MeSH tree.

mal subject headings used in these databases. This process is known as mapping. In contrast, searching by "keywords" or text words limits one to finding occurrences of the words you select anywhere in the database record. If a database uses "Decubitus ulcers" as a search term, searching on "Pressure ulcers" may or may not retrieve everything on this topic, but searching on "Decubitus ulcers" will retrieve everything indexed with this term.

DATABASE INDEXING

When a journal article or other information resource is included in a database, a record is created using a standard format for each type of published information indexed in the database (Allen, 1998). The database record has fields needed for the information that allows users to find the document needed, such as author, title, and the source. For example, the source field for journal articles includes journal title, date, and pages. The records also include fields for the subject headings used to describe the content. Subjects used in the record may vary based on the differences in the subject heading lists (thesauri) and individual human variation in selecting the subject headings for each indexed publication. The first consideration is that the indexer must choose terms from the database thesaurus, such as MeSH for MEDLINE indexing, or the CINAHL Subject Heading List for CINAHL indexing. Indexers are expected to use the most specific term available, and they may select as many subject headings as are required to describe the content of the article. Both major and minor subject headings are selected. Major subject headings are chosen to reflect the *main topics* covered in the publication.[2] Minor subject headings include common terms referred to as *check tags*, which indicate the populations studied (age groups and others), as well as additional subjects addressed in the article. They are useful when a user limits a search to a specific group, such as the aged. Subheadings such as diagnosis, nursing, or therapy may be used with both major and minor headings to better describe the content of the article. Indexing is an art, not an exact science. Given the same

[2] When a search interface asks whether to "Limit to focus," an affirmative response will limit retrieval to only those documents indexed with the term as a **Major** heading.

article, indexers will often differ in their selection of subject headings. Most of the time, however, they will agree on the key concepts in the article. Complete the first exercise for this chapter to compare MEDLINE and CINAHL indexing for an article.

Performing a Literature Review

Literature searches are a vital step in developing research-based practice. Subject headings are used to develop search strategies that will lead you to the most useful information on your topic. Although ideas for changes in clinical practice may come from regular reading of the literature, it is still necessary to search for more information to determine whether the information in the original article warrants a change in clinical practices. The Iowa group notes the importance of a critical review of the research literature, as found in a comprehensive literature search (Titler, et al., 1994; Titler, Mentes, Rakel, Abbott, & Baumler, 1999).

DEFINING THE TOPIC

The first step in developing a search strategy is to define the topic. It usually helps to write out the search question. As an example, to develop a research-based critical path for the care of patients undergoing a hip arthroplasty, articles from the biomedical and nursing literature must be found, as well as examples of critical paths from other organizations. The question might be, "What factors affect the recovery of patients undergoing hip replacement surgery?" The major concept in this question is hip replacement surgery. Other concepts could include age group or groups, length of stay, preoperative care, postoperative care, and rehabilitation. You could also look at potential complications, such as pressure ulcers. In this situation, the template from Chapter 15 would be modified to look like Figure 17-2.

SELECTING DATABASES

For most searches, nurses need to use the library catalog and the MEDLINE and CINAHL databases. Searches on many topics often require the use of additional electronic databases.

Psychosocial Questions

Because nursing is a holistic profession, some questions are best answered by adding searches of psychosocial databases such as PsycINFO and the CSA Sociological Abstracts. PsycINFO is produced by the American Psychological Association (APA; http://www.apa.org/). Libraries

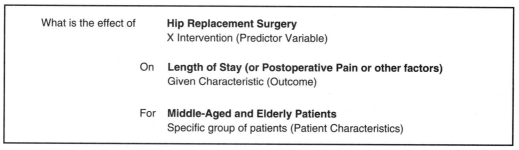

Figure 17-2 • Use of a template to develop a searchable question: outcomes related to hip replacement surgery.

may subscribe to the complete collection of PsycINFO databases, or subsets, including the ClinPSYC database, which contains the clinical literature indexed by PsycINFO.

Cambridge Scientific Abstracts produces CSA Sociological Abstracts (http://www.csa.com/detailsV5/socioabs.html). This database offers abstracts of information from more than 2,600 journals from sociology and related social sciences, as well as citations to books and book chapters, conference papers, dissertations, and reviews of books and other media.

Oncology Questions

For oncology questions, search CINAHL, MEDLINE and your library catalog, and also search databases from the National Cancer Institute for additional information (http://www.nlm.nih.gov/databases/databases_cancer.html; http://www.cancer.gov). Like CINAHL, CANCERLIT is a subject database that indexes information in *all* formats. It contains more than 1.5 million citations and abstracts from more than 4,000 different sources, including journals, proceedings, books, reports, and doctoral theses (http://www.cancer.gov/cancer_information/cancer_literature/). Physician's Data Query (PDQ; http://www. cancer.gov/cancer_information/pdq/) is an example of an authoritative full-text database. Its registries and directories can help patients as well as health professionals find cancer centers working with the latest research and drugs specific to their treatment needs.

Management Topics

A business database may be added to a search. Business methods are often applied in healthcare, with the latest research and innovations coming from outside the healthcare sector. Although MEDLINE includes journals selected for healthcare administration, it is wise to ask a librarian about business database availability. Many are produced with a large proportion of full-text articles so that the information is readily available.

Biomedical Research

Thorough searches for biomedical research should include other scientific databases. Although MEDLINE covers more than 4,600 journals, NLM estimates that between 13,000 and 14,000 biomedical journals are published worldwide (http://www.nlm.nih.gov/pubs/factsheets/j_sel_faq.html). EMBASE, the Excerpta Medica database, is an international biomedical and pharmacological database produced by Elsevier Science (http://www.elsevier.nl/homepage/sah/spd/site/locate_embase.html). It is particularly good for drug information. BIOSIS (http://www.biosis.org/) is another database that is important for basic science searches. Because of higher costs, these two databases are not as widely available as most of the other databases described in this chapter.

ISI Web of Science is the Web interface to several databases, including Science Citation Index (SCI) and Social Science Citation Index (SSCI). These databases cover more than 8,000 journals, including 42 nursing journals selected for SSCI (http://www.isinet.com/isi/products/citation/wos/index.html). These citation indexes include fields for the cited references in the indexed source articles. ISI citation databases are particularly useful when looking for works that build on key concepts in the literature; they provide cited work searching as well as key word searching of titles and abstracts. However, the ISI citation databases do not include subject indexes.

General Periodical Information

Many academic and public libraries and some states license "general" databases that index magazines and journals, which are commonly found in these types of libraries. These databases often include the full-text for many of the indexed titles. The *Reader's Guide to Periodical Literature* is a well-known example of a general periodical index. Like specialized databases, availability depends on the financial resources of the sponsoring library system.

Education Questions

For education questions, searching ERIC (Educational Resources and Information Clearinghouse) can also be useful. ERIC is an online index of articles, books, and reports related to education. Most academic libraries offer ERIC access using the search software from their primary database vendor, such as EBSCO or SilverPlatter. For free access, use the AskERIC program based at Syracuse University (http://ericir.syr.edu/). Because it is produced with government funding, the ERIC database subscription cost for libraries is relatively low. Many academic libraries also offer the ERIC reports on microfiche or electronically.

Patient Teaching

Patient and consumer teaching resources can be found in a wide variety of databases. Both MEDLINE and CINAHL index selected consumer health information resources. Because CINAHL has publication types for teaching materials and consumer/patient teaching materials (the latter beginning with 1997 indexing), it is easy to limit searches to this type of information. When information produced for the consumer cannot be found, articles in the nursing and allied health literature can be located that will help you with patient teaching. In 2002, NLM added "Patient Education Handout" as a MEDLINE publication type. See the NLM Technical Bulletin, *http://www.nlm.nih.gov/pubs/techbull/ma02/ma02_new_pt.html,* for more information on how to search for patient education resources in MEDLINE.

Several other commercial databases also index the consumer health literature, including EBSCO's *HealthSource: Consumer Edition, the Health & Wellness Center* from Gale, and *MDX.Health Digest,* which is produced by Medical Data Exchange. These databases contain both bibliographic and full-text information. Ask your librarians about availability—these databases are primarily marketed to organizations, not individuals. A free source worth searching is *CHID: Combined Health Information Database,* which contains records for pamphlets, kits, videos, articles, books, and book chapters on 18 major healthcare topics. CHID is a database constructed by health-related agencies of the federal government (http://chid.nih.gov). Other government agencies related to health and nutrition also offer databases of consumer resources, such as those linked from the Nutrition.gov website (http://www.nutrition.gov/).

In addition to bibliographic databases for consumer and patient health information, several publishers produce full-text patient education databases that can be licensed for access by organizations through their intranet, or sometimes through the Internet. One example is Clinical Reference Systems, available through various vendors and as the medical encyclopedia for MEDLINE*plus* (http://www.medlineplus.gov/). The Micromedex CareNotes System (http://www.micromedex.com/products/carenotes/) offers more than 3,000 customizable documents written for easy comprehension. Both these products feature patient education materials written in both English and Spanish.

Web-accessible resources from government organizations and nonprofit organizations are often free. As noted in Chapter 6, the problem with relying on the WWW for consumer and patient health information is that the information must be evaluated before using it in patient teaching. Several reliable Web sites review and index selected consumer health Web sites. Developed by libraries and government organizations, they offer a quality filtered road map to quality health information on the Web. MEDLINE*plus* (http://www.medlineplus.gov) is one of the best examples. Others may be linked from the Web site for this book.

Researchers

Sometimes one needs to locate nurse researchers for consultation, permission to use a research tool, or to identify studies that were never published. Nursing has two unique databases that can help:

▼ Sigma Theta Tau International (STTI)Registry of Nursing Research (http://www.stti.iupui.edu/library/)
  ▼ Information about researchers and their research projects, including citations to any published studies
  ▼ Researchers asked to index their entries with subject headings from approved lists
▼ Canadian-International Nurse Researcher Database (http://nurseresearcher.com/)
  ▼ Includes names, affiliation, research interests, and expertise
  ▼ Contact e-mail is "blinded" to protect privacy

Both these registries offer free access. They rely on the voluntary participation of those who register online. Nurses should encourage their colleagues to register and keep their entries up-to-date. Use of these registries supports collaborative research. Nurses should register their research in progress and search for others doing similar projects. The registries are examples of factual databases. The STTI registry is also bibliographic because it contains citations to published works.

MAKING THE SELECTION

From the listing of databases in this section, one can see that selecting the most appropriate database is just as important as the search strategy. If one is looking for peer-reviewed professional literature, use the online catalogs for libraries serving populations engaged in healthcare and education, and search databases and indexes such as MEDLINE, CINAHL, and ERIC. For patient teaching, one may be able to find what is needed on the Web or licensed databases on the local health system intranet. The important thing to remember is that a comprehensive search cannot be limited to online resources. Although a wide range of information resources may be found online, libraries, librarians, and bookstores are vital to help borrow or buy the knowledge-based resources needed for nursing education and practice.

 ## Search Strategy Development

The exact search strategy will depend on the databases that are selected and the search interface (software for searching, with underlying search engine) used to conduct the search, (e.g., Ovid or PubMed for MEDLINE). Just when a particular database search interface is mastered, the vendor's software typically will be upgraded or changed. There are, however, certain basic principles of database searching that, once mastered, will be useful in all situations. No matter which search interface is used, it is important to understand the nature of the database being searched, including its subject headings, so that the search can be tailored to the database. If the following questions can be answered, searching bibliographic databases using ever-changing search interfaces will not be a problem.

1. What is the default search mode? Some database search interfaces open with a screen that maps the user to approved subject headings, whereas the default in most is keyword searching (looking for particular words in the record). Mapping to subject headings is the default when using CINAHL*direct* and Ovid search interfaces. When subject mapping is not the default, some search interfaces offer an online thesaurus that one can select to find approved standard subject headings. Examples include the PubMed MeSH browser, EBSCO, and SilverPlatter.

2. How does a user switch from the default search option to other search modes, such as switching from subject heading searches to keyword (or text word) searches, or vice versa?

3. Can you use Boolean operators in your search? If yes, must AND and OR be capitalized? Is this done by filling out a form that automatically ANDs or ORs the information on each line, or by typing these operators between terms? Remember that AND narrows a search, whereas OR broadens it. In the diagram shown in Figure 17-3, use of AND will retrieve documents containing the condition specified in each circle, resulting in a relatively small group of records represented by the intersection of all three circles. Using OR will retrieve the records from all three circles—all of the records represented by circles A, B, and C. AND narrows your search, whereas OR broadens it.

4. Can separate search statements be combined with Boolean operators? If yes, how is this done? Example: In CINAHL*direct*, S1 represents the first search request, S2 the second, and so on. S1 AND S2 narrows the search, whereas S1 OR S2 broadens it. Search statements can be combined within parentheses: (S1 OR S2) AND S3. In PubMed, instead of S1 and S2, use the characters "#1" to represent the first search and "#2" to represent the second. In PubMed, Boolean operators must be capitalized.

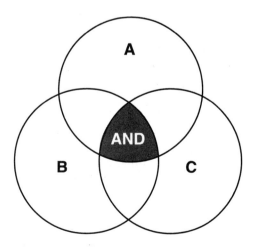

Figure 17-3 • Boolean operators: AND or OR.   OR = all circles "Or is more"

5. When searching databases with subject headings arranged in hierarchical trees (NLM and CINAHL databases), can subject headings explode to retrieve all the narrower terms included under a broader term? If yes, is this automatic, or can this feature be activated when the user decides it is needed?

6. Is phrase or multiword searching available? If yes, are operators such as ADJ needed for adjacent, or must the phrase be enclosed in quotes? Surprisingly, many search interfaces do not allow phrase searching. Instead, the words typed are automatically linked with an OR, which broadens the search rather than narrowing it.

7. Can terms be truncated to search on the root of a word? If yes, what symbol is used to indicate truncation? In many cases, but not all, an asterisk is used at the end of a root word, like psycholog* for psychology, psychological, and any other words beginning with psycholog. Although this system is useful for plurals and other word variations, be careful when truncating common medical terms because an unmanageable number of records (citations) may be retrieved.

8. When using keyword (or text word) searching, are *all* fields searched in the database record or only fields predetermined by the database vendor?

9. Can specified fields be searched? For example, how does a user search by author or title? Can an author and title searches be combined?

10. Can searches be *limited* (restricted) to particular populations, year or years of publication, publication types, language, or subsets? If yes, how?

11. What are the options for displaying and printing records?

12. Can records be downloaded or e-mailed for use in word processor or bibliographic management software? If yes, how does this work?

To learn about the search interfaces for the databases to be searched, look for tip sheets in libraries, either in print or on their Web pages. You should also consult the online help files that are part of most search interfaces. For *limiting* searches, it is helpful to know the age groups and publication types for the databases, particularly when the search interface does not list the options as part of a special limit function. Tip sheets listing MEDLINE and CINAHL limits and subsets are linked from the Web site for this book at http://connection.lww.com/go/thede.

 ## Search Examples

Searches vary by both topic and purpose. Additionally, to find all the required information about a topic, it may be necessary to approach the topic from different perspectives. To illustrate how searches for different purposes might be conducted, some sample strategies are outlined below. The MEDLINE searches were done using the PubMed search interface (http://www.pubmed.gov/), and the CINAHL database searches were done using the CINAHL*direct* Web search interface (http://www.cinahl.com).

CARE OF A HIP REPLACEMENT PATIENT: A GENERAL SEARCH

For the search question on care of the patient with a hip replacement, it was decided to search a library catalog and the MEDLINE and CINAHL databases.

In PubMed MEDLINE, look up *hip replacement* in the MeSH browser, which suggests using the MeSH term: Arthroplasty, Replacement, Hip. Searching on this MeSH term leads to more than 2,600 citations. The next step is to search for the term as a major MeSH heading (this is a choice on the Detailed Display screen). It is always a good idea to search for the main concept as a *major* subject. In some systems, this process is referred to as "limit to focus." The user can limit the result to English using the Limits screen (Language pulldown menu) or a search for English in the Language field. The number of citations retrieved, although reduced, still exceeds 1,800.

At this point, combine with other subject headings such as Length of Stay, or try the Clinical queries feature in PubMed. This feature, found under the MeSH browser on the PubMed search interface, helps narrow a search to quality studies, particularly clinical trials. Using Clinical queries, copy the MeSH heading "Arthroplasty, Replacement, Hip [MeSH]" word string from your first search and limit the search retrieval to the past 5 years. This strategy leads to a manageable result of about 60 citations, including several articles related to the prevention of deep vein thrombosis, and others related to pain management. Most of the articles are from medical journals, which is to be expected in a MEDLINE search.

In CINAHL, hip replacement also maps to Arthroplasty, Replacement, Hip. Limiting the focus, this search retrieved 317 citations in early 2002. This is still a large retrieval, so review the first citations (usually the most recently published) to find those of greatest interest, or limit the search to certain publication types, such as research, or use AND to combine with another subject, such as Length of Stay.

EVIDENCE-BASED PRACTICE SEARCHING: CARE OF A HIP REPLACEMENT PATIENT

In the Ace Star Model: Cycle of Knowledge Transformation (Figure 15-3), the steps include three types of literature that form the basis for Evidence-Based Practice:

▼ Discovery—original research literature, including quantitative and qualitative studies, as well as case studies
▼ Summary—evidence summaries, including systematic reviews, and meta-analysis
▼ Translation—translation literature in various published formats, including best practices, care plans, critical paths, practice guidelines, protocols, and standards, which provide for the translation of evidence to practice

MEDLINE and CINAHL publication types and subject headings can be used along with the evidence-based search strategies imbedded in PubMed to locate each of these critical types of literature. Given the task of developing a critical path for hip replacement patients, narrow your search using the steps described in the next sections. Table 17-1 summarizes these evidence-based search strategies.

Search for Translation Literature
Begin by looking for evidence-based examples of the various types of translation literature that serve to translate research findings into practice. Because MEDLINE offers just guideline and practice guideline as translation literature publication types, combine the first search (Arthroplasty, Replacement, Hip limited to major subject heading or "Focus," English, last 5 years) with the limit to guideline OR practice guideline OR the MeSH head-

TABLE 17-1 • *Useful Limits for Evidence-Based Searching*

	CINAHL	MEDLINE
Translation literature	CARE PLAN OR CLINICAL INNOVATIONS OR CRITICAL PATH OR PRACTICE GUIDELINES OR PROTOCOL OR STANDARDS Optional: CEU	GUIDELINE OR PRACTICE GUIDELINE OR **Clinical Protocols** OR **Critical Pathways** **Decision Trees** OR (systematic [sb] NOT REVIEW OR META-ANALYSIS)
Evidence summaries	SYSTEMATIC REVIEW OR **Meta-Analysis**	(Systematic [sb] AND REVIEW) OR META-ANALYSIS
Original research	RESEARCH	(CLINICAL TRIALS OR "Has abstract") NOT (REVIEW OR META-ANALYSIS)

Note: Limits are either *publication types* (SMALL CAPS) or **subject headings** (**bold**). Systematic [sb] is a special PubMed search strategy. It may not be available for use in other MEDLINE search interfaces.

ings describing other types of translation literature.[3] If using PubMed, try the Systematic subset, which is actually a search strategy designed to retrieve both evidence summaries and translation literature. Because the review and meta-analysis citations belong in the next step (evidence summaries), one can use the Boolean operator NOT to remove these two from the search result. Combine this with the previous search, again using OR. In early 2002, no recent practice guidelines were found in a MEDLINE search, but a total of 33 potentially relevant journal article citations were found.[4] At least seven described critical pathways related to hip replacement.

In CINAHL, several publication types are available as limits (see Table 17-1). Either limit the first search result to each publication type OR the results together, or combine the first result with a strategy that searches for these in the publication type field. In early 2002, the result of this search yielded nine citations, including a full-text example of a critical path included as full-text in the CINAHL database. Only one of these citations was identified in the PubMed searching, demonstrating the value of searching both databases.

Guidelines and other examples of translation literature may also be published on the web or in print by various organizations, including professional nursing associations. Links to websites offering or linking to Clinical Guidelines and other translation literature formats are included in the Evidence-Based Practice section of CINAHL*sources* Web Index (http://www.cinahl.com/csources/csources.htm), a free resource. See also "Finding and evaluating clinical practice guidelines" (McSweeney, Spies, & Cann, 2001), which can be found as an online continuing education (CE) article on the Lippincott Nursing-Center Website (http://www.nursingcenter.com/prodev/ce_online.asp).

[3] In PubMed, AND and OR must be capitalized—otherwise, search results include "and" and "or" as text words. Capitalization of Boolean operators is not necessary in most other search interfaces.

[4] If trying to replicate these examples, remember that the results will change over time, as additional publications are added to the database. They may even decrease as earlier years are dropped from the range of years selected for searching.

One can find articles that offer continuing education credit by searching CINAHL for your topic and limiting the publication type to CEU. Many publisher websites include articles with CE credit as freely accessible full-text, which is not true for most of their published content. The fastest way to find a journal website is to search in Google (www.google.com), putting the full journal title in quotes, and then search the site for the article using words from the article title.

Search for Evidence Summaries

Evidence summaries either use meta-analysis or descriptive methods to analyze and compare the results of selected research studies. They are often referred to as systematic or integrative reviews. Authors of these summaries search the literature for all relevant research on a topic. They then find and evaluate the published research to select studies for comparison. When offering a critique for an evidence summary, it is important to *evaluate the search strategy* as well as the published review (Brown, 1999). The search strategy for a valid evidence summary should include MEDLINE, CINAHL, other appropriate databases, and hand searching of potentially relevant journals. Hand searching is used to verify that no relevant articles were missed in the database searches, especially ones that were recently published or not selected for indexing. For example, although MEDLINE may index a journal, it does not index "brief items" such as abstracts from conference presentations. Producing high-quality evidence summaries is very labor intensive, so searchers should take advantage of the work of others before embarking on their own systematic reviews.

In CINAHL, simply search on the topic (broadly defined) and limit to the Systematic Review publication type. For hip replacement, the result is two citations, both from the Cochrane Library, which is a licensed full-text database available in most health sciences libraries or through interlibrary loan. However, approximately one third of the systematic reviews indexed in CINAHL are published in other sources, primarily journals, including two nursing journals currently devoted to publishing systematic reviews:

1. Online Journal of Knowledge Synthesis for Nursing (OJKSN; http://stti-web.iupui.edu/library/ojksn/)
2. Online Journal of Clinical Innovations (OJCI; http://www.cinahl.com/)

Extensive summaries of the articles in OJCI are available as Clinical Innovations (publication type) records in the CINAHL database.

As noted in the discussion about searches for translation literature, the PubMed "Systematic Review" search strategy is more of an evidence-based practice strategy that gets at all three types of literature used in evidence-based practice. It is *not* a search limiting retrieval to actual systematic reviews. However, it can be combined with topic searches and then limited to the Meta-analysis and Review publication types. This strategy identified 18 reviews in the last 5 years, including one of the Cochrane Library reviews found in the CINAHL search. None was published in nursing journals.

At this point, it is possible to use high-quality evidence summaries as the basis for some parts of the critical path for hip replacement patients, with a limited need to find recent research to supplement these published summaries. For example, several evidence summaries related to deep vein thrombosis prevention were published in 2001. Other topics, such as pain management and nursing care, require *current* searches for original research, because evidence summaries were not published. Additional searches are required to both *update* existing evidence summaries, and to *summarize* the original research related to those aspects of the topic not fully covered by evidence summaries found in your searches. By first searching for examples of translation literature and any evidence summaries on the topic, one can save the time required to do a complete multiyear systematic review of all original research related to a topic.

Search for Original Research

Searching for research in CINAHL is easy—simply limit the search result to the research publication type. This strategy is particularly useful for nursing, because not all studies are clinical trials. It allows relevant research to be identified, including potential research instruments to use in research replication or similar studies. To determine whether a study used a research instrument, review the Instrumentation field, which lists the research instruments used in a study. For Arthroplasty, Replacement, Hip, the CINAHL search result in early 2002 was 98 citations after eliminating those found in the first two steps. These citations can be sorted for review by specific topic (thrombosis prevention, pain management, and so on).

Searching for original research in MEDLINE is not as simple. The MEDLINE Clinical Trial publication type is useful for identifying randomized controlled trials (RCTs), often identified as the standard criterion of evidenced-based medicine, as well as other types of trials including the more specific randomized controlled trial publication type. Limiting to Arthroplasty, Replacement, Hip as the major topic identified more than 200 studies. Not all nursing problems are amenable to study using controlled trials, so additional methods are needed to identify this research. Instead of using the Clinical Trial publication type, one possibility is to limit to MEDLINE citations that include an abstract, as abstracts are included with most research articles. Unfortunately, the retrieval using this strategy is very large—more than 1,500 citations in the last 5 years. It makes more sense to use these two searches as the basis for narrowing the result to focus on specific aspects of care, such as pain management.

Often combining all the subject headings is too limiting. In an example of a search designed to develop a critical path for pressure ulcer prevention in hip surgery patients, narrowing the search to both concepts identified just a handful of articles (Allen & Levy, 2002), Instead, the authors looked at the broader concept of pressure ulcer prevention to identify original research, evidence summaries, and examples of translation literature. To summarize searching for resources that support evidence-based care, use the CINAHL and MEDLINE publication types and subject headings to limit retrieval to the three types of literature most useful for evidence-based practice. After searching for original research, findings can be summarized using meta-analysis techniques or comparison tables similar to those used in nursing journals publishing systemic reviews.

RELATED SEARCHES

There are times when one needs to look for information that is related to the main topic but may not be found in the initial search. Additionally, there may be a need to limit a search using other topics.

Research on Postoperative Pain

After reviewing the literature found in the searches for information on care of the patient undergoing hip replacement surgery, it was determined that postoperative pain is a major factor affecting length of stay, leading to a search for original research on postoperative pain in all hip surgery patients, with postoperative pain as the major focus.

To do this search in MEDLINE, the official subject heading is Pain, Postoperative. Because a search on this term retrieves more than 2,000 citations, combine it with Arthroplasty, Replacement, Hip OR Hip—surgery (subheading). This narrowed the result to 53 citations. Limiting to the Clinical Trial publication type OR articles with abstracts identified 46 potentially relevant studies. Only one was published in a nursing journal.

In CINAHL, Postoperative Pain as the major topic retrieved more than 1,100 citations. Combined with Hip Surgery, exploded to include the narrower term Arthroplasty, Replacement, Hip, the CINAHL search result was ten citations, including six Research (publication type) articles. Only two of these were identified in the MEDLINE search. Given the small number retrieved, the search was broadened to Pain, exploded to include all types, AND Hip Surgery, exploded as before. The result was 14 citations, of which seven were research articles, with four published in nursing journals. To find translation literature and evidence summaries on postoperative pain, search broadly, without limiting to a particular population such as hip surgery patients.

Age-Specific Pain Control

Instead of the hip or orthopedic surgery limitation to the postoperative pain search, one might want to try limiting the pain search to a specific population, such as the elderly. It is important to use the identical age group designations used in the indexing. Both databases use the same terms for age groups, but CINAHL uses Child for ages 6 to 12, whereas MEDLINE uses Child for the entire age range from birth to 18 (in MEDLINE, exploding the term Child retrieves all the smaller age ranges listed under Child). In MEDLINE, adding AND Aged AND (Clinical Trial [PT] OR "Has Abstract") to the search on Pain, Postoperative retrieved more than 500 citations published in the last 5 years. For effective review of this topic, consider how the result might be limited to surgical procedures related to hip surgery but without making the strategy too narrow. One possibility would be to limit the postoperative pain MEDLINE search to the Aged. This strategy retrieved 39 citations published in the past 5 years. An alternate strategy is to combine Pain, Postoperative with a second MeSH term, Length of Stay, which retrieved 31 citations published in the last 5 years, including five from the nursing journal subset. This has the effect of broadening the pain search to include all types of surgery while narrowing it to studies focused on length of stay.

In CINAHL, limiting the Postoperative Pain search to Aged, Research (publication type), English language, and last 5 years, retrieved 74 citations. Combining with the additional subject heading Length of Stay reduced the retrieval to six citations.

Patient Education Resources Related to Pain

Limit a CINAHL search to the Consumer/Patient Teaching Materials publication type:

- ▼ S1: Hip Surgery (exploded)—652 citations
- ▼ S2: S1 and publication type = Consumer/Patient Teaching Materials—nine citations

If not much is found, broaden the search to include all teaching materials for all audiences by limiting to the Teaching Materials publication type. For this question, also search other consumer and patient health information databases and databases for the virtual library, such as those described earlier in this chapter.

Nursing Classifications: Impaired Physical Mobility

In thinking about patients undergoing hip replacement, searches should include potential nursing diagnoses and interventions to consider in the critical path. A search on Impaired Physical Ability (classification from North American Nursing Diagnoses Association [NANDA]) in CINAHL was relatively successful, retrieving 64 citations. Unfortunately, combining this subject heading with Hip Surgery resulted in no references because nothing on this combination of topics had been indexed at the time the search was done. However, limiting this search to the Classification Record publication type provides a scope note that includes both the approved definition of the classification term and a search suggestion:

> CINAHL EDITORIAL SEARCH SUGGESTION: The term IMPAIRED PHYSICAL MOBILITY (NANDA) is used for indexing when articles specifically concern the term or research about the term. For citations that concern the general topic or topics related to the term, consider searching the subject headings: IMMOBILITY; PHYSICAL MOBILITY. (Extract copyright 2002 Cinahl Information Systems; used with permission.)

Using this strategy in CINAHL, combined with Hip Surgery (exploded) retrieve five citations, including one of the systematic reviews identified earlier.

FINDING ARTICLES SIMILAR TO A SPECIFIC ARTICLE

When a useful article is found, one often desires more information on the same topic. A good way to find this is to search for the article using the author and words from the title. For these searches, be sure you are searching the author field for the author's last name AND the title field for words from the title. After finding the online record, choose a display format that shows how the article was indexed—this approach helps identify subject headings, which can be used to find other articles indexed with the same or similar subject headings.

The PubMed search interface has a built-in shortcut to find articles similar to the one you selected. After conducting an author-title (or subject) search, you can select "Related Articles" from the Brief record format and retrieve a list of citations to articles indexed with the same or similar subject headings. This shortcut is not available in other search interfaces, but many interfaces allow you to click on subject headings in the record to find other articles indexed with the same terms. This is a good technique to use when unsure of the subject headings—search on keywords describing your topics and see how the most relevant publications are indexed.

AUDIOVISUALS ON NURSING THEORY

To search CINAHL for audiovisual programs about any of the nursing theorists, the best strategy includes these steps:

- ▼ S1: Explode Nursing Theory; limit to focus (major heading) = 3,026
- ▼ S2: Limit to publication type = Audiovisuals — 17 citations

A similar strategy can be used to find research based on a particular nursing model. Because the model is usually not the main focus of the research, do not limit to focus for this type of search.

BROADER SEARCHES

Sometimes, searches do not retrieve enough citations. A question may be too narrow, or there simply may not be a lot of information published on the topic. When searching for an in-depth research project, comprehensive literature searches must be performed to be sure no significant research has been missed. In these cases, broaden your search strategy. This can be done by searching additional databases or using broader or related search terms.

To find broader or related terms for searching, use the thesaurus function provided by each of the search interfaces used for searching the selected databases. The thesaurus will show where the term you select fits in the hierarchical tree structure so that a broader term can be selected. This is how the term Hip Surgery was found for the postoperative pain search in CINAHL. The online thesaurus often includes a scope note, which defines the term. It may also include related cross-references that point to other terms. Sometimes, it is easier to select search terms from a print version of the subject heading lists because related terms and cross-references can be viewed for a whole page of terms. The subject heading lists (thesauri) should be located in the reference section of your library—they are often kept with the print (index) version of the database. Annual volumes of *International Nursing Index* included a useful Nursing Thesaurus, which can still aid in the selection of MeSH terms for nursing topics.

SEARCHING FOR AUTHORS AND RESEARCHERS

To find nurse authors and researchers, try searching the nursing research registries noted earlier. In addition, search for their latest publications in CINAHL and MEDLINE. Along with the first author's organization, the Author Affiliation field in these databases often includes an e-mail address. If the e-mail address is not provided, search for the organization and look for a directory of faculty or staff. Search hints are provided via the Web page for this book (http://connection.lww.com/go/thede).

Search Strategy Review

In these examples, strategies used in broad searches were refined to limit retrieval to the most relevant citations. This method saves the time required to look at hundreds of citations and abstracts, which opens up more time for the next steps of retrieving and reviewing the documents found in your searches. As the articles and other information resources are read, additional database searches may be needed. Bibliographies can also be used for finding important citations missed in your database search. Perhaps the indexer did not assign the subject headings chosen for the search, or the journal was not indexed in the databases you searched. Sometimes, older, classic articles, which may still be relevant for clinical practice or research projects, are included in bibliographies.

Building Personal Bibliographic Databases

Given the vast amount of print and online knowledge-based information resources, many healthcare professionals have looked for tools that help organize and retrieve the information resources they encounter in the course of their ongoing reading and research. For many years, note cards or loose leaf binders were recommended for collecting information found in reading and literature reviews.

The problem with using note cards is the same problem faced by users of the library card catalog: a note card is a physical object that can only be filed in one place. Decisions have to be made on how to file cards (author, subject, or title), or multiple copies must be made for multiple points of access.

An alternative method would be for a user to create a personal database, so s/he can search and retrieve information by all the access points s/he might want. Commercial bibliographic management software, sometimes referred to as reference management software or **personal bibliographic reference managers**, is designed to save users the trouble of designing a database that is compatible with the records from online bibliographic databases. An additional advantage is that this software can output references according to a wide variety of publication requirements, such as the official style of the American Psychological Association. Nicoll, Oulette, Bird, Harper, and Kelley (1996) reviewed five of these software packages: EndNote Plus, Library Master, Papyrus, Pro-Cite, and Reference Manager. Like any other software, these packages are constantly evolving, so it is best to check current reviews before making a purchase decision. Librarians can provide helpful advice and instruction on this topic, including information on any bibliographic management programs supported by your organization.

FEATURES OF PERSONAL BIBLIOGRAPHIC DATABASE MANAGERS

Traditional bibliographic management software packages offer the following three functions:

- ▼ The ability to transfer bibliographic records into the personal database. This requires software filters, which may come with the package, or they may be available for an additional charge. In the latter case, the user must determine which filters to acquire, because they are programmed to conform to the record structure used by the database vendor (NLM, OCLC, Ovid, SilverPlatter, and so on.)
- ▼ A database manager to develop searchable personal bibliographic databases. This usually includes the standard bibliographic fields plus a notes field for adding comments on the information resource.
- ▼ Tools to output bibliographies formatted according to the needed publication format, such as APA or Modern Language Association style.

With this software, you can build a personal knowledge-based information database, which contains citations, abstracts, and—with some programs—links to online resources. You can choose to use call numbers and/or filing codes to link your references to a location for each of the resources you own. This system atic approach to managing knowledge-based information resources will enable you to refer to valued information resources, without the need to remember all the related details.

Good bibliographic management software also allows the user to add and edit records directly, without using the import filters or search interfaces. The user can copy and paste the data from any electronic document or simply type the information into the database. As a personal bibliographic database develops, the user will think of subject terms or keywords to add to the record, which will help retrieve information relevant to his or her personal interests.

Z39.50 COMPLIANT DATABASES

A Z39.50 compliant database is one designed in compliance with the Z39.30 bibliographic database standard. Some bibliographic management programs come with an interface for searching Z39.50-compliant databases and downloading the records directly into the personal database. When a program works with databases that are Z39.50 compliant, this means that they meet the requirements of this national standard for information retrieval. Officially known as ANSI/NISO Z39.50-1995—Information Retrieval (Z39.50): Application Service Definition and Protocol Specification, the Z39.50 standard establishes protocols for communication between two different computer systems. These protocols allow the client's software to search and retrieve records from databases residing on the server, which may be on a computer using a totally different operating system (Turner, 1997). Z39.50 compliant databases eliminate the need for filters in transferring downloaded records.

BENEFITS OF PERSONAL BIBLIOGRAPHIC MANAGEMENT SOFTWARE

The major advantage of this type of software is that the record structure allows the user to develop bibliographies for papers and publications that comply with the required publication style, without the need to retype the citations. This is particularly helpful if writing for courses or publications that have different style requirements. The record structure is designed to accommodate all information formats, so the databases developed are not limited to just one format, such as journal articles or books.

 ## Copyright

When searching knowledge databases, it is important to realize that much of the information you retrieve is subject to copyright. Although downloading and storing references in a personal database for research and study is usually considered fair use, copyright law covers the reproduction of this information for use by others. Only the bibliographic description—author, title, and other publication data—is in the public domain. For the most part, U.S. government information is not copyrighted, but one should check for any restrictions indicated on the actual document. Because MEDLINE is produced by the federal government, only the author abstracts are copyrighted. Otherwise, everything else you retrieve from knowledge databases is protected by copyright, including the subject indexing, abstracts, cited references, and full-text documents and images. Although some copying may be allowed under the much-deliberated fair-use doctrine, the best practice is to request permission for reproducing any copyrighted information resources.

 ## Databases for the Virtual Library

As the universe of knowledge-based information resources expands to include items in the virtual world such as Web sites and other Internet-accessible information resources, librarians and information scientists are applying subject-indexing principles to the development of databases that will index these new information formats. Web sites are now included in many online library catalogs. In the health sciences, the CINAHL database began indexing Web site records in 1998. For clinical medicine, there are now Web-based databases that use MeSH terms to index Web sites. Some examples include:

▼ CliniWeb from Oregon Health Sciences University (http://www.ohsu.edu/cliniweb/) uses MeSH terms from the Anatomy and Diseases trees to index approximately 10,000 clinically relevant Web sites. This database takes the terms a user enters and maps them to terms from the MeSH disease classification (Schloman, 1999). This site also provides links to the National Library of Medicine's PubMed database. It offers searching in five languages.

▼ Karolinska Institute Library: Diseases, Disorders and Related Topics (http://www.mic.ki.se/Diseases/index.html) is a MeSH based index; also in Swedish. Descriptions are from the actual Web content, which are similar to those retrieved by a typical Web search engine.

▼ OMNI (http://omni.ac.uk/) uses MeSH to index a growing database of more than 6,000 Web sites. From the United Kingdom, the records include original brief descriptions of the Web sites. OMNI includes NMAP, a database of Internet resources in Nursing, Midwifery and the Allied health Professions. Web sites are selected for OMNI and NMAP using established standards.

▼ SUMSearch, San Antonio Cochrane Center (http://sumsearch.uthscsa.edu/) uses MeSH headings to search for guidelines, systematic reviews, and other high quality evidence. It has clinical queries that add screening/prevention, adverse effects, and physical findings to the standard PubMed Clinical queries (therapy, diagnosis, etiology, prognosis).

▼ TRIP database (Turning Research Into Practice) http://www.tripdatabase.com/ searches more Web sites than SUMSearch, but does not offer standard subject headings. Search using all possible text word variations.

 ## Summary

Key databases for nursing include those produced by NLM, CINAHL, and the online catalog for your library. MEDLINE is now the primary NLM database for accessing journal articles. NLM provides free access to MEDLINE with PubMed, as well as access to other types of resources using NLM LOCATOR*plus* (books, audiovisuals, and journal holdings) and the NLM Gateway, which indexes both of these databases as well as NLM's web resources. CINAHL is more like the NLM Gateway, in that it provides access to information in all formats—not just journal articles, as in MEDLINE.

These key databases and many others are available from various vendors, each with their own search interface and underlying search engine. Even though some provide free access, those that are not produced by the government require either a personal or library subscription for access. Most search interfaces are web-based, but some libraries still offer CD-ROM searching. Search interfaces for online knowledge-based databases are constantly changing and evolving. It saves time to become familiar with the basic functions of search interfaces for frequently used databases.

A central feature of bibliographic databases is the added value provided by cataloging or indexing. In these processes, subject headings are assigned to the information resources cited in the databases. To obtain the best search results, use subject headings from the same approved subject heading list (thesaurus) used by the cataloger or indexer. Specialized bibliographic databases use specialized subject heading lists, whereas general library catalogs and databases use more general subject headings. Look for and use online thesauri to help you select subject headings. Keyword (or text word) searching should be reserved for situations in which subject headings do not match a need or when the user is looking for a very specific known item.

The knowledge-based online database record includes fields for specific types of information, such as author, title, source, publication type, and subjects. Limiting searches to terms in the appropriate field or fields leads to higher quality searches. Publication type limits are particularly useful for searches to support evidence-based practice.

Selecting the appropriate database or databases is just as important as devising a search strategy. Learn to match databases to information needs. Bibliographic management software can help you manage the hazards of information overload.

connection⎯⎯ **For definitions of bolded key terms, visit the online glossary available at http://connection.lww.com/go/thede.**

CONSIDERATIONS AND EXERCISES

1. Indexing an article:
   a. Find a peer-reviewed nursing journal article, either online or in your library or personal collection.
   b. Take a piece of paper and write the author, title, and source information on the top. Divide the rest of the sheet in three columns, with the headings My subjects, MEDLINE subjects, CINAHL subjects.
   c. Read the article and write the subjects you think it includes in the first column.
   d. Do an author/title search in MEDLINE and write the MEDLINE subject headings in the second column.
   e. Do an author/title search in CINAHL and write the CINAHL subject headings in the third column.
   f. Compare and contrast the three columns.
2. Finding Databases:
   a. Look for knowledge databases on your library and health system Web sites.
   b. Develop a three-column form and list those available in the first column, labeled databases.
   c. In the second column, note whether it is a bibliographic or factual database, or both.
   d. In the third column, briefly describe how you might use the database to support evidence-based practice.
3. Database searching:
   a. Choose a search topic related to a current patient care question.
   b. Plan a search strategy for MEDLINE, CINAHL, and one of the databases for Web sites described in this chapter. Note the subject headings on a worksheet similar to the one used in the first exercise.
   c. Execute the search in each of these databases.
   d. Compare and contrast your results.
4. Searching for evidence-based practice:
   a. Identify a nursing outcome that needs improvement in your health system.
   b. Plan search strategies to identify relevant translation literature, evidence summaries, and original research.

    c. Execute these searches and evaluate results.

    d. Discuss how the cited publications might help you prepare a local guideline to facilitate needed changes in practice.

5. Bibliographic management software:

    a. Read links on this topic on the Web site for this book, including information provided by the vendors.

    b. Read recent articles and reviews discussing bibliographic management software, both online and in journal articles that you retrieve through searching.

    c. Investigate the availability of local workshops and support for specific products.

    d. Based on your research, designate a bibliographic management software package that best meets your needs and discuss the rationale for the choice.

REFERENCES

Allen, M. (1998). Selecting keywords: helping others find your article. *Nurse Author & Editor, 8*(1), 4, 7–9.

Allen, M., & Levy, J. (2002). Evidence-based searching for nursing and allied health. *Bibliotheca Medica Canadiana, 23*(3), 90–5.

Arndt, K. A. (1992). Information excess in medicine. *Archives of Dermatology, 128,* 1249–1256.

Brown, S. J. (1999). *Knowledge for health care practice: A guide for using research evidence.* Philadelphia: W. B. Saunders.

Henderson, V. (1968). Library resources in nursing—their development and use, Parts I, II, and III. *International Nursing Review, 15,* 164–173, 236–146, 348–153.

Hospital and Health Administration index: Now quickly accessed by its subscribers at no cost. (2000). *NLM Newsline, 55*(1).

McSweeney, M., Spies, M., & Cann, C. J. (2001). Finding and evaluating clinical practice guidelines. *Nurse Practitioner, 26*(9), 30–49.

MEDLINE. (2001, May 22, 2001). [Website]. National Library of Medicine. Available at http://www.nlm.nih.gov/databases/databases_medline.html [Accessed March 10, 2002].

Nicoll, L. H., Oulette, T. H., Bird, D. C., Harper, J., & Kelley, J. (1996). Bibliography database managers: a comparative review. *Computers in Nursing, 14*(1), 45–56.

Nurses, librarians, and publishers making a difference: Celebrating 35 years of the International Nursing Index. (2002). *American Journal of Nursing, 102*(1), 103.

Schloman, B. (August 19, 1999). *Needle in a haystack? Finding health information on the Web.* Online Journal of Issues in Nursing Available. http://www.nursingworld.org/ojin/infocol/info_2.htm.

Titler, M.G., Kleiber, C., Steelman, V., Rakel, B., Barry-Walke, J., Small, S., & Buckwatter, K. (1994). Infusing research into practice to promote quality care. *Nursing Research, 43*(5), 307–313.

Titler, M. G., Mendes, J. C., Rakel, B., Abbott, L., & Baumler, S. (1999). From book to bedside: Putting evidence to use in the care of the elderly. *Joint Commission Journal on Quality Improvement, 25*(10), 545–556.

Turner, F. (1997, 1997). *Z39.50 Information retrieval standard: Overview and implementation.* National Library of Canada. Available at http://www.nlc-bnc.ca/publications/1/p1-207-e.html [2002, March 15, 2002].

Educational Informatics: e-Learning

Objectives

After studying this chapter you will be able to:

1. Describe different formats for computer-assisted-instruction.

2. Differentiate between the different educational methodologies for computer-assisted instruction.

3. Describe characteristics necessary for a good simulation.

4. Evaluate a computer learning program.

5. Interpret the factors affecting distance education.

6. Propose the use of e-Learning to a healthcare organization.

Educational activities are intended to increase the knowledge of learners. Resources for such activities appear in many formats, such as lectures, reading, and self-learning computer activities. Education itself can be looked at as the mental manipulation of data, information, and knowledge by learners to increase their knowledge. Learning only occurs in the learner, but it can be facilitated by a teacher, whether face to face, mediated by a medium ranging from paper to a digital visual disk (DVD), or through any combination of these. The job of an educator, whether as a parent, a nurse doing patient education, a teacher in a formal class, or a designer of educational aids, is to facilitate this process. These functions can be called educational informatics, and they may or may not involve technology. When they involve learning mediated by computer technology, they are termed **e-Learning**.

No matter which format is used for education, it is imperative that the primary focus be on learning, not the technology itself or lack of it. Informatics is about using the best methods to manage information, and e-Learning focuses on the appropriate use of computerized technology to achieve educational aims. As we move to using e-Learning, it is important to remember that simply moving a class or course to a computer format is not necessarily an improvement. Attention must be paid to how the technology is used, as well as to what it will add to the learning situation. Each technological method, from the early simple computer-assisted learning to virtual reality, possesses different attributes. An attribute is a factor, such as color or movement, that a medium implements. Their use may or may not add to learning. The type of learning desired and characteristics of the topic determine which attributes are needed to provide the best learning.

e-Learning Terminologies

e-Learning is another of the "e-words" that has crept into our language; it indicates a marriage between electronics, generally a computer, and educational software. It includes many different types of computerized instruction, from instruction using only the text portion of a computer to Internet-based **distance learning** using a multimedia-capable computer. There are many older terms that are used to refer to e-Learning such as **computer-assisted instruction (CAI)**, **computer-based learning (CBL)**, and **computer-based instruction (CBI)**.

Learning management is another concept that involves computer use in education. Terms such as **computer-managed instruction (CMI)**, **computer-managed learning (CML)**, and **learning management system (LMS)** describe software that assists in educational administrative tasks. The tasks this software performs can be as simple as presenting and scoring computer learning and printing a certificate to programs that register students and keep track of the courses that they have completed. A **learning content management system (LCMS)** extends services to instructors and training departments. It can help users to organize learning objects such as objectives, slides, video clips, illustrations, quiz questions, and even course modules; it can then present them in infinitely changeable combinations to meet an instructor's needs.

Computer Technology and Learning

Although educational informatics involves all facets of education, this chapter focuses on the use of computer technology formats. Use of this technology can be viewed from two different perspectives: from that of instructional methodologies and from the ways the technology is used.

INSTRUCTIONAL METHODOLOGIES

In any learning situation, it is important that four goals be considered. Information must be presented, students must be guided in their learning, they must be allowed to practice using the information, and some means of assessing the learning needs to occur (Alessi & Trollip, 1991). Some types of available e-Learning do not accomplish all these goals and must be supplemented with other modes of teaching. There are five different approaches to designing e-Learning: drill and practice, tutorials, simulations, instructional games, and tests. Many programs combine these approaches.

Drill and Practice

Drill and practice type software was among the first educational software introduced. It was relatively simple to produce and freed teachers from mundane chores and repetitive teaching. In one drill and practice format, the program emulates a teacher using flash cards. Other formats include multiple choice questions that students can use to review previously learned material. When well designed, these programs provide feedback on all of the answer choices. Another useful feature in this type of program is that it allows students to investigate the feedback for all answers, even when they get the right answer. This feature aids inquisitive students who want to use the program in a more tutorial mode.

The best use of drill and practice is to aid memorization. Although pure memorization is not a favored method of learning today, one needs to memorize basic medical terminology along with the rules for combining these terms to create other words, as well as anatomical terms. Additionally, although the goal in education is to develop critical thinking, there may be a place for a good drill and practice program in assisting a student to develop the cognitive structure necessary for the reflective thinking that produces critical thinking. When selecting a pure drill and practice program, however, keep in mind that there are sometimes more effective ways to develop this knowledge.

Tutorials

A *tutorial* is a program designed to impart information to learners. Most are patterned on the programmed learning model. Information is imparted, and the learner is asked questions about the material, often in a multiple-choice format. In one variation, if a wrong answer is given, the student is led back to the original information. In more sophisticated versions, a wrong answer leads the learner to a different approach to the information with the belief that this learner needs a different, or further, explanation before she or he will understand. Other features that may be included are an explanation for wrong answers, and the use of wrong answers as a springboard for correcting misinformation. The quality of a tutorial is evident in the use the program makes of branching techniques. At the low end of the continuum are programs that just inform the learner whether an answer is correct. Those at the high end will offer more than one explanation for the same phenomenon.

Tutorials do not have to "tell" learners what they need to know. Learners can instead be presented with a situation, given the tools necessary to discover the answer and then allowed to proceed at their own pace. In these situations, they are encouraged to experiment and draw their own conclusions. In one program of this type, learners input values that the program uses to create a fetal monitor strip representing the parameters the user entered. Learners then match their diagnosis of the strip against that of the experts. This type of tutorial tends to develop excitement and enthusiasm in the learner (Sweeney, 1985) and lends itself well to two or three learners working together.

Simulations

Simulations take the form of case studies. They are designed to allow the learner to practice a patient encounter by providing care to a simulated patient (White, 1995). The objective is to make the learner an actual participant in a patient care situation that would either be too difficult, dangerous, or time consuming to provide in a real clinical setting. An example of a very realistic simulation is one that is designed for nurses in a post-anesthesia recovery room. In this simulation, the learner has all the tools available that would be available in a real situation, including monitoring equipment. When a patient arrives in the recovery room, the learner is presented with the history, then care commences. A real-time clock is started to give the learner a guide as to when various monitoring activities should occur. The nurse is expected to perform as he or she would in a real-life situation, with no prompting from the computer. Results of all actions are seen in real time, whether it is a strip from a monitor or a readout of vital signs. The nurse is expected to base future actions on the results of assessments and standard recovery room protocols.

> **Display 18-1 • CHARACTERISTICS OF A GOOD SIMULATION**
>
> 1. No menus or guides to actions, allows user to make decisions as in real life.
> 2. Selection of the same choices as would be seen in the real situation (e.g., assessment, request laboratory values).
> 3. Provision for users to query the patient or others using standard English.
> 4. Free movement allowed between interviews to exams to actions, just as would occur in a real situation.
> 5. If time is a factor in the real situation, it should be part of the simulation.
> 6. Feedback pertinent to choices made.
>
> Adapted from White, J. E. (1995). Using interactive video to add physical assessment data to computer-based patient simulations in nursing. *Computers in Nursing, 13*(5), 233–235.

A simulation has many different uses. It could be used as part of an orientation or in-service, or with a computer projector in a classroom situation. There are, however, considerations that should be given when using a simulation (Display 18-1). The simulation should match the learner's knowledge background, or at least be only slightly above it, and the point of view in the simulation should be similar to what is being taught. Differences in point of view, such as a medical orientation instead of a nursing orientation, can cause frustration in learners who base their answers more on nursing philosophy than medical philosophy. Ideally, there would be no difference, but this is not always so.

Instructional Games

Games can be very similar to simulations, or they can be used in a drill and practice mode. Their purpose is to provide motivation to students to learn the needed information. Games are characterized by competition among opponents whose actions are guided by rules to achieve an objective (Abt, as cited in Ellington, Addinall, & Percival, 1982). There are many different types of games. Psychomotor games are intended to improve psychomotor skills. Intellectual skill games are often a form of drill and practice, whereas games of chance may add elements of psychomotor or intellectual skills to an a element of chance involved in achieving the goal (Ellington, et al., 1982). Games that are successful must meet instructional requirements and be enjoyable for players.

Computerized Tests

Computers have many different functions in testing. They can be used to score tests, create them, or administer them. Limited choice tests are easily scored by a computer, which can also provide statistics for the questions. Most test scoring software is also capable of providing a file for the instructor that can be imported into a database or spreadsheet and used as part of an electronic grading book.

Software exists that allows the creation of tests that can be printed or given online. One advantage of using online testing is the ability to create different formats for the test. One such format, **computerized adaptive testing** (CAT), designs an individual test based on the testees answers. Because testees do not spend time answering questions that are too easy or difficult for them, this process requires fewer questions than a paper test (Educational Testing Service, 1996). This is the format used by the National Council of Nursing State Board Examination. Another online testing format is a **clinical simulation test** (CST), which presents the examinee with a clinical care situation and evaluates the actions taken. For a more detailed discussion of computer testing, see the Web page for this chapter at http://connection.lww.com/go/thede.

THE TECHNOLOGIES

Although the various formats that e-Learning takes are discussed as separate entities, as the power of computers increases, the lines between categories are becoming increasingly blurred. In this chapter, the term computer-assisted-instruction (CAI) will be used to denote all these technologies—from plain CAI to virtual reality.

Plain Computer-Assisted-Instruction

Plato (Programmed Logic for Automatic Teaching Operation), a text only program designed to allow creation of educational software, was used in the late 1960's by Bitzer, Boudreaux, and Avner (1973) at the University of Illinois Urbana to put together a maternity course. Plato only generated text. Besides being the first recorded use of computers in nursing education, this CAI set a standard that even today is rarely seen. The approach used an inquiry approach in which learners had maximum control. The teaching logic was based on the ideas of the famous educational psychologist, Brune; students, instead of having information delivered to them, were led to figure things out for themselves, a process that improves the ability to retrieve information from memory. To complete the program, learners sought needed information, sorted it, then organized, interpreted, and applied it. Instead of answering multiple choice questions, learners gave free text natural language responses to questions that were parsed and compared with a list of acceptable answers. The results were that students using this CAI learned the content just as well as their counterparts who learned in a classroom, but they completed their learning in 23.5 hours compared with the 66.5 hours for classroom learning. Additionally, the students using the CAI had excellent long-term retention of the information. Although it is tempting to credit this success to the computer, the real reason for its success was the teaching methods it employed.

For the past several decades there have been hundreds of research studies that attempted to support the premise that computer learning was somehow superior to "traditional teaching." A meta-analysis of 29 studies reported in the literature from 1966 to 1991 studied the results of using CAI in nursing education; it revealed that in most studies, CAI was favored over so called traditional education (Cohen & Dacanay, 1994). These researchers also found that in those studies in which learner attitude was reported, learners had a more positive attitude toward CAI than toward traditional instruction. This study supported a previous meta-analysis of studies in all branches of education that had also found a slight overall factor in favor of CAI (Kulik, Kulik, & Cohen, 1980). There are several difficulties with these studies. In most of them, "traditional teaching" is poorly defined (Thede, 1995). The only clear comparison is generally the type of medium used, not the educational methods employed.

Multimedia—Interactive Video, CD-ROM, DVD

The original meaning of the term **multimedia** was the combination of visual and audio from different sources. It was used in the 1970s to describe theater and slide-show productions (Multimedia, 2002). It is now used to describe any combination of hardware and software that displays images or plays sound. Today's computers are capable of being multimedia players, but given the huge size of many of these files, it took the addition of CD-ROM and DVD players to make this use feasible. Multimedia is also obtainable over the Internet, but it requires special add-ons to one's browser, not only to play the multimedia, but often to provide the **streaming** download necessary to make its use feasible.

There are multimedia tools that automate the teaching of cardiopulmonary resuscitation (CPR). The system uses CAI for didactic training but connects a mannequin to a computer to teach the psychomotor skills. The mannequin enables the timing and effectiveness of chest compressions and breathing to be recorded and counted. The system is approved by the American Heart Association for CPR certification.

Virtual Reality

Virtual reality (VR) is based on illusions (Pimentel & Teixeira, 1992). It is the use of technology to allow the participant to exist in another reality, experiencing an event that although it appears real does not physically exist. The objective is to create a scene in which the participant is free to concentrate on the tasks, problems, and ideas that he or she would face in a real situation. The primary criterion is that the participant be surrounded by an environment and be "inside" the information.

There are two main components to VR. One is the model or visualization that resembles reality and allows manipulation of the environment; the second is an interface that resembles the three-dimensional world (Robertson, 1997). During the VR experience, the "environment" reacts just as it would in the real world.

There are many formats that use the term VR as a label. The most advanced type of VR is a flight simulator. At the opposite end of the spectrum is a very simple type of VR, sometimes called desktop VR. In this system, a scene on a computer display is used to portray the virtual world. A higher level of VR is created by the use of special gloves, earphones and goggles all of which receive input from a computer. These devices not only feed sensory information to participants, but they also monitor their activities. For example, the goggles track eye movements and respond with appropriate video input (Webopedia, 2002).

In another type of VR, called *video mapping* or *projected reality*, a video input of the user's silhouette is merged with a two-dimensional computer graphic of the environment. On the monitor, the user sees the interaction of his or her body with the world. A higher level, sometimes labeled an *immersive system*, completely immerses the user in the virtual world. These systems often use a head-mounted display that the user wears as a helmet or mask. This mask holds the visual and auditory displays. The power of this VR is derived from its ability to focus a participant's perceptions on a specific problem or experience (Pimentel & Teixeira, 1992).

Given the practice-based nature of nursing and other healthcare education, VR may eventually become a very popular training method for the healthcare professions. One application that has been developed is as a method of teaching intravenous puncture, in which virtual tissues are used. A virtual tissue is one that has been programmed to behave just like real tissue when it is cut, tugged, stretched, or punctured. In this application, the tissues are programmed to resemble a rolling vein, sclerosed vein, and a vein in an obese patient (Merril & Barker, 1996).

As designed, this simulator integrates clinical decision making with learning the procedure by using various patient situations in the program. The learner's first task is to read a patient's situation and base his or her actions on it. After the facts of the situation have been assimilated, the user selects an appropriate site for the venipuncture, places the tourniquet, and manipulates the needle (Merrill & Barker, 1996). Penetrating the skin produces in the user approximately the same feel as when one actually performs the procedure. The user also receives feedback that simulates how the pressure of venous wall resistance feels. During the simulation, the screen shows the user the position of the needle in relation to the vein. When the needle is inserted appropriately, blood is seen flowing from the vein into the needle. Simulations like this, which can be used to teach invasive procedures that need a high degree of skill if patient discomfort is to be minimized, can revolutionize how skill teaching is done.

Web-Based Instruction

In addition to providing a virtual encyclopedia, use of the World Wide Web has also been incorporated into formal education. It is used in many diverse ways, from augmentation of a regular class to a full online class. Many instructors in traditional courses are experimenting with placing syllabi, class notes, or even "lectures" online. Additionally, the Web is often used for discussion. There are many software products available today that make it easy for faculty to use the Web to either supplement a course or teach the full course online.

As more education moves online, the need to make Web sites available to those with physical disabilities becomes more pronounced. The Equal Access to Software and Information Association (EASI), an organization affiliated with the American Association for Higher Education, is trying to raise awareness of this issue (Kiser, 2001). A survey of the home pages by this organization in December 2000 found only 15% of accredited distance education programs' Web sites that were free from serious usability problems. Any school that wishes to make courses available to government employees will need to update their online offerings to meet disability standards.

INTEGRATING E-LEARNING INTO AN EDUCATIONAL PROGRAM

Like Web-based instruction, other forms of e-Learning can be used in a multitude of ways, as an adjunct to a class, as a substitute for a class, or as an entire course. Web-based instruction has found uses in all educational venues, including degree programs and continuing education. Healthcare agencies that find it difficult to release employees at given times for classroom classes have found that CAI in its many formats can meet the need for mandatory and continuing education. Although there are up-front costs for the technology and software, there are also savings. The costs of instructors and materials, the difficulties in releasing employees at set times, and the clerical costs of keeping necessary records can all be greatly reduced with appropriate learning management software. Many vendors now offer CAI that meets the criteria for the Joint Commission on Accreditation of Healthcare Organization's (JCAHO) mandatory educational programs.

CAI is also useful in patient education. Office or clinic waiting rooms are an excellent location for the use of any of the e-Learning formats. Patient educators can design CAI to be used in a waiting room, as part of a one-on-one session, or in group teaching. One example is a program designed to teach asthmatic children. Using a combination of a simulation with a tutorial and a motivational game, the program was found to significantly increase children's knowledge of self-regulation, prevention, and treatment strategies, as well as to increase their beliefs that they had control of their disease (Shegog, Bartholomew, Parcel, Sockrider, Masse, & Abramson, 2001).

ROLE OF INSTRUCTOR

The role of an instructor who uses CAI varies. Some instructors assign a CAI program just as they would a chapter in a book. They may or may not discuss the content in class. Another approach is to integrate the CAI with another assignment, such as a short paper, to help the student to integrate the content with other information. The CAI may also be used as part of a class presentation that uses a computer screen projection device. Some CAI lends itself to group learning. In this mode, learners often contribute to each other's learning by discussing the various options; they use investigative behaviors that would not have been tapped in single learning.

Effective use of CAI requires that it be part of a total educational plan. It is important that as much thought go into the use of CAI as it does into assigning readings or other learning activities. CAI that is assigned as an afterthought because it is available is generally not conducive to producing learning outcomes in keeping with class or course objectives. Innovative use of CAI can create a learning environment different than that promoted by CAI alone. For example, software using more of the behaviorist principles discussed in Chapter 1, together with appropriate activities, could be part of the constructivist teaching approach addressed in Chapter 1. Constructivist software can be given more structure by preparing the learners with appropriate activities. It is not the labeling of educational philosophy that is important; it is how one chooses to integrate it into a teaching situation that determines the type of learning that occurs. Identifying the different teaching approaches used by the software, and compensating when necessary, often makes the difference between whether learners find success or experience frustration.

EVALUATING CAI

Determining which CAI to use and how to use it will depend on the objectives of the instructional material. When considering using CAI, one needs to consider the type of objective. Does it involve a psychomotor skill, critical thinking, memorization, or just knowledge assimilation? VR, if available, would best meet the needs of a psychomotor skill, whereas a program using the behaviorist principles discussed in Chapter 1 would best meet the needs for memorization. Critical thinking needs can best be met by software that uses more of the constructivist philosophy.

When evaluating CAI, the primary characteristic to be considered is whether it meets a learning need. When considering this factor, keep in mind that learners are at a different educational level than the individual selecting software and may have a different point of view. One of the best ways to evaluate CAI involves having potential users with three different learning abilities (low, average, and high) preview the software. One should also consider whether the offering would be just as effective in a different medium. Electronic page turners are a waste of computer abilities and lose some positive attributes of reading material, such as ease of review.

The one characteristic that elevates CAI above all other teaching mediums, with the exception of a human teacher or live experience, is interactivity. How effective an interaction is depends on the mental processing required and the nature of the learner's inter-action with the content (Thede, 1995). The relative quality of the questions will deter-mine the level of learning that is required. Simply phrased questions may discourage deep learning, whereas questions requiring analysis or syntheses encourage a deeper process-ing (Ross & Tuovinen, 2001). In considering the quality of an interaction, look at both the methods used to solicit input and the way the computer reacts to inputs. The lowest level of user input occurs when a user answers a multiple choice question, and the high-est level occurs when the user enters free text with no clues provided by questions. In a simple tutorial, a high-level reply includes feedback that attempts to assist the learner to correct misinterpretations. In a high-quality simulation, the user sees the results of ac-tions and needs to give input based on those results.

When evaluating CAI, examine the graphics and animation to determine whether they are used to facilitate learning a concept or as extras. Investigate whether the learner is en-couraged to be passive or expected to provide input. If the learner has the ability for in-put, evaluate whether it is more than the rote answering of questions. Other factors to consider are: Can the learner determine the flow of instruction? Exit the program at will? Request more information? When the student is allowed to have control, learning be-comes more interactive (Bolwell, 1988).

It is very tempting to develop a form to use in evaluating CAI. Generally, however, as with the evaluation of Web resources, there is such a great difference in the types of programs, as well as in learning needs, that the one-size-fits-all approach is difficult to support. The col-lection and evaluation of 87 CAI evaluation forms by Sparks and Kuenz (1993) reveals some of the difficulties of trying to create an objective evaluation form. Those authors found a great variation in length of the tool (from one to eight pages) and approach to evaluation (from the appearance and appeal of the program to mechanical function) in what was included in the evaluation. A more effective approach is to consider the items that have been discussed above as well as others that are pertinent to educational needs (Display 18-2).

Pros and Cons of CAI

CAI is neither a panacea nor something that will replace teachers. Like all innovations, it has advantages and disadvantages. Advantages include the availability of CAI outside reg-ular classroom hours and the patience of a computer as a teacher (Ball & Hannah, 1984;

Display 18-2 • QUESTIONS TO ASK WHEN EVALUATING COMPUTER-ASSISTED INSTRUCTION (CAI)

1. Is the learning active or passive?
2. Does the program provide prompt, constructive feedback?
3. Is the user's time used productively?
4. Are different ways of learning the material available?
5. Does the program support collaborative learning?
6. What level of learning is supported?

Adapted from Jeffries, P. (2000). Development and test of a model for de-signing interactive CD-ROMs for teaching nursing skills. *Computers in Nursing, 18*(3), 118–124.

Rouse, 1999). Perhaps one of the greatest advantages is that computers can be used to allow learners to participate in learning experiences that otherwise are not available outside real life. They also permit the learner to set his or her own pace. Another advantage is that, unlike a traditional lecture, exactly the same material is presented each time. Properly designed CAI is accessible by students who are physically unable to attend class. It can also be designed to accommodate hearing-impaired students. Some difficulties that may be encountered are the initial cost of the software, anxiety related to a lack of familiarity with the technology, lack of support staff, and resistance to change (Caputi & Dreher, 1997, as cited in Rouse, 2000).

Teachers are still searching for the most effective ways to use CAI in learning. Entrenched educational ideas, held by both students and faculty, such as believing that teachers should deliver information in a classroom rather than facilitate learning using other techniques, may interfere with creative use of CAI. As more people become comfortable with computers and are able to experiment with different learning methods, the many formats of CAI will find a major role in quality education.

Creating CAI

The introduction of CD and DVD burners, **digital cameras**, and software for editing allows anyone with garden-variety hardware and software to create multimedia programs. This may tempt some to want to create their own CAI either for online use or as a CD-ROM. This is not a task to be undertaken lightly. It is one thing to present information in person but it is quite another to design something that stands alone. In a classroom or one-on-one situation, teachers have the ability to see the reaction of learners to a presentation and to answer questions. When developing a stand-alone module, such feedback is completely absent. If software that could be used to meet the learning task exists, the wisest course is to purchase it. Developing CAI is labor intensive and costly. Estimates of the time required to develop 1 hour of instruction vary from 100 to 750 hours, depending on the desired quality and complexity involved.

Distance Learning

Distance learning is a phenomenon that has been with us since Roman times and whenever and wherever reliable postal service was available. In the United States, correspondence courses have been available since the 18th century. Although correspondence courses are still the primary mode of distance learning in most of the world, technology is used more and more in this endeavor. Some distance learning uses one- or two-way video and one or two way audio. With the spread of the Internet and Web technology, the move toward technology is continuing, especially in areas of the world that have reliable communication systems.

Two terms are used to label this type of learning: **distributed learning** and **distance learning**. Distributed learning describes education that uses technology and does not occur face to face (Boschmann, 2001). Distance learning describes a situation in which teachers and students are in different locations. Distance education formats differ in the time frames that they use; some are **synchronous** and others **asynchronous**. In synchronous learning, class is held at set times and all participants are "present," either online or with the use of microwave or other technology. This method resembles traditional edu-

TABLE 18-1 • *Time Criteria Continuum in Distributed Learning*		
Functions	**Synchronous**	**Asynchronous**
Meeting times	Set meeting times	No set meeting times.
Assignments (includes quizzes and tests)	Set due dates	Students complete assignments when they have time, there is no due date beyond that of the end of the course.
Time period of course	Starts and ends on a given date	Starts and ends at convenience of student (Most have a given time length from beginning to end of course)
Type of learning	Instructor-led/class discussions	Independent, only feedback is on assignments.

cation; the students may gather in small groups at set locations in various places or alone at home.

In the asynchronous format, learners use the learning resources at a time and place that is convenient for them. They may or may not have a set time for completing the learning requirements. The most extreme form of asynchronous learning is the correspondence course. The Internet can also deliver asynchronous courses, but with the advantage that the communication between the learner and an instructor is much faster. The Internet has another advantage over correspondence courses; it permits collaboration by learners as if they were in a classroom. Combinations of either synchronous or asynchronous conditions are also employed, including requiring students to be physically present in one location for a given number of sessions (Table 18-1). Generally, the more asynchronous features that an educational offering uses, the less structured it is and the more it requires independent learning.

Distance learning requires skills that students educated in traditional classrooms may need to develop. Some of these skills involve using technology. Even those who routinely use the computer often need an orientation to the software that is used to manage the online portion of a class. Skills like using e-mail may need to be reviewed and reinforced. Learners often need to be reminded to use a subject line and a signature with all their messages. Additionally, they need to know how to organize their email messages into folders.

If the learning is complete distance learning, the learners may need help in signing up with an **internet service provider** (ISP) and establishing an e-mail account. The policies of an ISP need to be checked. Those who use e-mail accounts at work need to check with their information services department to be sure that they can send and receive attachments. Some organizations have been forced to ban attachments because of concerns about computer viruses. In these cases, sometimes a student can get a free offsite e-mail address, and messages with attachments can be sent there.

Discussions, whether in a forum, in an electronic mailing list, or as part of an online "chat," are often a part of an online course.[1] The protocols of the discussion format need to be learned. The student also needs to learn functions such as how to reply to a person, how to reply to the group as a whole, and how to archive messages. Learners may also

---

[1] Online chats today are conducted in writing, but as the bandwidth of the Internet improves, these will eventually be verbal.

need to learn how to preserve the **thread** of a discussion. Some of these methods may seem confusing at first. In an online "chat," the arrival of a proliferation of messages as the student is trying to reply to an earlier message may cause a learner to become disorganized until familiarity with this method is achieved.

Given today's requirements for life-long learning and the specialization seen in today's healthcare, it is probable that everyone with 20 years or less experience will at least once, if not routinely, take an online course. Online courses require an additional set of skills not always required in a regular classroom (Display 18-3). Most distance learning uses more active learning activities than regular classroom education. Many students are not prepared for this type of learning. When there is no regular classroom lecture to supplement readings, students need to read differently. Taking notes while reading, just as they would if the reading were a lecture in a regular class, underlining key points and ideas, and noting material that is not understood are required skills for distance learning. When writing, students need to be cognizant that their audience does not share their situation or agency policies or know the acronyms they use. They also need to realize that the informality used in speaking often produces lack of clarity in written messages.

USES FOR DISTANCE LEARNING

Internet-based distance learning has found many uses in healthcare. One of the most widespread uses is in continuing education. This type of learning is available in different formats. Some sites offer online articles and questions that can be read by anyone but require a fee if the answers are submitted for credit. Others provide an abstract but require a fee to retrieve the actual learning material and questions. Some sites provide the ability to print out a certificate after a credit card number has been submitted. Staff educators may find that many of these offerings could be made a part of a staff education program for career ladder programs or other necessary learning.

Full degree-granting programs are also offered online. Although in some quarters there are still doubts about the legitimacy of these programs, accreditation of distance learning

---

Display 18-3 • SKILLS REQUIRED IN DISTANCE LEARNING

Students engaged in distance learning will find it helpful to:

1. Have and reserve adequate time for the course work and meetings (if any).
2. Concentrate fully while reading.
3. Identify what is important in a reading.
4. Identify what is not understood and ask for clarification.
5. Develop collegial relationships related to education in their environment, both online and in their community.
6. Identify and find needed resources.
7. Use written communication effectively.
8. Be very comfortable using the required technology.
9. Work independently.

is offered by the major college accrediting bodies in the same way as it is given to programs held in a regular classroom.

Several certificate programs are also offered online. The various programs vary in their requirements for a presence on campus during the program; some require none, others may require a week-end presence during each course or an on campus presence sometime during the program.

EFFECTIVENESS OF DISTANCE LEARNING

Most of the research studies that compared distance learning with regular classroom learning have found that course objectives and learning outcomes are achieved (Billings, Ward, & Penton-Cooper, 2001). In addition, there is no significant difference in academic achievement between distance learning and traditional education. As is the situation with all new technologies, there are negative and positive aspects to distance learning (Display 18-4). Perhaps the greatest drawback is lack of personal contact. Many instructors, as well as students, miss this. Encouraging students to share something about themselves is one activity that can at least give all participants the feeling that they know something about a colleague and the professor. The two biggest advantages of distance learning are the ability of students in rural or remote areas to take advantage of continuing learning and the ability of students to schedule learning at times convenient to them.

Distance and/or distributed education is a growing field. As Internet infrastructure improves, expect to see visual contact and hear audio during distance education meetings. Cameras about 4 inches in size that sit on top of a PC monitor and allow the computer user to send pictures of himself or herself are available for less than $100. The use of these in addition to a microphone and software such as Net Meeting can create a classroom atmosphere.

Nightingale Tracker

One innovative use of computer communication technology is the Nightingale Tracker, developed by FITNE, Inc. (formerly the Fuld Institute for Technology) for use in com-

---

Display 18-4 • ADVANTAGES AND DISADVANTAGES OF DISTANCE LEARNING

Advantages of Distance Learning

1. Depending on the structure, students can participate on their schedule.
2. Students without easy access to a college can participate.
3. Some agencies have found that offering distance learning as a perk increases retention.
4. Classes in a limited specialty can be offered because of an expanded audience.
5. Access to class is available 24 hours a day, 7 days a week.
6. Learners must think before they express their ideas, thus cannot speak impulsively. Organizing one's ideas increases learning.
7. All learners must participate.

Disadvantages of Distance Learning

1. Additional resources are needed to assist instructors and students.
2. Lack of face-to-face contact.
3. May not be suitable to all content.
4. The technology may contribute to frustration.

munity nursing. The tracker system uses a client-server architecture, consisting of field clients that are personal digital assistants (PDAs) which use regular telephone lines and a central server. The Tracker facilitates clinical communication functions such as the generation and transfer of clinical assignments. It also permits students to develop a plan of care using the Omaha System, one of the American Nurses Association (ANA) recognized standardized terminologies. Students may also transfer their documentation to instructors and clinical agencies and be in telephone contact with their instructor during a home visit. The PDA also provides the user with communication features such as e-mail, faxes, and access to the Web. In addition, information collected by the server can serve as a long-term clinical data repository (FITNE, 2000). The Tracker is an example of a system that was designed with a great deal of user input (Nightingale Tracker Field Test Team, 1999).

 ## Summary

In the information age, it is imperative that one of the aims of formal education be to prepare learners to be active independent learners and problem solvers. When it is used appropriately, e-Learning can assist in this process and provide a venue for the continued learning necessary in today's world. CAI can be classified in two ways, either by the methodology used or the technology. There are five different approaches to CAI: drill and practice, tutorial, simulation, gaming, and testing. The technology includes simple CAI, multimedia, VR, and the Web. Each modality meets different needs.

Using e-Learning successfully depends on how it is integrated into the total learning program. Selecting appropriate software is best accomplished by using the viewpoints of different levels of learners. The level of interactivity also needs to be considered and matched with program goals. Like all teaching methods, CAI has advantages and disadvantages. Advantages include interactivity and the accessibility of the medium. Disadvantages may include lack of familiarity with the technology and expense. Although the equipment for creating one's own CAI is commonly available, the least costly choice is usually to purchase software.

With the advent of the Internet, distance learning has become a popular method for educational offerings. Programs offered through distance learning vary from correspondence courses and magazine articles to full degree programs. Distance learning requires the development of skills that are not always needed in traditional education, such as the ability to discipline oneself to set aside time for the program and the ability to communicate effectively in writing.

connection For definitions of bolded key terms, visit the online glossary available at **http://connection.lww.com/go/thede.**

CONSIDERATIONS AND EXERCISES

1. Describe simple CAI, multimedia, and VR.
2. Differentiate between the characteristics of the following software programs:
   a. Drill and practice
   b. Tutorial
   c. Game

3. List and briefly describe the characteristics necessary for a good simulation.
4. Describe the different modes of computerized testing.
5. Evaluate a computer educational program.
6. Briefly discuss the:
   a. Uses for distance education
   b. Skill sets needed in distance education
7. One of your functions in a 100-bed hospital is to provide staff education. You wish to integrate e-Learning into your organization. Write a proposal that:
   a. Interprets the various choices for e-Learning
   b. Discusses the advantages of each choice
   c. Provides reasons for using one or two of these methods

REFERENCES

Abt, C. C. (1968). Games for learning. In S.S. Boocock, & E. O. Schild, (Eds.). *Simulation games in learning.* Beverly Hills, CA: Sage Publications.

Alessi, S. M., & Trollip, S. R. (1991). *Computer-based instruction* (2nd ed.). Englewood Cliffs, NJ: Prentice Hall.

Ball, M., & Hannah, M. J. (1984). *Using computers in nursing.* Reston, VA: Reston Publishing Company.

Billings, D., Ward, J. W., & Penton-Cooper, L. (2001). Distance learning in nursing. *Seminars in Oncology Nursing, 17*(1), 48–54.

Bitzer, M. D., Boudreaux, M., & Avner, R. A. (1973). *Computer-based instruction of basic nursing utilizing inquiry approach.* (CERL Report X-40). Urbana, IL: University of Illinois.

Bolwell, C. (1988). Evaluating computer assisted instruction. In T. Lochhass (Ed.), *Proceedings of the Third International Symposium on nursing use of computers and information science.* (pp. 825–830). St. Louis: C. V. Mosby.

Boschmann, E. (2001). *What is distributed learning?* Retrieved March 14, 2002 from http://www.indiana.edu/~iude/frameset-de-def.html.

Caputi, L., & Dreher, M. (1997). *The design and development of computer-assisted instruction.* Oak Brook, IL: C*D Computer Enterprises.

Cohen, P. A., & Dacanay, L. S. (1994). A meta-analysis of computer-based instruction in Nursing Education. *Computers in Nursing, 12*(2), 89–97.

Educational Testing Service. (1997). *Tests and services directory.* Retrieved March 12, 2002 from http://www.ets.org/search97cgi/s97_cgi.

Ellington, H., Addinall, E., & Percival, F. (1982). *A handbook of game design.* New York: Nichols Publishing Company.

FITNE, (2000). One view of the present. Retrieved March 26, 2002 from http://www.nightingaletracker.com/nursing/08_nursing.html.

Jeffries, P. (2000). Development and test of a model for designing interactive CD-ROMs for teaching nursing skills. *Computers in Nursing, 18*(3), 118–124.

Kiser, K. (2001). Web-enabled? *Online Learning, 5*(6), 28–30, 32–33.

Kulik J. A., Kulik, C. C., & Cohen, P. A. (1980). Effectiveness of computer based college teaching: A meta-analysis of findings. *Review of Educational Research, 50*(4), 525–544.

Merrill, G. L., & Barker, V. L. (1996). Virtual reality debuts in the teaching laboratory in nursing. *Journal of Intravenous Nursing, 19*(4), 182–187.

Multimedia definition. (2002). Retrieved March 14, 2002 from http://www.scala.com/multimedia/definition.html.

Nightingale Tracker Field Test Team. (1999). Designing an information technology application for use in community-focused nursing education. *Computers in Nursing, 17*(2), 73–81.

Pimentel, K., & Teixeira, K. (1992). *Virtual reality.* New York: Intel/Windcrest/Intel.

Robertson, C. (1997). *VRML and QuickTime VR technology.* Retrieved March 14, 2002 from http://www.nlc-bnc.ca/9/1/p1-247-e.html.

Rouse, D. R. (1999). Creating an interactive computer-assisted instruction program. *Computers in Nursing, 17*(4), 171–176.

Ross, G. C., & Tuovinen, J. E. (2001). Deep versus surface learning with multimedia in nursing education. *Computers in Nursing, 19*(5), 213–223.

Shegog, R., Bartholomew, L. K., Parcel, G. S., Sockrider, M. M., Masse, L., & Abramson, S. L. (2001). Impact of a computer-assisted education program on factors related to asthma self-management behavior. *Journal of the American Medical Association, 8*(1), 49–61.

Sparks, S. M., & Kuenz, M. A. (1993). *Interactive instruction in nursing and other health sciences: Review of evaluation instruments.* Lister Hill Monograph LHNCBC 93-1. Washington, DC: U.S. Department of Health and Human Services.

Sweeney, M. A. (1985). *The nurse's guide to computers.* New York: Macmillan.

Thede, L. Q. (1995). *Comparison of a constructivist and Objectivist framework for designing computer-aided-instruction.* Dissertation Abstracts International, UMI #9612383.

Webopedia (2002). *Virtual Reality.* Retrieved March 14, 2002 from http://www.pcwebopedia.com/TERM/v/ virtual_reality.html.

White, J. E. (1995). Using interactive video to add physical assessment data to computer-based patient simulations in nursing. *Computers in Nursing, 13*(5), 233–235.

Informatics:
Challenges and Issues

Objectives
After studying this chapter you will be able to:

1. *Describe issues involved in implementing the National Health Information Infrastructure plan.*

2. *Apply the three elements involved in data security.*

3. *Describe current needs for data standardization.*

4. *Describe issues surrounding decision support systems.*

5. *Explain legal issues involved in healthcare informatics.*

6. *Apply ergonomic principles.*

7. *Interpret ethical principles in informatics issues.*

8. *Analyze human issues in applying healthcare informatics.*

9. *Describe the CPRI-HOST vision of an electronic patient record.*

The ultimate aim of clinical informatics is to create information systems that are integrated with one another and also to provide a universal, birth-to-death healthcare record. This system would not only allow a person to be treated anywhere in the country using this record, but it would also incorporate knowledge-based systems as both **factual databases** and **decision-support tools**. Additionally, it would be linked to community, state, and national databases to provide a current picture of the public health status.

Such a tool would make the following situation commonplace. A woman with a heart problem who is visiting a national park experiences stomach and chest pains. She activates her wireless medical alert system and a global positioning device pinpoints her location. The system notifies the nearest emergency team who access her medical records while going to the scene. They transfer her to the nearest emergency department where the doctor on duty has retrieved her health record. The doctor diagnoses gastroenteritis and tells her to drink lots of water, clears her to continue her trip, and updates her medical records. The medical record system alerts her home cardiologist about the incident and sends the local health department information about the gastroenteritis. This information is added to the health department's database of local park incidents. Seeing an unusual number of such incidents that afternoon, they locate a broken sewer line in the park that is contaminating park drinking water.

This vision is based on the National Committee on Vital and Health Statistics' (NCVHS) proposal for a National Health Information Infrastructure (NHII). The overall goal of the NHII is to make it possible to share information and knowledge appropriately to facilitate the best possible healthcare decisions by consumers, providers, and public health personnel (NCVHS, 2001). In effect, the NHII plan would integrate information and knowledge about healthcare from many sources and provide it on an as-needed basis. The technology that would make this possible is available. The issues that need to be resolved before this becomes a reality are challenges not only to our system of healthcare but to our views about healthcare data. Many of the issues provide more questions than answers, and many must be addressed today even with our limited use of electronic healthcare records.

 ## The Electronic Health Record

The starting point for transforming this vision into reality is the electronic health record (EHR). The terms used to designate electronic patient records vary. Besides EHR, some institutions use computer-based patient record (CPR); others, electronic patient record (EPR). The meaning of the term varies according to the user's vision. The vision of the Computer-Based Patient Record Institute (CPRI-HOST) that would permit the scenario already described is an "electronic record" that maintains lifetime information about an individual's healthcare (Vision, n.d.). Instead of being one record, the EHR will consist of independent systems at individual care sites. Connectivity standards will make it possible to access needed data by authorized users, including the patient. Besides providing complete, accurate patient data, regardless of the location of the patient, the system will provide decision support, contain clinical reminders and alerts, and provide links to related knowledge bases. The use of one integrated patient record for each patient in today's large healthcare enterprises is the first step in achieving this vision.

The benefits to society from such an EHR can be many. Given the mobility of our population, having up-to-date access to healthcare information from any location in the country will add to patients' peace of mind and facilitate the provision of quality care. Patients who need to visit more than one specialist can be assured that each one will have access to the complete record. Emergency admissions of unconscious patients will not need to rely on either no history or possibly sketchy information from the accompanying person. Patients can check their own medical records for errors, but they will not need to take the full responsibility for keeping the record current. When researchers can easily access aggregated data to look at a client's drug interactions, unknown incompatibilities will be able to be identified much earlier than they are today.

This type of system can also assist in meeting the demands for more healthcare information by those who ultimately pay the bills: third-party payers, business organizations, and labor unions. It will provide answers to questions that are not feasible to answer with paper records or individual enterprise systems. Information will be provided for questions such as:

▼ Why is the rate of surgeries for a given condition in one city greater than in another?
▼ Why does this variation seem to correlate with the number of specialists available?
▼ Which new technologies are effective?
▼ Why do costs for the same procedures vary even within the same community? (Shortliffe, Tang, Amatayakul, Cottington, Jencks, Martin, et al., 1992).

The reasons for adopting an EHR go beyond the convenience of healthcare professionals to access individual records in an acceptable format and the needs of the third-party payers for information to justify costs. Providing the best possible patient care requires access to the data generated in patient care situations and systems that can monitor for known problem areas and anticipate others (Display 19-1). Many barriers must be broken down before this becomes a reality.

 ## Concerns About Healthcare Data

In the present healthcare system, patient care records are seen as the property of the organization or healthcare provider that created them, as is the responsibility for their accuracy (Dick & Steen, 1991). The result is a multitude of medical records for each patient with no integration between them. If there is to be one record for each person and data are to be added from multiple sources, the issue of responsibility for the record will need to be resolved. Should the consumer be ultimately responsible for the contents of the record? Should there be a healthcare professional designated by the consumer to work with the consumer in carrying out this responsibility? This issue will be encountered as large healthcare enterprises create one record for each of their clients. To meet the requirement of client access to personal records, it will be necessary for consumers to have access to their electronic records. How will this be arranged? How will conflicts regarding errors discovered in the record be resolved? It is clear that solutions to these problems will not be perfect and will require compromise on the parts of all parties.

PROTECTION OF HEALTHCARE DATA

When paper records were used, healthcare providers sealed them away in file cabinets and prohibited others from seeing them. State laws that governed the use and disclosure of

---

Display 19-1 • SOME BENEFITS OF A FULLY INTEGRATED ELECTRONIC HEALTH RECORD (EHR)

To clinicians
- Availability of information when and where it is needed. This information includes patient data and bibliographic resources.
- Decision support.
- Organization of information specific to the discipline so that it can be easily located.
- Facilitation of the process of preparing reports for internal and external entities.
- Ease of order entry.
- Elimination of multiple entries of the same data.

To patients
- Knowledge of who has access to their data.
- Individualized treatment anywhere the computer-based patient record is available.
- Ability to check the accuracy of their record.
- One location for all healthcare data.
- Evidence-based healthcare.

To researchers and policy makers
- Time savings in obtaining data.
- Large databanks yielding more valid and precise research.
- Ability to answer questions on local, state, national, and possibly worldwide levels.

this information left many gaps that became evident when computerization arrived. As a result, this information has sometimes been shared inappropriately, such as with medical and drug suppliers who used this information to target their marketing efforts. It was also shared with researchers, most of whom used it responsibly under the guidelines of the agency facilitating the research.

The protection of patient data, both for privacy reasons and to preserve records of care, has three parts: privacy, confidentiality, and security. **Privacy** refers to allowing the patient to decide which items shared with a healthcare worker will become known to others. This includes other healthcare workers and can be described as those items the patient will allow to be included in a medical record or discussed with others. **Confidentiality** refers to those who have access to healthcare information in a medical record, whereas **security** deals with protecting data from errors, either from input or system errors. Security also means safeguarding the data from destruction and prying both inside and outside the institution. Meeting the requirements to provide for each of these entities requires a combination of individual, organizational, and technical practices.

Privacy

Protecting patient privacy is an important professional responsibility. Being sick does not make intrusions into one's personal life justifiable. In some instances, people have been denied employment because of known medical conditions. This can make patients hesitant to share their health history when they know that it will be entered into a record for anyone with access to read. Patient privacy also needs to be considered when interviewing a patient. The environment should be such that the interview cannot be overheard. Another item to consider is the placement of computers on which charting is done. Ideally, the computer screen will not be visible to anyone except the person doing the charting. Additionally, information that is routinely asked of clients should be scrutinized to be sure it is pertinent to the care that can be rendered in the agency.

Confidentiality

Confidentiality is a constant balancing act. The more confidential we make a record, the more difficult it becomes to use it. Before computerized records, we gave minimal concern to confidentiality. We believed that the record was safe. Yet in most institutions, anyone with a white coat and a name badge that read "Dr. X" could pick up a record and read it. Additionally, when a patient was sent to another area, such as the operating room, the chart was tucked under a corner of the gurney where anyone could easily remove it. This made it easy for staff in another area to view the record, but it also raised questions about confidentiality that were seldom addressed.

Computerized records have brought the issue of confidentiality to the forefront. Even with the flaws in paper records, it was difficult to obtain information from more than one or two records at a time. When records are computerized, if one gains entrance to the system, it is easy to access many records. Hence, the first line of protection is to defend against unauthorized access or entrance to the system. This is achieved with a login process that authenticates that the person using the system is permitted access. The most secure method of authentication is **biometrics**, or the use of physiological characteristics such as fingerprints, retinal or iris scan, or a voice print that is presumably unique to the particular person. Of these, the iris scan seems to hold the most promise and return the least number of false "no matches." There are 266 unique spots on the iris, compared with the 13 to 60 that characterize other biometric measurements (Daugman, 1999). Additionally, the iris remains the same during one's lifetime, but it deteriorates very quickly at death due to lack of oxygen. The second most secure method is the use of a card or key given to authorized users that must be inserted into a terminal in the system and is accompanied by a password. The least secure system is the user id and password.

Most systems today, however, rely on a **user id** and a **password** for authentication. Various systems of designating user ids are used, such as first initial and last name, most of which are fairly easy to guess. Thus, the rules for passwords are much more stringent and vary from agency to agency. The best passwords involve a combination of upper and lower case letters and numbers in a manner that will not form a word, (e.g., "Sec9uR7ity)." This prevents someone with an electronic dictionary from trying various passwords until the right one is found. Additionally, making passwords case sensitive (i.e., one must use lower and upper case letters in the same way each time the password is used) also makes them more difficult to guess.

Policies on how often to change passwords are based on the premise that after a given length of time one's password has been compromised, either purposely or accidentally. This length of time is determined by the system administrator. Additionally, most systems prohibit users from reusing a password. Forcing a change too frequently can result in users' writing the password down and pasting it either near the computer or on the back of an ID badge. Not changing frequently enough leaves users open to having the security of their account breached. There also must be a system in place to close access to users as soon as they leave their positions in the company or institution.

Automatic log-out is another function used to preserve data confidentiality. Knowing that emergencies do arise that involve calling a nurse away from the computer, most systems will time out after a given length of time with no input. If the time interval is too short, this can be annoying to users who have to go through the entire login process again. If it is too long, it could allow someone else to perform unauthorized activities on the login of the original user.

Confidentiality of computerized records starts with the users. They need to understand the need for protecting their account; they must tailor behaviors to guarantee this protection. Users need to understand that between the time they log in and out, they are responsible for anything that is done from their account. This is another reason passwords should not be shared and should be difficult to guess. Using a pet or a child's name or birth date makes it easier for someone to guess a password. Besides memorizing and guarding passwords, users need to be sure to log off after using an account.

Another confidentiality issue concerns how healthcare data are transmitted. A growing trend exists for data to be exchanged electronically, either by fax or computer data transfer. When data are faxed, care must be taken to provide a cover sheet that hides confidential information. Additionally, the sender must be careful that the correct number is dialed. Using a pre-entered and checked phone list can help here. Notifying the recipient that medical information is being transferred is also good. The sender should know what happens to the fax that is being sent. Does the receiving fax machine sit where anyone could pick up the incoming messages? What policies does the third party agency have for protecting data?

When data are exchanged outside an institution using a computer, a method of **encryption** is necessary. Encryption involves translating the data into a code that requires a password by the recipient to **decrypt** it. There are two types of encryption, symmetric, and asymmetric. In symmetric encryption, the same key is used to encrypt and decrypt a message. In asymmetric encryption, different codes are used to encrypt and decrypt a message. Using this method, also called public-key encryption or public key infrastructure (PKI), a sender uses the recipient's public key to encrypt a message. The recipient then decrypts the message using his or her secret code. It is virtually impossible to deduce the private key from the public key. The key used to encrypt the message is called the public key because it is known to senders.

Most breaches of confidentiality come from inside. For this reason, it is imperative that an agency has written policies regarding the confidentiality of information, both paper and computerized. These policies should include information about the consequences of breaches of confidentiality which may include termination of employment. Most healthcare institutions today require in-service training on this topic. Users are also required to sign a confidentiality agreement that clearly states their responsibilities in using data and may contain information about the consequences of not abiding by these practices. To be sure that employees remain aware of confidentiality, many agencies require a yearly in-service session on this topic, as well as the resigning of the confidentiality agreement.

Data Security

The third element in this group, data security, is mostly the purview of the information systems team. Data security have three aspects. The first deals with ensuring the accuracy of the data, the second with protection of the data from unauthorized eyes inside or outside the agency, and the third with internal or external damage to the data.

Accuracy of data can be improved with methods that check the data during input. For example, when a user chooses phrases for input from a list, the person needs to be sure that only recognized terms are entered. To check that the desired phrase was chosen before leaving the page, the user can be presented with a screen that shows the items that will be entered into the record. Another item that must be considered is how to handle incorrect entries. Generally, provision is allowed for the entry to be corrected within a given time period, but a record of all entries is kept.

Accuracy of the original data is also the responsibility of users. There have been situations in which clinicians have entered anything in a mandatory field just to continue in the system (Magistro & Smith, 1998). Not only does this put patient care at risk, but it compromises the integrity of the database. This cavalier attitude can be attributed to a multitude of factors: a lack of awareness of what is done with the data, an unwieldy system for entering data, time pressures, and inadequate training in using the system. Regardless of the cause, it presents a very real problem that needs to be addressed if data are to be valid.

Protecting data from prying eyes involves not only **audit trails**, but decisions about how much access individual users should have. Who has access to what information differs from agency to agency. For pure ease of use, all professional healthcare workers would have access to any patient record in the system. This is very helpful when patients are transferred from one department to another, and it is allowed in some institutions. Its use must be backed up by audit trails, or by a record of which individual worker accessed which record at what time and where. Additionally, these audit trails must be routinely examined to determine whether breeches of security are occurring. Most institutions provide access only to records of those patients on the unit where the healthcare worker is stationed and they index these by job description. Limiting access too severely will prohibit holistic care and can put patients in jeopardy.

Protection From Outside Intrusions. With the rise of the Internet and the actuality that most agencies are now connected to it, preventing outsiders from accessing institutional information has become a major responsibility of the information services department. One of the first lines of defense for protecting against unauthorized outside access is a firewall. Firewalls can be either hardware or software or a combination of the two. A **firewall** operates in one of two ways. Either it examines all messages entering or leaving the system and blocks those that do not meet specified criteria, or it allows or denies messages based on whether the destination port is acceptable. Firewalls require constant maintenance. To ensure that the system is safe from prying eyes, some agencies hire **white hat hackers** to try and penetrate their systems. Protection is then devised for any breaches in security that are found.

Systems also need to be protected from outsiders who gain physical entrance to the agency and from insiders intent on gaining unauthorized access. The first line of defense against this type of breach includes staff education in the importance of data security and encouragement of the staff to demand identification from unfamiliar persons and refuse access to anyone without a recognized authorization (Jackson & Numbers, 2001). Determining the level of security in this area can be learned by a **security audit** (Display 19-2). In a security audit, outsiders are hired to enter the agency and attempt to gain access to patient information. The

---

Display 19-2 • ITEMS FOR A SECURITY AUDIT

Here are some sample indicators that can be used as a guide for a security audit:

1. Could an unidentified visitor obtain an employee lab coat and/or hospital ID?
2. Were data readily available on a vacant PC screen, vacant printer, or waste receptacle?
3. Was an unidentified visitor allowed to remove hardware (e.g., PC equipment) without being questioned or detained?
4. Was a telephone caller (auditor who identified self as an information services [IS] staffer) able to obtain a user logon ID and password? For example: "My name is Sue, I'm from IS and I'm working on your department's system configurations. I need your login and password to check it."
5. Was an unidentified visitor left alone while sitting at a terminal?
6. Did an unidentified visitor:
   a. Obtain access to system?
   b. Receive logon assistance?
   c. Obtain access to locked area (such as Marketing, or Stock Room)?
   d. Receive a copy of a patient bill?
   e. Receive access to a patient medical record?
   f. Receive a copy of a lab result?

Adapted from Jackson, C. & Numbers, T. (2001). Is it time for a security audit? *Informatics Nurses From Ohio Newsletter, 1*(3), 1:3–4.

outsider may be asked to impersonate a physician, nurse, or information services employee. The auditors use various subterfuges, such as saying that they are from information services and need a password to check something in an account. Or the outsider may pretend to be a physician who forgot to change his or her password and needs to see a specific patient referred to them by Dr. Y, a physician well-known to the unit. Results of the audit need to be shared with employees. Those who correctly followed agency policy need to be acknowledged, at the same time counseling should be provided to those who did not.

Protection From Data Loss. Computer data need to be protected from being lost due to either a system problem or a disaster, natural or otherwise. This latter element has taken on new importance since the events of September 11, 2001. To provide this protection, back-ups of data must be routinely created and stored off site in a secure place. These back-ups should be periodically examined to make sure that they are accurate. Additionally, a disaster recovery plan needs to be devised and tested. This plan should be made in conjunction with key people in the agency to ensure adequate protection. The objective in disaster recovery is to allow work to resume at the same standards as before the disaster with the least amount of effort (Poker, 1996). One of the first tasks in planning for disaster recovery is to do a risk analysis. This analysis will determine vulnerabilities and appropriate control measures. By identifying weaknesses in the system, disasters can also be prevented. Once a disaster plan is formed, it should be tested at least twice a year.

Health Insurance Portability and Accountability Act

In 1996, Congress passed a bill that is having a great affect on healthcare, the Health Insurance Portability and Accountability Act (HIPAA). Unlike the problems that had been anticipated for the turn of the millennium, this act affects an entire healthcare entity and not just information technology. This act addressed several areas pertaining to healthcare information, including simplifying healthcare claims, providing standards for health data transmission, and the security of healthcare information. The aim of this act is to improve the effectiveness and efficiency of healthcare and to combat medical fraud by standardizing the electronic exchange of financial and administrative data (Services, 2000).

The area that has generated the most public attention has been the privacy and security rules that address many of the privacy, confidentiality, and security issues already explored earlier in this chapter. There have been many areas of disagreement among the stakeholders about these rules, and legitimate concerns exist on both sides. One rule requires that a specific person be assigned the responsibility of overseeing efforts to secure electronic data. The rules imply that the individual in this position has the authority to implement policies to secure data and protect privacy. This person must be proficient in information technology, auditing, agency policies and practices, ethics, state and federal regulations, and consumer issues.

Although the data privacy issues generate the most media attention, HIPAA also mandates "technology neutral" methods for the transmission of data among healthcare organizations. "Technology neutral" means that any computer system can import and read the data. (This is similar to the rich text format [RTF] that permits most word processors to read documents created by other word processors.) To simplify and encourage electronic transfer of administrative and financial healthcare data among payers, plans, and providers, HIPAA requires national code standards to replace the many nonstandard transfer formats now in use (DOH Medicaid Update, 2001).

This act also requires the use of specific identifiers such as a national provider identifier, national employer, and third-party-payer identifiers and possibly unique patient identifiers for use in filing electronic claims with private and public insurance programs (Services, 2000). Currently, different plans assign each entity a different ID number, which results in slower payments, increased costs, and lack of coordination (HHS Fact Sheet, 2002). Although proposals for a national provider and employee identifier are currently being considered, because of the many issues surrounding a unique patient identifier, this has been put on hold indefinitely.

Whatever the final outcome of all the rules promulgated under HIPAA, this act will create a fundamental change in how healthcare is conducted (Goerdert, 2000). If the full intent of the act is implemented, it will be another step on the road to a fully integrated healthcare system. Because this is such a contested area and implies great change in healthcare, expect to see these issues debated for many more years.

Data Standardization

Healthcare data are used in many ways. Although clinicians are generally aware of how it is used with individual patients, it also provides information on populations of patients for epidemiology; public health; quality assurance; information about healthcare agencies for planning, management, and remuneration; and information about the current state of medical practice (Rector, 2001). This information has many users: direct care providers, managers, billing departments, researchers, health information managers, and patients, who are increasingly demanding to see their own records. When data need to serve all these different uses, it is imperative that decisions be made about which data need to be used and what terminology should represent the chosen data. Identifying the core set of data elements requires participation by representatives of all patient-record user groups. Devising the actual terminology is usually the province the most affected group. These efforts need to be national and international in scope.

An obstacle to data standardization often comes from healthcare providers who do not see enough value in the data to warrant a change in documentation. Other difficulties include deciding which data represent healthcare to the many users and the need for terminologies to be coordinated with medical record and messaging standards (Rector, 2001). There are also conflicts between the users' needs for ease of data entry and the requirements of rigorously developed terminologies. However, the needs of standardized data outweigh the encountered difficulties. All those involved must realize that any data that are not standardized will not be in the database for any use beyond individual patient care.

Health Level 7 (HL7)

One of the biggest difficulties faced by today's institutions is integrating the data from their **legacy systems**, or older systems, with new and other systems in the agency. This often involves entering data more than once, a process that can easily introduce errors. To facilitate solving this problem, standards known as **Health Level 7 (HL7)** are being developed. The group responsible for HL7 carries the same name and is one of the American National Standards Institute (ANSI) accredited groups. HL7 is a vendor- and provider-supported organization with a mission to provide standards for the exchange, management, and integration of healthcare data (Dolin, Alschuler, Beebe, Birion, Boyer, Essin, et al., 2001). Although well known for their efforts in developing healthcare messaging standards, the HL7 group is also developing standards for the representation of clinical documents, such as progress notes and discharge summaries.

The term HL7 means that the message standards are at the seventh, or highest, messaging level, which is concerned with the end-user view of information exchange. The lower layers are concerned with more mundane issues such as hardware and actual transmission of the data (Vargo & Hunt, 1996, as cited in Smith, 2001). At levels five and six, concern moves to the interaction between two processors, converting code, and data reformatting.

 ## Ergonomics

Ergonomics is the consideration given to designing a product, or work environment, so that it is convenient to use and does not prove injurious to health. Ergonomics is an important consideration for preventive health in terms of placement of terminals and keyboards, but it goes beyond the immediate physical environment and touches on the virtual environment or user **interface** of a system.

PHYSICAL LAYOUT

Paying attention to ergonomics when designing a computer system saves money by preventing repetitive strain injuries, or injuries associated with any repetitive activity, such as typing. Computers are supposed to facilitate data recording, not impose additional burdens on healthcare personnel. When planning a system, walk a day in the shoes of a user or several days in the shoes of several users before making firm decisions about computer placement. Nurses who have spent the better part of a day standing may appreciate being able to sit while using the computer. If the computer is also used by those standing, an adjustable computer stand could be employed so that a user who is standing does not have to stoop. Additionally, if it is necessary to place the computer at a fixed height for those standing, a stool should be provided for the nurse who uses the computer extensively. **Touch screens** and **light pens** may be ideal for quick entry, but for extended entries, they are very tiring to the arm. Providing dual means of entry may solve this situation. **Resolution** of a screen is also important. The higher the resolution, the easier the screen is on the eyes. It is also important to prevent glare on the screen. In situations where this is impossible, it is possible to purchase screen filters that will cut down the glare.

More thought needs to be given to how a workstation is designed for those who will use a computer for the better part of the day. Consideration needs to be given to the posture the user will be forced to adopt. The best chairs have adequate support for the outward curve of the lumbar spine and the inward curve of the thoracic spine. The user should be in a slightly reclined position (about 110 degrees), and the feet should be flat on the floor, or a footrest should be provided (Figure 19-1). Wrists, knuckles and the top of the forearm should fall into a straight line while typing (Bailin, 1995). To promote circulation to the lower arm and hand, the elbow angle should be open. Both of these are can be accomplished with a **negative tilt keyboard** (CUErgo, 2002). The monitor should be placed directly in front of the user to avoid neck twisting. Studies have found that the best position for the monitor is for the center of the screen to be about 17-1/2 degrees below eye level and about an arm's length away (CUErgo, 2002). The ideal placement of a

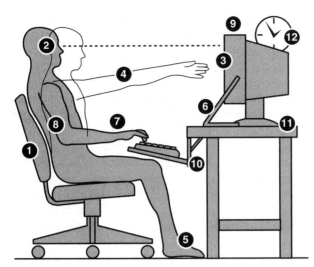

1. Use a good chair and sit back
2. Top of monitor 2-3" (5-8 cm) above eyes
3. No glare on screen
4. Sit at arms length
5. Feet on floor or footrest
6. Use document holder
7. Wrists flat and straight
8. Arms and elbows close to body
9. Center monitor and keyboard in front of you
10. Use negative tilt keyboard tray
11. Use a stable work surface
12. Take frequent breaks

Figure 19-1 • Ideal computer posture. Used with permission of Professor Ann Hedge. From a class project of the DEA651 class of 2000. Found at http://ergo.human.cornell.edu/dea6512k/ergo12tips.html.

mouse is on a flat, movable mouse platform positioned one to two inches above the numeric keypad. Users should look at something more than 20 feet away for a minute every 15 minutes to let the muscles inside the eye relax. Using good ergonomic fundamentals will prevent repeated stress injuries (RSI) and reduce fatigue.

USER INTERFACE

The skill sets needed for coding a workable informatics system are not the same as those needed to produce a system that is user friendly. Design of the user interface, however, influences the acceptance it receives from users. Software designed from the point of view of the programmer, although technically sound, often proves hard to use. To be user friendly, it must be designed to allow users to accomplish their everyday goals, something that can be elusive because users may be aware of the tasks they need to accomplish but may not be consciously aware of their goals (Cooper, 1995). Some of these goals involve not looking stupid or making any big mistakes, accomplishing their work, and excelling in their jobs.

A well-designed system will reduce training time, affect productivity, and prevent errors. The system is affected by many factors, such as having a consistent user interface (Ambler, 2002). If users double click on an item to open a screen, this principle should be followed throughout the entire system. Error messages should provide concise information and suggest a solution constructively. Colors should be used consistently, and they should have a secondary indicator for those who are color blind. Adequate color contrast and easily readable fonts should be a part of good screen design. Too much information on a screen can be as disconcerting as too little. Progressive disclosure, in which more information on a topic is available with a mouse click, can serve the desires of both those who only seek immediate information and those with more extensive information needs. Data that are needed to accompany other data should not require the user to memorize the information on a prior screen or to switch between screens. Acronyms or abbreviations can also be confusing. They may cause errors or confuse the novice.

A system needs to accommodate both novices and experts. New users may require menus, but those who have mastered the system should have a shortcut available, such as a key press, to accomplish the same tasks. Providing easy exits for the inevitable wrong selection also adds to user friendliness. When mistakes are made, such as entering the wrong information on a patient, making the change should involve the same principle as using the undo icon in a word processor (Staggers, 1995). Errors in inputting information, such as entering the number 204 for a temperature, should be met with a clear message about the error and how to correct it. When possible, it is even better to assist the user to avoid the error in the first place. In short, being concerned about human factors makes a system much easier to use and more likely to be successful.

 ## Legal Issues

A patient's medical record documents a plan of care and serves as a legal document. The move to electronic record-keeping has changed the record format and added some legal problems. The security issue, something that has changed with electronic records, was already explored earlier in this chapter. There are, however, other issues. State laws regulating medical records can create problems in implementing an information system. They are often obsolete, ambiguous, and non-uniform (Dick & Steen, 1991). They vary in what may be automated and what may not. Many state laws still assume that paper records are used, so there is sometimes a legal limbo surrounding electronic patient records. Additionally, legal experts accustomed to reviewing paper records in malpractice suits are often confused when confronted with an electronic record. Most paper records have a fairly well known structure, with items classified by area of origin, for instance, laboratory, nursing, and the like. Electronic records, conversely, are often combined with paper records, making it even more difficult to follow the course of a patient's progress. When electronic documentation follows a critical path, the course of a condition becomes much clearer. Legal experts, outside the agency, need to be oriented to the documentation as well as provided with access to the record.

Clinical decision support systems are another area where liability could arise. Harm can occur either by following or ignoring the suggestions. Although practitioners who use the system in place of a consultant or to supplement the library (Dick & Steen, 1991) are expected to evaluate the information or suggestions, in emergency situations this may not occur. In cases in which harm is done, depending on the situation, anyone or all of several parties including the computer programmers, system developers, manufacturers and users could be held culpable.

Electronic signatures represent another legal issue. A digital or electronic signature is a code that uniquely identifies the sender and is attached to an electronically transmitted message. An electronic signature must be unique to the individual, capable of verification, under the sole control of the individual, and linked to the information so that when the data are changed, the signature is invalidated (Real Legal E-Transcript, 2002).

Although HIPAA does not specifically require the use of digital signatures, it says that if the use of an electronic signature is required by an HIPAA-specified transaction, HIPAA standards must be used. The HIPAA standards for a digital or electronic signature require three things: message integrity, non-repudiation, and authentication (Cassidy, 2000). Message integrity means that the message sent is the same one that is received. Non-repudiation means that assurance exists on the part of the recipient that the message came from the sender and that the sender cannot claim that they did not send the message. Authentication ensures that the "signature" belongs to the person who uses it.

Ethics

All relationships between two or more people are subject to certain ethical principles, depending on the situation. Healthcare personnel, and those involved in informatics who may have access to a great deal of confidential information, have a special obligation to abide by legal statutes and to be ethical in their handling of information. Conflicts creating dilemmas in interactions with others within and without the agency may arise about access to and disposition of data. The Code of Ethics of the American Nursing Association (2001) addresses issues concerned with privacy and confidentiality and acknowledges the conflicts that nurses often feel from competing loyalties. The Health Information Professionals Code of Ethics (2001) holds that all people have a duty to facilitate the good of others in keeping with their fundamental values and to avoid harming others.

Aggregated patient care data are used in quality improvement programs. In the past, it has been used for research without the need to acquire permission from each person involved (Peck, Nelson, Buxton, Bushnell, Dahle, Rosebrock, et al., 1997). Increasingly, however, a distinction between research and quality improvement is becoming more difficult to draw. The ethics of using patient data for quality management will need to be resolved. Healthcare data, outside of research studies, has the ability to facilitate improvements in patient care, not just within one agency, but as a part of regional and national databases. It may be necessary to educate healthcare professionals, individual patients, and governments about the value of aggregated data. Still, ethical conflicts will arise about which data should be included in the aggregated data.

Factors Related to Acceptance of Information Systems

Just build it and they will use it is not a theorem that works with information systems. Despite the overwhelming need to manage healthcare information more efficiently, many barriers still exist to achieving this end, especially in regard to clinical documentation. Data standardization and privacy concerns have been examined already. Attitudes towards accountability are another area that needs to be examined. Present nursing documentation tends to be task oriented. It does not promote practitioner accountability (Ball, Douglas, & Newbold, 1995). Using standardized terminology can increase accountability and make nursing input more visible. This is a wonderful opportunity; the challenge is for nurses to embrace this new step as an advance in their profession.

A piecemeal approach to informatics and a failure to appreciate the need for an overall strategic information plan have resulted in wasted money and user frustration. Effort needs to be expended to educate system designers about the importance of screen design and planning a system around work flow. Given the time pressures of modern day healthcare, clinicians will only embrace those things that do not impede their work flow. Costs for information technology are high and will continue to be. As healthcare providers, we need to realize the value of information for patient care and worldwide healthcare.

As long ago as 1993, far-sighted individuals set standards for the "next-generation" nursing information system (Zielstorff, Hudgings, & Grobe, 1993). They argued that nursing is essentially an information processing activity, that information is a critical resource in the healthcare environment, and that a nursing information system exists as part of an enterprise-wide integrated patient-care system. They foresaw that atomic level data captured by the nursing information system would have many uses, from patient care to global healthcare. They also described various functional requirements for these systems: the system must promote productivity and efficiency, it must facilitate care by assisting clinicians to make the best possible patient care decisions, and it must be designed to embrace usability concepts. Their design is based on the assumption that there will always be a need for humans to interpret computer output. Informatics can provide us with the data, information, and knowledge to improve patient care, but nurses and other healthcare professionals will always be needed as the final arbiters who provide the wisdom needed to transform the knowledge into successful patient care.

Summary

Healthcare informatics exists in the world of healthcare and affects its culture. Today, many visionaries envision a nationally accessible database of healthcare information that uses data from patient care and research to improve the health of the nation. Technologically, even today, this is possible. First, however, many human issues need to be resolved. These include a patient's right to privacy versus the public's right to data that could save lives, data standardization, and legal issues.

Before large decision support systems can be built, data from actual clinical situations need to be captured in standardized format and shared across many venues. If systems are to be useful and efficient, ergonomics, including both the physical and interface issues, need to assume greater importance in the design of systems. Perhaps the greatest change that needs to occur is for healthcare to move from an insular approach to care to an approach that considers that the best patient care will occur when data and information from all specialties, both intradisciplinary and interdisciplinary, are synthesized for individual care and aggregated to provide more information and knowledge.

The main challenge today is to resolve the many issues that impede the institution of a full EHR. The opportunities for improved healthcare that the CPRI-HOST vision of an EHR provides make this a priority. This will involve a spirit of cooperation and many compromises among all those responsible for healthcare, including practitioners, administrators, and legislators.

connection For definitions of bolded key terms, visit the online glossary available at http://connection.lww.com/go/thede.

CONSIDERATIONS AND EXERCISES

1. Describe two of the issues involved in implementing the National Health Information Infrastructure.

2. In nursing's quest to provide complete care, patients have been asked questions about their sexual life. When is this information pertinent to care and when might it be considered an invasion of privacy? Explain your conclusions.

3. What activities pertaining to patient data are the responsibility of the:
   a. User
   b. Information Services Department
   c. Administration

4. You have just started work in a home care agency that uses computerized records. Access to records is permitted only to the nurse who is responsible for a given patient and to the supervisor. Your login name is your first initial and your last name. You are told to also use the same "word" for a password so that your patient's records can be accessed by another nurse if you are not available. How should this be handled?

5. The establishment of unique individual identifiers would greatly improve the climate for the establishment of a lifetime electronic healthcare record. This could prevent deaths by making information about allergies and other life-threatening conditions immediately available to healthcare workers anywhere. This number could also be misused. What proposal would you make regarding the establishment of such a unique identifier?

6. Investigate the legal status of electronic signatures in your state.

7. Using the 12 tips for an ergonomic computer workstation, evaluate a workstation.

8. Evaluate the user interface of an information system in terms of productivity and efficiency and make suggestions for its improvement.

9. While testing the security of closed laboratory reports in your position as an informatics nurse specialist, you accidentally become aware that Jim has tested positive for HIV. A close girlfriend of yours is dating him and has no knowledge of this. What will you do?

10. What benefits can you see from the CPRI-HOST vision of a electronic patient record?

REFERENCES

Ambler, S. (2000). *User interface design: Tips and techniques.* Retrieved April 8, 2002 from http://www.ambysoft.com/userInterfaceDesign.html.

American Nurses Association (2001). *Code of ethics for nurses with interpretive statements.* Washington, DC: American Nurses Publishing.

Baillin, J. (1995). *Ergonomics & computer injury: FAQ.* Retrieved April 8, 2002 from http://www.netsci.org/Science/Special/feature01.html.

Ball, M. J., Douglas, J.V., & Newbold, S. (1995). Integrating nursing and informatics. In M.J. Ball, K.J. Hannah, S. K. Newbold, & J. V. Douglas, (Eds.). Nursing informatics: Where Caring and technology meet (2nd ed; pp. 3–9). New York: Springer-Verlag.

Cassidy, B. S. (2000, September). HIPAA on the job: Get ready for digital signatures. *Journal of AHIMA.* Retrieved December 28, 2001 from http://www.ahima.org/journal/features/feature.0009.3.html.

Code of ethics for health informatics professionals (2001). Retrieved April 10, 2002 from http://www.imia.org/pubdocs/Code_of_ethics.pdf.

Cooper, A. (1995). *About face: The essentials of user interface design.* Foster City, CA; IDG Books.

CUErgno. (2002). *Ideal typing posture: Negative slope keyboard support.* Retrieved April 8, 2002 from http://ergo.human.cornell.edu/AHTutorials/typingposture.html.

Daugman, J. (1999). *Iris recognition: The technology.* Retrieved May 19, 2002 from http://www.iris-scan.com/iris_technology.htm#The Iris.

Dick, R., & Steen, E. V. (Eds.). (1991). *The computer-based patient record.* Washington, DC: National Academy Press.

DOH Medicaid update (2001). Retrieved April 6, 2002 from http://www.health.state.ny.us/nysdoh/mancare/omm/2001/mar2001.htm.

Dolin, R. H., Alschuler, L. Beebe, C., Birion, P. V., Boyer, S. L., Essin, D., et al. (2001). The HL7 clinical document architecture. *Journal of the American Medical Association, 8*(6), 552–561.

Goedert, J. (2000). The dawn of HIPAA. *Health Data Management 8*(4), 84–86, 90, 94, 97–98, 104, 106.

Health and Human Services Department Fact Sheet.(2002). *Administrative simplification under HIPAA: National standards for transactions, security and privacy.* Retrieved April 6, 2002 from http://www.hhs.gov/news/press/2002pres/hipaa.html.

Jackson, C., & Numbers, T. (2001). Is it time for a security audit? *Informatics Nurses From Ohio Newsletter, 1*(3), 1, 3–4.

Magistro, D., & Smith, K. (1998). Defining Nursing Informatics. *Capital Area Roundtable on Informatics in Nursing, 13*(4), 2, 5.

National Committee on Vital and Health Statistics (2001). *A strategy for building the national health information infrastructure.* Washington, DC: U. S. Department of Health and Human Services.

Peck, M., Nelson, N., Buxton, R., Bushnell, J. Dahle, M., Rosebrock, B., & Ashton, C. (1997). On the scene: LDS Hospital, a facility of intermountain health care, Salt Lake City. *Nursing Administration Quarterly, 21*(3), 29–49.

Poker, A. M. (1996). Computer system failure: Planning disaster recovery. *Nursing Management, 27*(7), 38–39.

Real Legal E-Transcript (2002). Retrieved April 8, 2002 from http://www.reallegal.com/sigsindepth.asp.

Rector, A. I. (2001). Clinical terminology: Why is it so hard? In R. Haux & C. Kulikowski (Eds.) *Yearbook of medical informatics* (pp. 286–299). Stuttgart, Germany: Schattanuer.

Services. (2000)Retrieved April 6, 2002 from http://www.anthem.com/anthem/affiliates/anthembcbsnv/services/medicalpro/edi/HIPAA.html.

Shortliffe, E. H., Tang, P. C., Amatayakul, M. K., Cottington, E., Jencks, S. F., Martin, A. MacDonald, R., Morris, T. Q., & Nobel, J. J. (1992). Future vision and dissemination of computer-based patient records. In M. J. Ball & M. F. Cohen (Eds.). *Aspects of the computer-based patient record (pp. 273–293).* New York: Springer-Verlag.

Smith, K. (2001). Technical standards used in health care informatics. In S. Engelbardt & R. Nelson (Eds.) *Health care informatics: An interdisciplinary approach* (pp. 361–394). St. Louis: Mosby.

Staggers, N. (1995). Connecting points. Evaluating usability: Essential principles for evaluating the usability of clinical information systems. *Computers in Nursing, 13*(5), 207, 211–213.

Vargo, J., & Hunt, R. (1996). *Telecommunications in business strategy and application.* Boston: Irwin, 152–154.

Vision (n.d.). Retrieved April 1, 2002 from http://www.cpri-host.org/about/vision.html.

Zielstorff, R. Hudgings, C., & Grobe, S. (1993). *Next-generation nursing information systems: Essential characteristics for professional practice.* Washington, DC: American Nurses Association.

Devices for the Input of Data Into a Computer

Device	Explanation
Keyboard	Device that resembles a typewriter keyboard, but with many more keys, that allow a user to input data. These include alphanumeric keys (the letters and numbers); punctuation keys; function and control keys; arrow keys; keys to delete, insert, and move the insertion point; and shift and caps lock keys. Some of the keys react differently than on a typewriter. Lower case "L" cannot be substituted for a 1, nor can the letter "O" be used for a zero. A computer interprets an upper case letter "L" as ASCII code 76 and the number 1 as ASCII code 49, thus making these two characters significantly different to the computer. The FN keys at top of keyboard perform preprogrammed functions that vary somewhat with different programs. Although caps lock capitalizes all letters, when a number key is tapped with the caps lock depressed, the symbol above the number is not output. The shift key is required for any characters printed on top of a numeric or other key.
Mouse	Device for locating, selecting, and making changes to objects on the screen. There are many varieties, but all work on the principle of a physical movement by the user to move the mouse pointer and "clicking" one of the buttons on the mouse to evoke a command. Generally, a left click signifies acceptance of a choice and a right click opens a menu that depicts those functions that can be applied to the selected object.
Joystick	A device that affects objects on the screen. Consists of a stick that protrudes vertically from a box. Moving the stick in any direction causes a pointer on the screen to move in that direction. Used primarily for playing games.
Touch screen	A special screen covered with a touch sensitive transparent panel, on which a user makes selections by touching an object on the screen.
Light pen	User moves a pen with a light-sensitive detector to the desired choice and selects it by clicking the pen.
Scanner	A device for inputting text or pictures on paper into a computer. Quality is measured by resolution or the dots per inch that are used in the input process. May be handheld, part of a printer, or flatbed. The latter type resembles a photocopy machine.
Bar codes	A printed pattern of wide and narrow bars that represent numerical codes that are recognizable by bar code readers. The output can be directed into a computer system for uses such as billing or inventory.
Voice	See Chapter 3.

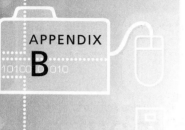

Devices That Output Computer Information

Device	Explanation
Monitor (may function as input device for mouse, touch screen or light pen)	Box that contains the display screen for your computer. Characteristics include screen size, resolution, the dot pitch, the refresh rate, video adapter (card) and **interlacing**. The monitor interfaces with the computer through a video adapter, or a board that plugs into the motherboard in side the computer. Display capabilities are influenced not only by monitor characteristics, but the video adapter. The ability of the monitor and the video board must be coordinated.
	Screen size is measured diagonally. **Resolution** is a factor of the number of pixels, or dots of light that make up the basic picture element of the screen. Computer screens are made up of thousands (in those with very high resolution, millions) of dots arranged in a series of rows and columns like a table with very small squares. As the number of dots per line increases, so does the resolution and the ability to create round circles and other shapes that are not perfectly square. The clarity of letters and other objects improves with the resolution. The terms below are used to denote this resolution. The numbers indicate the number of pixels on the screen, the first the horizontal, the second, the vertical.
	▼ VGA — 640 × 480 resolution ▼ SVGA — 800 × 600 resolution ▼ XGA — 1024 × 768 resolution ▼ SXGA — 1280 × 1024 resolution ▼ UXGA — 1600 × 1200 resolution
	Dot pitch refers to the amount of vertical distance between pixels. The smaller the dot pitch, the sharper the image will be. If, however, the distance is too small, the screen brightness and contrast will be reduced. On color monitors a range from 0.22 mm to 0.42 mm is seen. The 0.22 mm dot pitch gives a better picture.
	The **refresh rate** refers to how often the screen is redrawn. Measured in hertz (Hz), monitors of all resolutions listed require that the screen be redrawn at least 75 times per second for a refresh rate of least 75 Hz. A lower refresh rate will result in screen flicker.
Flat panel monitor	A very thin monitor. Is different from a flat screen monitor, which is a regular-sized monitor with a flat screen.
Dot matrix printer	Dot matrix printers produce characters by striking pins against an ink ribbon that prints closely spaced dots in the appropriate form. They are inexpensive to use, but their output quality is low. They are noisy and can easily become jammed if the paper feed is not perfectly aligned with the tractor feed device. Largely replaced today by the ink jet printer.

Device	Explanation
Ink jet printer	The most popular printers today, ink jet printers work by spraying ionized ink at a sheet of paper in the desired shapes. Produces a page almost equal to the quality of a laser printed page. Initial cost is considerably lower than that of a laser printer, but a special type of ink is required that can smudge on inexpensive copier paper. Ink jet printers that produce color are available relatively inexpensively. Today many are combined with a copier, a fax, and/or a scanner. The output often needs time to dry or it will smudge. Additionally, output can be more expensive per page than a laser printer.
Laser printer	Laser printers use the same technology as a photocopy machine; a laser beam that produces an image on a drum which is rolled through a reservoir of toner. The toner is transferred to the paper through a combination of heat and pressure. Laser printers produce the highest quality printing. Because of the way a page is prepared for printing laser printers need RAM. A graphic that is only partially printed indicates a printer with insufficient RAM. The ink cartridges can be made to last longer if, once printing becomes faint, they are removed and shaken, then replaced.
Plotters	A device that draws pictures on paper as directed by a computer. Used most often in computer-aided design.
Voice	See Chapter 3.

Devices That Both Input and Output Computer Data

Device	Explanation
Disks	See Chapter 2.
Port	A **port** is a socket, generally in the back of a computer, to which specially designed plugs that connect a device to a computer can be attached. Ports can be serial, parallel, Universal Serial Bus (USB), or Firewire. Cables, specific to the type of port, are attached to the port to make the external connection. Connectors used to attach these cables are designed so that they will only fit the port for which they are designed, thus leading to "worry-free" connections.
Parallel port	A port that transmits data 8 bits at a time. Often used to connect a printer, or external Zip or Jaz drive.
Serial port	Serial ports are referred to as RS-232C ports. They transmit data one bit at a time. Often used to connect mice and modems (device to allow computer data to be sent over a telephone line).
IEEE 1394 (Firewire)	A port that supports very fast connections and will allow many external devices to be connected to that one port. Supports plug-and-play and hot plugging. Is expensive. (This same name is given to a very fast external bus.)
Universal Seria Bus (USB) port	A port for connecting the universal serial bus. This bus supports data transfer rates of 480 megabits per second. It can connect up to 127 peripheral devices such as mice, modems, and keyboards. Also supports plug-and-play and is replacing serial and parallel ports. One can buy devices such as electronic "multi-plugs" that allow more than one device to be connected to one USB port.
Modem	See text, Chapter 4.

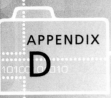

Universal Windows Key Presses

Task	Tap
Copy a selected object	Ctrl + C
Cut a selected object or text	Ctrl + X or Shift + Delete
Delete a character when the insertion point is to the left of the character	Backspace
Delete a character when the insertion point is under or to the right of the character	Delete
Help	F1
Move back one blank on a form	Shift + Tab
Move to a cell to the left in any table including spreadsheets or databases	Shift + Tab
Move to a cell to the right in any table including spreadsheets or databases	Tab
Move to the next blank on a form	Tab
Open a document	Ctrl + O
Paste an object or text on the clipboard in another location	Ctrl + V or Shift + Insert
Redo the deletion	Ctrl + Shift + Z
Save a document	Ctrl + S
Search for text	Ctrl + F
Select text	Shift + Arrow keys
Select an entire document, or all objects	Ctrl + A
Undo a previous action	Ctrl + Z

Note: When instructions are written with more than one press, hold down the first key, tap the second, release the second, and release the first key.

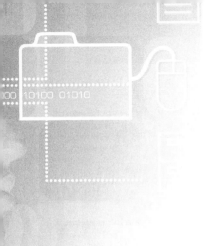

Index

Note: Page numbers followed by "f" indicate figures; page numbers followed by "t" indicate tabular material.